Evaluating Research in Speech Pathology and Audiology

Second Edition

Evaluating Research in Speech Pathology and Audiology

Second Edition

Ira M. Ventry

Nicholas Schiavetti
State University of New York, Geneseo

with a chapter by Teri A. Denson
School of Medicine, University of Southern California

Macmillan Publishing Company
New York
Collier Macmillan Publishers
London

Macmillan Publishing Company
866 Third Avenue, New York, New York 10022

Collier Macmillan Canada, Inc.

Library of Congress Cataloging-in-Publication Data

Ventry, Ira M.
    Evaluating research in speech pathology and
audiology.

    Includes bibliographies and indexes.
        1. Speech, Disorders of—Research.   2. Audiology—
Research.   I. Schiavetti, Nicholas, 1943—
II. Denson, Teri A.   III.   Title. [DNLM: 1. Evaluation
Studies.   2. Hearing Disorders.   3. Language Disorders.
4. Research.   5. Research Design.   6. Speech Disorders.
WM 475 V467e]
RC423.V45   1985   616.85′5′0072   85–17926

Printing: 2 3 4 5 6 7 8   Year: 7 8 9 0 1 2 3 4 5

ISBN   0-02-422940-7

Dedicated to the Memory of

Ira M. Ventry

1932–1983

Preface

The original impetus for the first edition of this book arose from the authors' attempts to teach a course for master's degree students in the evaluation of research in speech pathology and audiology. There was no single textbook that fit the needs for the course, and we both struggled for several semesters to assign readings from different books in psychology and education that covered various topics we wanted to incorporate in the course. It was difficult to find texts that were written at the appropriate level, provided appropriate coverage of the material, and dealt with the evaluation of research rather than the conduct of research. In addition, the examples in these books were seldom relevant to students in speech pathology and audiology. We finally decided that the only way to fill this void was to write a book ourselves.

The vast majority of professionals in speech pathology and audiology are not *producers* of research but most of them are *consumers* of research in their professional activities. Therefore, this is *not* a book which describes *how to do* research. It *is* a book about how to *read, understand,* and *evaluate* research that someone else has done. It should be apparent, however, that the ability to read, understand, and evaluate the research done by others is a basic prerequisite to doing good research. It is sometimes difficult to write about research for the consumer without discussing some of the considerations that face the producer of research and we tried to limit our treatment of these considerations.

The main audience for the first edition of this book proved to be master's degree students preparing for a clinical career in speech pathology or audiology. The original intent was to help such students prepare for a clinical career that would be guided by a reasonable assessment of developments in the field as reported in the research literature published in the professional journals. We also hoped to introduce those master's degree students who planned to pursue doctoral study to some of the basic concepts and terminology that they would encounter in the more rigorous research training which doctoral programs provide for potential producers of research.

Two main kinds of revision have been incorporated into the second edition. First, the text has been revised in places where reviewers, students, or colleagues have suggested improvements. These will be particularly evident in the first part of the book. Second, many of the examples have been changed, particularly the excerpts in the second part of the book. Some examples were replaced by newer examples that illustrate points more clearly. A new example is not necessarily better than an old one. Some examples had to be dropped because an author could not be located to grant permission for the second edition.

The second edition, like the first, is divided into three parts. Part I includes basic information on types of research, evaluation criteria, design considerations, and organization and analysis of data. Part II reflects the four typical parts of a research article: introduction, method, results, and dicussion and conclusions. The excerpted examples in Part II are intended to illustrate many of the points made in Part I. Our intent in both editions was to select good examples of the points we wished to make and to avoid extensive criticism of examples of poor research. Part III contains two complete research articles reprinted with our annotations concerning various features of research discussed in Parts I and II.

Ira Ventry died in April 1983, six months after we had begun work on this second edition. Although I finished the revision alone, his influence on the second edition will be obvious to those who read the first edition and to those who knew him or his work. He remains as the senior author of this book in many ways. Because he never had the chance to read or write the final version of the second edition, however, the responsibility for any errors is mine alone.

I wish to thank the many colleagues, students, and reviewers who have offered suggestions for both the first and second editions. Three people who helped make the second edition possible deserve special thanks. Ray O'Connell of John Wiley & Sons guided me through the administrative and editorial processes of revision. Nona Ventry graciously afforded me access to Ira's notes and files that were needed for the revision. My wife, Carolyn, provided the encouragement and support needed to complete this edition.

Nicholas Schiavetti
Geneseo, New York

Acknowledgments

We gratefully acknowledge the kind permission granted by the Acoustical Society of America, *Acta Otolaryngologica*, the *American Annals of the Deaf*, the American Speech-Language-Hearing Association, and the *Journal of Auditory Research* and by the many authors and coauthors to reprint selections from the journal articles. We are especially indebted to Margaret Lahey, Arlene Neuman, Irving Hochberg, Dale Metz, and John Folkins for allowing us to reprint their articles *in toto*. Credit lines for all reprinted material in Chapters 1 to 5 are found in the APA-style references at the end of each of these chapters. Credit lines for all other reprinted material appear within each excerpt in Chapters 6 through 9 and at the beginning of the articles reprinted in Chapters 10 and 11 and Appendix A.

Contents

Part I
Basic Considerations in Evaluating Research　　　　**1**

Overview　　　　1

1. Who Can Read Research?　　　　**3**

Introduction　　　　3
The Clinical Enterprise in Speech Pathology and Audiology　　　　4
The Research Enterprise in Speech Pathology and Audiology　　　　8
The Clinician–Researcher Dichotomy　　　　13
The Editorial Process in the Publication of a Research Article　　　　15
Some Myths and a Caveat　　　　18
Journals Dealing with Normal and Pathological Aspects of Speech,
　　Hearing, and Language　　　　20
Summary　　　　20
Study Questions　　　　21
References　　　　22

2. Types of Research in Speech Pathology and Audiology　　　　**25**

Introduction　　　　25
Common Steps in Empirical Research　　　　25
　　Statement of the Problem　　　　26
　　Method of Investigation　　　　26
　　Results of Investigation　　　　27
　　Conclusions　　　　27
Variables in Empirical Research　　　　29
　　Independent and Dependent Variables　　　　29
　　Active and Attribute Variables　　　　32
　　Continuous and Categorical Variables　　　　33
Experimental Research　　　　35
　　Bivalent Experiments　　　　37

Multivalent Experiments 40
Parametric Experiments 43
Descriptive Research 49
Comparative Research 51
Developmental Research 55
Correlational Research 57
Survey Research 61
Case Study and Retrospective Research 62
Combined Experimental–Descriptive Research 64
Summary 67
Study Questions 67
References 68

3. Criteria for Evaluating Research Designs 72

Introduction 72
Meaning and Purpose of Research Design 73
Internal Validity and Factors That Affect It 75
History 75
Maturation 77
Testing or Test-Practice Effects 79
Instrumentation 81
Statistical Regression 83
Differential Selection of Subjects 84
Mortality 86
The Hawthorne Effect 87
Interaction of Factors 89
External Validity and Factors That Affect It 89
Subject Selection 90
Reactive or Interactive Effects of Pretesting 92
Reactive Arrangements 92
Multiple-Treatment Inference 93
Reliability and Validity of Tests and Measurements 94
Reliability of Tests and Measurements 94
Validity of Tests and Measurements 97
Summary 100
Study Questions 101
References 102

4. Evaluation of Research Designs 104

Introduction 104
General Research Design Considerations 105
Between-Subjects Designs 105
Within-Subjects Designs 113

Mixed Designs   117
External Validity of Research Designs   117
Evaluation of Some Experimental Designs for Studying the
  Effectiveness of Therapy   121
  Weak Designs   121
  Stronger Designs   125
  Meta-analysis of Therapy Research   135
  Ethics of Using Control Groups in Therapy Research   137
Protection of Human Subjects in Research   138
Summary   139
Study Questions   139
References   141

5. Organization and Analysis of Data by Teri A. Denson   143

Introduction   143
  Rationale for the Use of Data-Manipulation Techniques   143
  Levels of Measurement   144
Organization of Data   146
  Characteristics of Data   146
  Tabular and Graphic Presentation   146
  Basic Summary Statistics   149
Analysis of Data   155
  Basic Concepts of Data Analysis   155
  Methods for Analyzing Relationships   162
  Methods for Analyzing Differences   172
Summary   185
Study Questions   185
References   187

**Part II
Evaluation of the Components of a Research Article   189**

Overview   189
Reference   191

6. The Introduction Section of a Research Article   193

Introduction   193
Title of the Article   194
The Abstract   195
General Statement of the Problem   197
The Rationale for the Study   200
Review of the Literature   207

Statement of Purpose, Research Questions, and Hypotheses   210
Miscellaneous Considerations   214
Summary   215
Evaluation Checklist   216
Reference   216

7. The Method Section   217

Introduction   217
Subjects   217
    Sample Size   218
    Criteria for Subject Selection   222
Materials   231
    Hardware Instrumentation and Calibration   231
    Reliability and Validity of Behavioral Instruments   241
    Other Measurement Considerations   249
Procedures   264
    Within-Subjects Experimental Design   265
    Between-Subjects Experimental Designs   266
    Mixed (Between-Subjects *and* Within-Subject) Design   273
    Within-Subjects Time-Series Experiments   275
    Between-Subjects Comparative Design   281
    Developmental Research Designs   284
    Correlational Research   290
    Retrospective Research   294
    Survey Research   295
    Case Study Research   300
Summary   301
Evaluation Checklist   302
References   304

8. The Results Section   306

Introduction   306
Organization of Results   306
    Frequency Distributions: Tabular and Graphic Presentations   307
    Summary Statistics: Central Tendency and Variability   315
    Some Characteristics of Good Data Organization   323
Analysis of Data   324
    Correlational Analysis   325
    Analysis of Differences   337
    Some Characteristics of Good Data Analysis   350
Summary   351
Evaluation Checklist   352

9. The Discussion and Conclusions Section   353

Introduction   353

Relationship of Conclusions to Preceding Parts of the Article   353
 The Research Problem   354
 The Method of Investigation   355
 The Results of the Investigation   359
Relationship of Results to Previous Research   362
Theoretical Implications of the Research   368
Practical Implications of the Research   374
Implications for Future Research   382
Summary   389
Evaluation Checklist   389

Part III
Evaluation of the Complete
Research Article: Two Examples   **391**

 Overview   391

10. Annotated Article: Speech and Language   393

11. Annotated Article: Audiology   410

Appendix A
Protection of Human Subjects in Speech and Hearing Research   425

Author Index   439

Subject Index   443

Part I
Basic Considerations in Evaluating Research

Overview

The five chapters of Part I introduce the reader to the basic principles we have employed in generating guidelines for evaluating research articles. Part I lays the foundation for the detailed analyses of research articles that are presented in Parts II and III of the book.

Chapter 1 discusses the reasons for the book and the need for critical evaluation of the research literature. Emphasis is placed on the fact that clinical practice is modified and improved primarily by incorporating the findings of adequate and relevant research into the clinical setting. The clinician–researcher dichotomy is discussed along with the process by which an article sees (or does not see) the light of day. We also stress, in Chapter 1, that an intelligent consumer of research must be reasonably knowledgeable about the subject that has been researched. It is difficult to evaluate a research article dealing with vocal pathology without a solid background in anatomy and physiology and a more than casual acquaintance with the literature on voice disorders. We have assumed throughout that our readers have the substantive knowledge or are in the process of acquiring it.

The primary focus of Chapter 2 is on the types of research most frequently encountered in the speech pathology and audiology literature—experimental research, descriptive research, and combinations of experimental and descriptive research. True experimental research is differentiated from descriptive research and three major types of experiments are described:

bivalent, multivalent, and parametric experiments. The major types of descriptive research—comparative, developmental, correlational, and survey—are discussed.

Using the framework described by Campbell and Stanley (1966) for assessing the adequacy of experimental research, Chapter 3 presents an extended discussion of the threats to the internal and external validity of experimental studies. If uncontrolled, factors such as history, maturation, subject selection, and instrumentation can confound results, affect the interpretation of the data, and sorely limit generalizations drawn from the data. It is these threats to validity that good research designs, whether experimental or descriptive, attempt to minimize. How well the researcher succeeds in minimizing the threats to validity determines, to a large extent, the adequacy of the research reported. Because researchers (and clinicians) in speech pathology and audiology often employ a variety of measurements and tests in their research, the last part of Chapter 3 deals with some basic considerations related to the reliability and validity of tests and measurements.

Chapter 4 is devoted to a discussion of some general principles of research design and presents some examples of strong and weak designs for studying therapy. The weak designs are weak because they do not account for the various threats to internal or external validity; the stronger experimental designs do minimize these threats. Specific examples of many of the points discussed in Chapters 3 and 4 may be found in Chapter 7. It may be useful to read Chapter 7 immediately after completing Chapters 3 and 4.

The organization and analysis of data are treated in Chapter 5. The chapter covers such material as levels of measurement, tabular and graphic presentations of data, and basic summary statistics as well as such concepts as levels of significance, Type I and Type II errors, and degrees of freedom. The more commonly used methods for evaluating differences and describing relationships are also discussed. The purpose of Chapter 5 is to familiarize readers with some of the terminology, some of the concepts, and some of the statistical treatments they will encounter in reading and evaluating the research literature. The material in Chapter 5, in conjunction with the illustrations and discussion in Chapter 8, is intended to assist students in the reading of the Results section of research articles. It is beyond the scope of this book to teach statistics per se, but it is assumed that graduate students in speech pathology and audiology will have at least a one-semester introductory course in statistics. Chapters 5 and 8 will review the major terms and concepts of a semester's survey of statistics and provide relevant examples from the speech pathology and audiology literature as an illustration of the specific application of statistical procedures to speech pathology and audiology data.

1
Who Can Read Research?

Simply understanding journal reports of research is not sufficient; we must be able to evaluate them critically.
Minifie, Hixon, and Williams (1973)

Introduction

The purpose of this book is to help practitioners and students in speech pathology and audiology to become critical readers of the research literature in the field. Here and throughout, the word "critical" is used to mean ". . . involving skillful judgment as to truth, merit, etc. . . . as in critical analysis" (*American College Dictionary*, 1965). "Critical" is not used here to mean "inclined to find fault or to judge with severity" (*American College Dictionary*, 1965). The book, then, facilitates the practitioner's use of the research literature to improve, modify, and update clinical practice through a reasoned assessment and evaluation of the literature relevant to clinical practice. Our goal stems from the basic premise that sound clinical practice should be based, in large part, on the relevant basic and applied research rather than on pronouncements by authorities, intuition, or dogma. The whole point of the text is to assist the clinician and student to arrive at reasoned decisions about the adequacy of the research reported in our journals and to make independent judgments about the relevance of the research to their clinical activities. In the process, we hope to dispel some of the more common myths about the research article, myths such as "You must be a statistician to read the literature" or "If it is in print, it must be good" or "The more difficult to read, the more scholarly an article must be."

In addition to our goal of helping clinicians develop the critical skills required in reading research, we have two additional goals: we hope the book serves as a bridge between clinician and researcher; and we view the

3

text as a foundation, as a *first* course for the student who plans a career in research or for practitioners interested in conducting research within a clinic or school setting. It must be emphasized, however, that this is not a book on how to do research; it is a book on how to *read* research. It will become apparent, however, that intelligent evaluation of research has much in common with the intelligent conduct of research.

The Clinical Enterprise in Speech Pathology and Audiology

Most speech pathologists and audiologists are clinicians and most students currently in training will become involved in the clinical practice of speech pathology and audiology. In a recent report, Punch (1983) noted that about 70% of the members of the American Speech-Language-Hearing Association (ASHA) provide direct clinical services. If we add another 4% who do supervision and 3% who teach the handicapped, it is obvious that over three fourths of the speech pathologists and audiologists who are members of ASHA are involved in the diagnosis and remediation of communication problems. In sharp contrast, only 1% of ASHA members reported research as their principal employment activity.

It can be argued, then, that the clinical enterprise constitutes the heart of the speech pathology and audiology profession. That this is the case is reflected in the various certification and accreditation activities of ASHA. These include the certification of clinical competence of the individual clinician, the accreditation of both clinical service programs and academic programs, and the activities of the Ethical Practice Board. The publication program of ASHA also recognizes the clinical focus of the profession through two important journals, the *Journal of Speech and Hearing Disorders* and *Language, Speech, and Hearing Services in Schools*. In addition, the house organ, *Asha*, contains many articles relevant to the practitioner. In sum, then, the work activities of speech pathologists and audiologists, the accreditation and certification activities of ASHA, as well as its publication program, and attest to the primacy of the clinical enterprise in speech pathology and audiology.

How does the clinical enterprise grow? How is it modified to reflect changing client needs and to take into account new and important information emerging from the laboratory? Many forces act on the profession to change its shape, to alter its course. Federal and state legislation have an important impact on the development and growth of a profession. Technological advances play a significant role in affecting clinical practice. Advances in theory create new models of diagnosis and therapy. Even economic conditions can play a crucial part in determining the future of a clinical profession. But most relevant for our purposes is that clinical practice also changes, or should change, as the empirical foundation, on which the practice rests, develops and expands.

How is the student or practitioner exposed to such knowledge—to this information base? It happens in a variety of ways. Professional conventions at the national, regional, and state level play an important part in helping the clinician to keep abreast of significant new developments. Interaction with colleagues is also of value. But three of the most important ways of maintaining contact with new developments are through formal course work taken in an academic program, through reading texts, and through ongoing exposure to the periodical literature, that is, the journals relevant to the profession of speech pathology and audiology.

The student's knowledge about clinical practice and the scientific basis of that practice come primarily through exposure to academic course work offered in the formal setting of a college or university. The student, in a very real sense, sees the profession through the eyes of the professor. Theory is presented, principles are expounded, practice is described, and clinical performance is evaluated under the close supervision of an academic staff member. The student depends, to a very large extent, on the knowledge, the wisdom, and the experience of the mentor. Ideally, the mentor provides the framework and the tools that enable the students to arrive at independent decisions once they become practicing clinicians. How successful the process is depends not only on the skills and the talents of the professor but on the skills and talents of the students.

In addition to the interaction that takes place within the confines of academe, the student and the practitioner look toward textbooks for new learning and new information. Textbooks obviously can contribute substantially to our knowledge and provide an excellent impetus to professional growth. But a text is basically a secondary source. That is, the author of a text has distilled, synthesized, organized, and clarified for the reader that theory and research the author believes is important and essential. The reader of the text, again, sees the world of speech pathology and audiology through the eyes of the writer. The reference lists and the bibliographies in textbooks identify many, if not all, of the *primary* sources used by the author. On occasion, the reader may check on a primary source but more often than not, relies on the author's interpretation of the source rather than evaluating both the original source *and* the author's interpretation of the original data. Of course, a textbook can also describe and report the author's own research and then it becomes a primary source. Bloom's (1970) early work on language development is a good example. Because it is a report of research, such a text requires the same critical evaluation as would be given to a research article published in a periodical.

It is not easy to assess the adequacy of a textbook. Logical organization, clear and precise writing, comprehensive coverage, the extent and thoroughness of the bibliography, and the frequency with which the text is referred to in other texts or articles are some of the factors that need to be considered in the evaluation of a textbook. Book reviews are also helpful. *Contemporary Psychology*, a journal devoted exclusively to book reviews, is an excellent source of reviews of texts and books in psychology and related disciplines. Books on normal and disordered aspects of communication are often reviewed here. *Asha* has a section devoted to reviews of books in speech pathology and audiology, but these reviews are frequently less critical and less scholarly than those appearing in *Contemporary Psychology*. And the coverage of new books is more limited than it should be. It should come as no surprise that textbooks contain errors, have misprints, promote the author's biases, and, at times, are simply poorly written. Given sufficient problems, a poor text will disappear from the marketplace. Perhaps, that is the final judgment of the adequacy of the text.

Although the textbook can make a valuable contribution to the growth and development of clinical practice, the original research, the primary source for change in scholarly practice, makes an equally important contribution. For example, many of the tests that are used in speech pathology and audiology are first described in the periodical literature. Follow-up studies and continued evaluation of the tests are reported in subsequent years. The test, if it withstands careful scrutiny, is gradually incorporated into clinical use and eventually becomes a routine part of a test battery. The current emphasis on acoustic impedance measurement and its widespread adoption in the audiology clinic is an excellent example of the way in which a "new" test becomes part of the clinical test battery (see Jerger, 1975). Similar examples can be cited from the speech pathology or language disorders literature. Diagnostic techniques and therapy approaches, the tools of the trade, often first see the light of day in the periodical literature.

At some point in time, sometimes early and sometimes late, the clinician must make a decision on whether to incorporate the test, the therapy approach, the rating scale into his or her clinical practice. The student clincian may have little choice; the student's supervisor or professor, presumably after a careful evaluation of the available data, recommends the procedure and the student accepts the recommendation, at least for the present. The professional, on the other hand, will probably no longer seek the professor's advice. Rather, the clinician may turn to colleagues in the clinic, to texts, to information obtained at professional meetings. Or the professional may go to the primary sources, the journal articles themselves, to help arrive at a decision based on a careful evaluation of the relevant research. It is to this evaluative process, this critical review, that we address ourselves in this text.

It is interesting to note, and also somewhat surprising, that there is little available to guide the practitioner or student in this evaluation process. There are a number of texts in the behavioral sciences that deal with research methodology and there is certainly no dearth of books on statistics. There are far fewer texts and articles on evaluation of research, and in speech pathology and audiology, this literature is nearly nonexistent. As an example, Auer's (1959) text, *An Introduction to Research in Speech* first appeared almost 30 years ago and is only one of three books of its kind remotely related to our interests here. The Auer text, however, deals primarily with the conduct of research; considerable space is devoted to research methodology in general speech, rhetoric, and the like. Fewer than five pages of the book are devoted to the evaluation of experimental research (see pp. 39–40 and 201–203). Also, the relevance of Auer's book to today's speech pathologist and audiologist is limited in view of the dramatic changes that have taken place in the profession in the last 25 years. The book by Silverman (1977) on research design is intended for professionals interested in *doing* clinical research; another work by Shearer (1982) is mainly aimed at students preparing theses.

The periodical literature on the evaluation of research in speech pathology and audiology is equally limited. There are only a few current articles relevant to the research evaluation process. For example, Adams (1976) describes several problems in stuttering research; Young (1976) suggests alternative approaches to ex post facto research; and Duffy, Watt, and Duffy (1981) discuss path analysis for investigating multivariate causal relations. The point is that remarkably little has been written about research design and methodology in speech pathology and audiology per se and that there is virtually nothing available on evaluation of research in speech and hearing.

There is, however, one often-overlooked source of evaluation material that does appear in the periodicals. That source is the "Letters to the Editor" section found in many journals. In many research-oriented journals, the letter to the editor is usually a critique of a published article and, in most instances, the researcher is given the opportunity to respond to the criticisms. These letters make interesting and educational reading. A case in point is the criticism by Giles and Giles (1976) of an article on "Speech fluency fluctuations during the menstrual cycle" written by Silverman and Zimmer (1975). Giles and Giles criticized methodological and statistical aspects of the study as well as the interpretation of the results. They concluded that Silverman and Zimmer's "... finding that women's speech at premenstruation is more disfluent than at ovulation seems to be methodologically biased, statistically dubious and perhaps socially meaningless" (p. 188). In their response, Silverman and Zimmer (1976) dismiss the Giles and Giles arguments and state, in summary, that "... our study is methodologically and statistically sound ... our statement of our findings is both reasonable and unbiased" (p. 190). Is the study methodologically sound or is the design flawed? Are the statistics adequate or not? Are the results subject to equally plausible alternative explanations or not? Can the results obtained on these subjects be generalized to other women? The intelligent consumer of research must be able to answer these questions. These questions, and their answers, again reflect the essence of our book.

In summary, we see the profession of speech and audiology as primarily a clinical enterprise. It is an enterprise that is changing, growing, and developing. For growth to be truly substantive, it must rest, we believe, on a scientifc and research basis, a basis that must be understood and incorporated into clinical practice.

The Research Enterprise in Speech Pathology and Audiology

As implied above, all professions, including speech pathology and audiology, are based on one or more scientific disciplines. It is these disciplines that constitute the scientific underpinning of the profession. Physics, biology, and psychology, in general, and speech science, hearing science, and psycholinguistics, in particular, are examples of disciplines and subdisciplines that provide the knowledge and tools required to attack and solve clinical problems in speech and hearing. Further, if we accept the definition of a discipline as consisting of a common core of knowledge, common knowledge-gathering techniques, and a special vocabulary (American Speech and Hearing Association [ASHA], 1963, p. 27), then speech pathology and audiology can be considered as a legitimate academic discipline in and of itself. What definition of a discipline is employed it is clear that the *practice* of speech pathology and audiology must depend on the *scientific discipline* of speech pathology and audiology.

To understand the research enterprise (i.e., common knowledge gathering) in speech and hearing, it is necessary to understand the general framework of behavioral science within which these research activities operate. *Science* is a search for knowledge concerning general truths or the operation of general laws, and it depends on the use of a systematic method for the development of such knowledge. The *scientific method* includes the recognition of a problem that can be studied objectively, the collection of data through observation or experiment, and the drawing of conclusions based on an analysis of the data that have been gathered. *Behavioral science*, which has been differentiated from the physical and natural sciences in the past, is that branch of science that deals with the development of knowledge concerning human or animal behavior. In recent years, physical and natural sciences (e.g., physics and biology) have been combined with the traditional behavioral sciences (e.g., psychology and sociology) for interdisciplinary research on many aspects of behavior. Areas of study such as sociobiology, neuropsychology, psychoacoustics, and vocal physiology illustrate considerable overlap among behavioral, physical, and natural sciences in the study of human or animal behavior.

Scientific research may be directed toward the development of knowledge per se, in which case it is called "basic research," or it may be undertaken to solve some problem of immediate social or economic consequence, in which case it is called "applied research." In recent years, professionals in many disciplines have realized that basic and applied research are not entirely separate or opposed activities. A piece of research that was done for the sake of basic knowledge may turn out to have an important application; a piece of research done to solve an immediate problem may provide basic information concerning the nature of some phenomenon. In the past, there have been instances of acrimonious opposition between people identified with the so-called basic and applied schools, and such opposition has resulted in communication failures that have retarded rather than advanced the development of knowledge. Today, many people recognize the importance of both basic and applied research as well as the need for clear communication between researchers with more basic orientations and professionals with more applied orientations.

Within the framework of behavioral science, two major types of research may be identified: *descriptive* and *experimental*. Descriptive research examines group differences, developmental trends, or relationships among variables through the use of laboratory measurements, various kinds of tests, and naturalistic observations. Experimental research examines causation through observation of the effects of the manipulation of certain variables on other variables under controlled conditions. These two types of research are different empirical approaches to the development of knowledge. Scientific endeavor depends on a complex interplay of empirical *and* rational inquiry, so it is important to understand the relationship between these two modes of inquiry in behavioral science.

Empiricism is a philosophy that assumes that knowledge must be gained through experience. Empiricists generally rely on inductive reasoning, that is, the use evidence from particular cases to make inferences about general principles. To be accepted into the realm of knowledge, explanations of phenomena must be based on evidence gained from observations of phenomena, and critical evaluation of the accuracy of observations is necessary before the observations can be accepted as evidence. This critical, self-correcting activity of empiricism is the core of scientific endeavor and is a necessary requisite of sound behavioral science research.

Rationalism is a philosophy that assumes that knowledge must be gained through the exercise of logical thought. Rationalists generally rely on deductive reasoning, that is, the use of general principles to make inferences about specific cases. Rationalism is often referred to as a *schematic* or *formal* or *analytic* endeavor because it deals with abstract models, and the logical criticism of propositions is necessary for the acceptance of explanations into the realm of knowledge.

Various schools of thought within the behavioral sciences differ in the extent to which they rely on empirical and rational endeavors. In linguistics, for instance, Chomsky (1968) insists that rational consideration rather than empirical inquiry is necessary for the development of a theory of language. In psychology, Skinner (1953) has relied on empirical evidence for a functional analysis of behavior and eschewed the exclusively rational approach. Although these two examples illustrate the extreme ends of the continuum of rational and empirical thought, many positions regarding the integration of empirical evidence and rational inquiry exist along this continuum. Stevens (1968, p. 850) suggested the term "schemapiric" for the "proper and judicious joining of the schematic with the empirical," and concluded (p. 856):

Science presents itself as a two-faced, bipartite endeavor looking at once toward the formal, analytic, schematic features of model-building, and

*toward the concrete, empirical, experiential observations by which we
test the usefulness of a particular representation. Schematics and
empirics are both essential to science, and full understanding demands
that we know which is which.*

Empirical and rational inquiry lead to the development of theories that are
statements formulated to explain phenomena. Kerlinger (1973, p. 9) stated
that theory is the "ultimate aim of science" and defined a theory as:

*a set of interrelated constructs (concepts), definitions, and propositions
that presents a systematic view of phenomena by specifying relations
among variables, with the purpose of explaining and predicting the
phenomena.*

Rummel (1967) discussed the relationship of rational and empirical inquiry in theory construction and stated that empirical facts alone are meaningless unless they are linked through propositions that confer meaning on
the facts. According to Rummel (1967, p. 454):

*A scientific theory consists of two components: analytic and empirical.
The analytic component is the linking of symbolic statements through
chains of reasoning that obey logical or mathematical rules but that
have little or no operational-empirical content . . . . this analytic
component of theories can be the creation of the scientist's imagination,
the distillation of a scholar's experience with the subject matter, or a
tediously built structure slowly erected on a foundation of numerous
experiments, investigations, and findings. The empirical component of
theories is operational. It fastens the abstract analytic part of a theory
to the facts.*

Theories generally fall into one of two broad categories (Sidman, 1960).
First, they may be generalizations, developed after the facts are in, that try to
synthesize the available empirical evidence into a coherent explanation of a
phenomenon. Skinner (1972, p. 100) has called such a theory "a formal
representation of the data reduced to a minimal number of terms." Second,
theories may be tentative generalizations or conjectures that can be subjected
to future empirical confirmation—as such, they are often called "hypotheses." The first kind of theory looks back at available data and employs a
formal logic to synthesize this empirical evidence; the second kind looks
ahead to future empirical and rational inquiry for verification of the theory.
Empirical and rational inquiry are necessary for verification of a theory or for
its modification if observed facts do not fit the theory. A knowledgeable
consumer of research should recognize the theoretical organization of empirical evidence and the empirical confirmation of theories as two activities
that coalesce to form the "schemapiric view" in the behavioral sciences.
More detailed consideration of these issues may be pursued by interested
readers in references such as Marx (1963), Chaplin and Krawiec (1968),
Kerlinger (1973), and Stevens (1968).

It is extremely difficult to paint a complete picture of the research enterprise in speech and hearing. No one has done it and we will not do it here. The data that would form the basis of such a picture are simply not available at the present time. A few generalizations should help, however, in understanding the broad scope of research activities that impinge, either directly or indirectly, on speech pathology and audiology.

Although relatively few speech pathologists and audiologists are involved in fulltime research (Punch, 1983), the research enterprise in speech and hearing is much broader than would appear from surveys of the ASHA membership, One obvious reason is that not all people who are involved in speech and hearing research are members of ASHA. More important, though, is that many people are involved in research activities on less than a fulltime basis. Perhaps the best example of such a person is the academician whose primary job responsibility is teaching. Such an individual is often involved in his or her own research or supervises doctoral dissertations or master's theses. The same person publishes the results of his or her research not only to advance knowledge but also to advance his or her own standing in the academic community because, unfortunately, the "publish-or-perish" phenomenon is still commonplace in university life. Other part-time researchers include doctoral students and clinicians working in a variety of clinical settings. Finally, much of the research appearing in the periodical literature is done by people working on the periphery of speech pathology and audiology. These include individuals such as otolaryngologists, experimental psychologists, psycholinguists, and neurophysiologists. The numbers of published articles that relate directly or tangentially to the interests of the speech pathologist and audiologist attest to the numbers and different interests and backgrounds of individuals involved in the speech and hearing research enterprise.

The areas investigated are equally diverse, ranging, for example, from the study of the effects of noice on the hearing sensitivity of chinchillas to the study of hearing-aid evaluation procedures, from a study of infant respiration to a study of the most efficient way to teach esophageal speech to a laryngectomee, from the study of how children acquire language to the study of how aphasics relearn speech and language. The areas studied are almost as numerous as the people involved in their study.

The settings in which research is conducted are equally varied. Language acquisition of a normal child is studied in the naturalistic environment of the child's home; the efficiency of an auditory site-of-lesion test is evaluated in the audiology clinic. The chinchilla's hearing sensitivity is investigated within the confines of a laboratory; the effects of noise on human hearing sensitivity may be studied in a factory setting. Stuttering behavior may be investigated in a laboratory, a clinic, or a school. In broad terms, normal processes are usually, but not always, studied in a laboratory setting; the study of disordered communication is frequently, but not always, carried out in a clinical setting.

Finally, as we will see in Chapter 2, the types of research strategies in

speech pathology and audiology are also diverse, ranging from survey studies performed in the field to experimental research performed in the laboratory.

This section would be incomplete without some mention of the responsibilities incumbent on the researcher. In addition to doing "good" research,
the researcher has two major responsibilities: to communicate and to be
relevant. Fox (1969) has pointed out that the researcher needs to inform a
relevant audience about the nature of the problem studied and the need for
studying it, the way the study was done, the nature of the results, and the
writer's interpretation of those results. The reader needs to judge how well
this communication was accomplished. Fox (p. 710) emphasized that the
researcher

> must reach the practitioners in language clear enough for them to
> understand not only the results of the research but the potential
> implications . . . . this responsibility is the researcher's and it is a
> responsibility that researchers have clearly ignored in the social
> disciplines.

Although few would dispute the need for communication scientists to
communicate clearly about their research, the issue of relevance is another
matter. Clinicians complain about the lack of relevance; yet, what is seem-
ingly irrelevant today may have major clinical implications tomorrow. The
examples in speech pathology and audiology are almost too numerous to
cite. The research done in the early 1950s on delayed auditory feedback,
conducted originally to obtain a better understanding of normal speech and
hearing processes, has found its way into stuttering therapy and the audiology clinic. The ear's ability to detect changes in intensity, first studied in
the 1920s and 1930s, gave rise to the clinical techniques developed in the
1950s and 1960s for measuring differential sensitivity. The study of normal
language acquisition provides a better understanding of the language problems of children seen in the clinic. The problem is not that our basic research
is irrelevant to clinical practice but rather that the researcher may have failed
to discuss the relevancy, or potential relevancy, of the research to the practitioner. Even a disclaimer noting the lack of immediate relevancy or application is better than ignoring the issue altogether. J. D. Harris, in his report on a
portion of the proceedings on graduate education in speech and hearing
(ASHA, 1963), wrote (p. 30):

> However unlikely an approach we may feel a scientist's efforts to be,
> from the point of view of revitalizing the clinical practices of speech
> pathology and audiology, our justification for and faith in those efforts
> must be that they may one day do so.

Harris, after noting that scientists are human beings who have human
concerns and empathy and sympathy for the handicapped, stated (p. 30):

thus all speech and hearing scientists are led from the laboratory to the clinic, perhaps to their own clinic, or at least to the clinical sessions and discussions of their professional organizations.

But in the long run, as one conferee (p. 29) put it:

Basic science has to be justified on the basis of its application. This is peculiar to our field; when we study a process for the sake of study, we then become other specialists.

In addition to having a responsibility to communicate relevant findings, the researcher has other important ethical responsibilities—responsibilities that are inherent in the research process. Several professional associations have codes of ethics that specify the ethical constraints placed on investigators who do research with human subjects. For example, subjects must have the freedom to decline to participate in a research project or to withdraw from the project at any time. The welfare and dignity of subjects must be protected at all times. The investigator must protect the confidentiality of information obtained during the course of the study. The investigator must protect subjects from physical and mental discomfort, harm, and danger. Investigators must honor all agreements and committments made to subjects. More complete description of these ethical obligations can be found in such sources as *Ethical Principles in the Conduct of Research with Human Participants* (American Psychological Assocation [APA], (1973) and in Part III of the November 23, 1982, *Federal Register.*

The ethical responsibilities placed on the researcher are as stringent as those required of clinicians, especially when the researcher is using human subjects. In fact, researchers have both ethical *and* legal responsibilities to protect the rights of both human and nonhuman living subjects. Many institutions are required to have an Institutional Review Board that studies research proposals to ensure that the welfare of subjects is scrupulously maintained, especially if the institution is interested in obtaining governmental funds for the conduct of the research. Suffice it to say that researchers have important obligations to a varied constituency—to their audience, their subjects, their institutions, their profession, and themselves.

The Clinician–Researcher Dichotomy

Much has been written about the differences and similarities between the clinician and the researcher. In actual fact, few would deny that the clinician should be an *applied* scientist and Perkins (1977, p. 5), for one, views speech pathology (and probably audiology) as an "applied interdisciplinary behavioral science." Emerick and Hatten (1974), in their book on diagnosis and evaluation in speech pathology, emphasize the applicability of the scientific method to diagnosis. They point out (p. 10):

the scientific method directs the diagnostician to observe "all" of the available factors, formulate testable hypotheses to determine their validity, and formulate conclusions based upon the tested hypotheses. The method demands rigorous adherence to standardized procedure and has as its favorable characteristics objectivity, quantifiability, and structure.

The same note was struck by a participant at a conference on graduate education in speech pathology and audiology (ASHA, 1963, p. 34). The participant is reported as saying:

There can be no dichotomy as to what material is or is not appropriate as scientific material. Anything may be. The important point is to treat the material in a reputable, repeatable, rigorous, quantified fashion.

Ringel (1972), in an attempt to bridge the gap between clinician and researcher, highlighted the similarities between therapy and research activities. He noted that the diagnostic evaluation is akin to the researcher's definition of a problem, that the treatment rationale is comparable to the working hypothesis of the researcher, that the clinician's evaluation of progress is similar to the scientist's analysis of the data, that the therapeutic result can be likened to the conclusions drawn by the researcher and, finally, that the clinician's case report is analogous to the published report of research. Ringel concluded that there are more similarities than differences in the approaches used by the researcher and clinician and that the dichotomy between the two is artificial.

In comments appended to the Ringel article, two reviewers offered their reactions to the Ringel outline. One reviewer pointed out that Ringel's basic premise was incorrect and that clinicians do indeed ". . . stress data-oriented, empirical approaches with behavioral objectives"; further ". . . that current clinical-research teaching . . . emphasizes the experimental analysis of behavior via the single subject design"[1] (p. 352). The other reviewer said, in essence, that although, presumably, all researchers use the scientific method, not everyone who uses the scientific method is a researcher. Ringel countered by stating that research goes beyond the walls of a laboratory and that "when 'scientific clinicians do indeed approach clinical problems in a scientific manner' they are conducting research of the most important type, with the result being the intent 'of delivering the best clinical management possible'" (p. 353).

This same issue, in a somewhat different context, was addressed by Jerger in 1963. Jerger—in an editorial, "Viewpoint: Who Is Qualified to Do Research?"—contended that not everyone is competent to do research and that research is the province of the trained researcher, just as clinical work is the province of the trained clinician. Both Spriestersbach and Wood (see Jerger, 1964) took exception to Jerger's stance. Spriestersbach pointed out that the

---

[1]There are entire books written about single-subject experiments. See, for example, Davidson and Costello (1969) and Hersen and Barlow (1976).

clinician uses the scientific method in clinical work and asked, "At what point does the application of the scientific method to problems stop being Research?" Wood took a stronger position and accused Jerger of expressing a separatist attitude toward research and clinical practice. "It is all right to encourage better research," Wood wrote, but ". . . it is not all right to encourage compartmentalization by separating those who do research from those who do clinical practice. Research is not only an activity; it is a state of mind, an attitude." And further, Wood contended, "A great deal of helpful research has come from very busy clinicians." In response, Jerger (1964) continued to assert that research needs to be done by those who are qualified to do it and that being research minded was not the same as doing research.

Is the clinician an applied researcher? In the sense that all good research adheres to scientific methodology, the case can be made that the clinician is involved, on a day-to-day basis, in a research enterprise. Is the clinician a researcher in the traditional sense? The answer is probably no, in that some of the basic components of research are, out of necessity, missing. That is, the clinician has little control over the many variables that can affect outcome or behavior, the sample size is usually too small and nonrandom to permit meaningful generalizations to larger samples or populations, the contribution to theory may be minimal, the treatment of data is oftentimes less precise, and the end product is a case report and not a publication. Although Ringel (1972) noted the similarity between the case report and a publication, the former is less likely to receive the same kind of critical peer review that a published article will receive.

In summary, then, we see the clinical practitioner as an applied scientist who uses the clinic or school as a laboratory for the application of the scientific method toward the end of providing the best clinical services possible. The scientific method, we think is at the heart of the clincal enterpise. We agree with Harris (ASHA, 1963, p. 34) who wrote:

> It is a cancerous attitude which strikes at the very life of the profession to assert that there is something immiscible about the clinical and the research philosophies.

The Editorial Process in the Publication of a Research Article

One common myth that needs to be dispelled early is that if an article appears in print, it must be worthwhile, valuable, and a significant contribution to the literature and to our knowledge. This is simply not the case! Inadequate research is reported, trivial problems are investigated, and articles vary tremendously in quality and value. Perhaps a brief description of the publication process will help the reader understand how an article gets published and how the quality of research can vary from one article to the next.

Although the editorial process differs from journal to journal, there are commonalities in the review process that cut across most journals. (For a description of the editorial process for articles published by the American Psychological Association, the reader should consult the Association's Publication Manual [American Psychological Association, 1983, pp. 165–173].) Let us use, as an example, a clinical research article submitted for publication to the *Journal of Speech and Hearing Disorders (JSHD)*, one of the journals published by ASHA. At the time of writing, the journal was directed to professionals who provide speech and hearing services to people with communication disorders. Manuscripts that deal with the nature, assessment, and treatment of communication disorders were invited. Note that the *Journal of Speech and Hearing Research (JSHR)*, also published by ASHA, "invites papers concerned with theoretical issues and research in the communication sciences."[2] Manuscripts submitted to *JSHD* are considered on the basis of clinical significance, conformity to standards of evidence, and clarity of writing. The journal welcomes philosophical, conceptual, or synthesizing essays as well as reports of clinical research. The details are contained in the Information for Authors section, of each issue, a section that defines, in a general way, the scope and emphasis of the journal, thus helping potential contributors to decide if *JSHD* is the appropriate journal for their manuscript.

The editorial staff of *JSHD* consists of an editor and several associate editors in areas such as motor speech disorders, stuttering, phonology, rehabilitative audiology, clinical audiology, acquired aphasia, voice disorders, and orofacial anomalies and nonvocal communication. In addition, there are approximately 160 editorial consultants, all of whom are knowledgeable in one or more areas of speech, hearing, or language disorders. Overall editorial policy is established by the editor and must be consistent with the general guidelines set by the Publications Board of ASHA.

On receipt of a manuscript, a decision is made into whose purview the manuscript falls. An associate editor is then assigned to oversee the review process and to serve as a reviewer. Next, the manuscript is forwarded by the associate editor to two editorial consultants who, after careful evaluation of the manuscript, recommend one of four alternatives: (1) accept for publication as is, (2) accept contingent on the author agreeing to make certain revisions recommended by the reviewers, (3) defer decision pending major revisions and another review by two different editorial consultants, and (4) reject outright.[3] No matter which alternative is recommended, the final deci-

---

[2]There is no point here in discussing at length what type of article appears in which journal, a subject that has aroused considerable controversy over the years. In addition, publication policy changes and what is true today may not be the case tomorrow. For our purposes, the important point is the *JSHR* and *JSHD* are two journals that are important to speech pathologists and audiologists and that both contain research articles relevant to clinical practice.

[3]Sherman (1960) has identified the following reasons for rejecting manuscripts submitted to *JSHR*: insufficient new material; unsuitable for publication in *JSHR*; inappropriate statistical procedures; incorrect information, inferences, or generalizations; poor reporting; and faulty designs.

sion to accept or reject lies with the editor. If a decision to reject is reached, the evaluations by the reviewers are forwarded to the author, sometimes with a marked copy of the manuscript. The editorial consultants are not identifed to the author and the editorial consultants do not know the name of the author or the author's institutional affiliation. That is, manuscripts are subjected to a "blind" review in which reviewers are ostensibly unaware of the identity of the author.

Although every effort is made to arrive at a publication decision quickly, the review process can be time consuming, especially if extensive revision is requested. The revisions may require considerable work on the part of the author, data may have to be reanalyzed or displayed differently, tables and figures may have to be added or deleted, and portions of the manuscript may have to be rewritten. Obviously, the more revisions required, the less likely is a manuscript to be accepted, particularly if a journal has a backlog of manuscripts already accepted for publication. All of this necessitates considerable correspondence between the author and the editor and, perhaps, even another review by two more editorial consultants. It is for these reasons that considerable time may elapse between the date the manuscript is received and the date it is finally accepted. The information on date received and date accepted is appended to articles appearing in *JSHD* and can give the reader some clue about how long the review process was for a given article.

It should be noted that some manuscripts have undergone a sort of pre-review process. These are manuscripts that are based on doctoral dissertations or master's theses. In these instances, especially for dissertations, the prereview process may have been rigorous because it was conducted by faculty members skilled in research and often by faculty who have no personal commitment to a doctoral candidate (the "outside" reader). Thus, the approval of the dissertation by the examining committee constitutes an endorsement of the quality of the candidate's research. But again, not all dissertations are equal in quality, and it is no simple job to translate a dissertation into a good journal article.

Knowing the rather thorough scrutiny that a manuscript receives, the reader may simply assume that the published article is free of error. That this is not the case can be determined by perusing the "Letters to the Editor" section of the journal. Knowledgeable readers may find statistical errors that were overlooked by both author and reviewers, may identify design and methodological shortcomings, may cite an inadequate rationale or overgeneralizations, and the like. Other problems may also be noted by sophisticated readers who do not take the time to write a letter to the editor.

How do inadequate or marginal manuscripts end up being published? Despite the care that is taken to select knowledgeable and informed editorial consultants, not all editorial consultants have the same level of expertise, not all have comparable research or evaluative skills, not all are equally familiar with a given area, not all use the same standards in evaluating a manuscript, and not all give the same amount of time and energy to the evaluation process. In addition, a biased review may result in those instances in which the identity of the author is discerned by the reviewer. That is, a manuscript submitted by a person known to have a good research track record may receive a rather cursory review, but the manuscript of an unknown author may be subject to a more rigorous evaluation. One reason for doing "blind" reviews is to reduce these biasing effects.

Other factors can affect the quality of articles appearing in a journal. The overall editorial policy and the policies of a given editor may change publication standards, or the demand for publication space may require a higher rejection rate leading to an improvement in the articles published. Note the following excerpt from a memorandum from an editor of a journal:

> We are developing a backlog of papers, and even if we publish additional pages . . . . our rejection rate is going to have to increase. Sometimes we've had to reject outright papers which one or both consultants tended to favor. . . . In recommending a questionable paper for revision or perhaps publication, please do develop a statement indicating what positive features of the paper warrants its further development.

Such a policy, which may seem severe to potential contributors, can help to upgrade the contents of a journal. Of couse, the more scholarly the journal, the more likely scholars will want to publish in that journal. Finally, the research sophistication found among members of a profession or discipline can have a pronounced effect on the character and excellence of its journals.

To summarize, the publication of an article in a reputable professional or scientific journal is no mean feat. This is reflected, in part, by the fact that relatively few members of ASHA do any publishing at all. For example, Castle, Newman, and Johnson (1967) reported that less than 20% of ASHA members had published one or more journal articles, and the recent data of Seaton, Cosker, and Weinrod (1981) indicated that about 2000 articles were published in the entire field of speech–language–hearing in 1978, at a time when there were about 30,000 ASHA Members. Be that as it may, great care must be taken by the author in conducting and reporting research and great care must be taken by the journal staff to ensure a high degree of excellence. Despite everyone's devotion to quality, journal articles do indeed differ in excellence, and educated consumers of research have the responsibility of being able to identify those differences.

Some Myths and a Caveat

One of our goals is to explode some of the myths surrounding research and the evaluation of research. We have noted already that the appearance of an article in a journal is no guarantee of the article's quality. There is good research and there is poor research, both of which may be published. The objective of the critical evaluation is to discern which is which. A stance of healthy skepticism is good for both the reader and, in the long run, for the researcher and the profession.

A major obstacle standing in the path of the consumer of research is the attitude that one must have a solid background in statistics before one can read intelligently the research literature. A similar attitude is that research and statistics are synonymous. Nothing could be further from the truth. Data analysis is only one segment of a research report and statistical treatment is the tool used in the analysis. As Binder (1973) has pointed out, statistical analysis serves only as a bridge between research design and interpretation; it has no independent status. Binder (1973, p. 50) stated that, "while many writers of statistical texts and editors of journals have tried to elevate statistics from servant to master, the overwhelming tendency at the present time is in the reverse direction." Plutchik (1974) supported this view by noting that statistical analysis is not an end in itself and cannot ensure meaningful conclusions simply by its application to experimental data. And, as Drew (1976) has noted, courses on statistics devote little attention to how statistics relate either to the research problem or the meaning and interpretation of the results. No matter how excellent and sophisticated the statistical treatment, a major weakness in any other part of the research study or article vitiates the value of the statistical analysis. A trivial problem is still trivial no matter how sophisticated the statistical analysis. A poorly conceived research design remains poorly conceived, despite a complex statistical approach. The inferences and generalizations drawn from the data may be appropriate and fair but the statistical analysis does not ensure this.

Statistical analysis is an essential tool for the researcher, but research and statistical treatment are not the same. A serious weakness in *any* part of a research article—introduction (rationale), method, data analysis, or discussion—weakens the whole.

Another myth, perhaps less widely held, is that the researcher is characteristically a recluse in a white coat isolated in the ivy-covered laboratory working on problems that have little relevance to human life, no less to the practicing clinician. Again, this is not true. Most researchers in speech pathology and audiology are concerned about people with speech and hearing problems, and it is this concern that continues to motivate their research. In fact, many of today's researchers have strong clinical backgrounds and extensive clinical experience. Many researchers, while perhaps not involved in research that has immediate application, are doing research that tomorrow may have considerable relevance to clinical practice. Researchers usually do not go out of their way to be obtuse or uncommunicative; some may not write well, but the poor writing is unintentional. A number of leading researchers have played important roles in the nonresearch professional aspects of speech pathology and audiology. Some researchers are haughty and aloof; so, too, are some clinicians.

Now for the caveat. Although we are attempting to lead the interested clinician through the process of research evaluation, a fundamental prerequisite to intelligent consumership is the fund of substantive information possessed by the reader. To illustrate, let us take a research article on stuttering and, further, let us consider the introductory section devoted to developing the need for the study and the purpose of the study. How can one evaluate the author's rationale without some knowledge of the literature on stuttering? Have important citations been omitted because they are inconsistent with the author's purpose? Can the reader understand the theoretical framework within which the author is operating? Has the author misinterpreted or misunderstood previous research? The only way the reader can answer these questions is to have a strong background in the subject of stuttering. The identical problem exists for the editorial consultant; that is why journals have large rosters of reviewers. The information explosion in speech and hearing has made it almost impossible for one person to be truly knowledgeable in all substantive areas.

This is not a book on stuttering, or aphasia, or cleft palate or audiometry, therefore, we have made the assumption that practitioners and students will approach a journal article with some background on the topic dealt with in the article. Although we have provided a framework for evaluation, the framework must rest on a substantive foundation and the reader must have this. Wood (1974, p. 6) summed up the point quite well:

> Although to understand and judge research in some areas of the social sciences requires specific technical knowledge, numerous research findings can be thoroughly understood, and in many cases critically evaluated, through a knowledge of general research methodology.

We will focus throughout on the *evaluation* of such research methodology.

Journals Dealing with Normal and Pathological Aspects of Speech, Hearing, and Language

In the first edition of this book, we attempted to identify, in list form, some of the more prominent journals in which articles on communication sciences and disorders were published. The list became hopelessly outdated immediately. New journals appeared; old ones disappeared. Journal names changed. Journals merged or split to form new ones. We have, therefore, decided not to try to list the primary source material in this second edition. Instead, we suggest that speech pathologists and audiologists who wish to find a list of journals that publish articles on communication sciences and disorders should consult the current-year October issue of *dsh Abstracts* and examine the section on Sources of Abstracts for a list of the journals abstracted in any one year.

Summary

The profession of speech pathology and audiology is composed primarily of individuals whose main responsibility is to provide clinical services—both diagnostic and therapeutic—to children and adults with communication disorders. Although a variety of forces can influence clinical practice, one of the most important is the knowledge and information gained through basic and applied research. To modify and improve clinical services, scholarly practitioners must be able to evaluate critically the research literature relevant to their clinical practice. The major purpose of this book is to allow the clinician to do just that. In addition to improving clinical practice, the educated consumer of research can help bridge the gap between the clinician and the researcher, can stimulate an improved research product, and can help raise the scholarly standards of the entire profession. An understanding of how to evaluate research can also be the first step in understanding how to do research. It is emphasized that one need not be a statistician to read the research literature. What is more important is the ability to think logically and to have a strong background in the various substantive areas of speech pathology and audiology. Finally, it is stressed that the publication of a research article is no simple matter and that the mere fact that it appears in print does not ensure that the article is perfect.

Study Questions

1. Read the following article: Ringel, R. L. (1982). Some issues facing graduate education. *Asha*, *24*, 399–403.
   (a) What are the major issues that Ringel raised regarding graduate education of researchers?
   (b) What did he say about the innovation and creativiy of young scientists?

2. Read the following article: Goodwin, P. E. (1982). Ratings of professional journals by ASHA members. *Asha*, *24*, 185–189.
   (a) Which journals do you find most important in your academic study or clinical practice?
   (b) How do your selections compare to the results of Goodwin's survey?
   (c) Are there journals in Goodwin's lists that you have never read before but that might be of interest to you in the future?

3. Read the following articles: Goldstein, D. P., & Hayes, C. S. (1965). The occlusion effect in bone conduction hearing. *Journal of Speech and Hearing Research*, *8*, 137–148. Shipp, T., & McGlone, R. E. (1971). Laryngeal dynamics associated with voice frequency change. *Journal of Speech and Hearing Research*, *14*, 761–768.
   Examine the overlap of physical and behavioral measurements in the investigation of speech and hearing phenomena in these two articles.

4. Read the following studies: Jerger, J., Speaks, C., & Trammel, J. L. (1968). A new approach to speech audiometry. *Journal of Speech and Hearing Disorders*, *33*, 318–328.
   Examine the reference list at the end of the article for references to

previous articles on this same topic by these same authors. Follow these articles chronologically and examine the interplay of so-called basic and applied research considerations in the development of this program of research concerning synthetic sentence identification.

5. Read the following article: Stevens, S. S. (1968). Measurement, statistics, and the schemapiric view. *Science, 161,* 849–856.
   Summarize Stevens's viewpoint on the relationship between the schematic and empirical aspects of science. What is the meaning of Stevens's reference to the two faces of Janus?

6. Read the following articles: Siegel, G. M. (1970). Punishment, stuttering, and disfluency. *Journal of Speech and Hearing Research, 13,* 677–714. Schwartz, M. F. (1974). The core of the stuttering block. *Journal of Speech and Hearing Disorders, 39,* 169–177.
   Discuss the manner in which each author deals with the relationship of empirical evidence to theory. Are theories cited that represent a synthesis of previous evidence? Are new theories advanced that need to be confirmed by future empirical evidence?

References

Adams, M. R. (1976). Some common problems in the design and conduct of experiments in stuttering. *Journal of Speech and Hearing Disorders, 41,* 3–9.

American college dictionary. (1965). New York: Random House.

American Psychology Association. (1973). *Ethical principles in the conduct of research with human participants.* Washington, DC: Author.

American Psychological Association (1983). *Publication manual of the American Psychological Association* (3rd ed.). Washington, DC: Author.

American Speech and Hearing Association. (1963). *Graduate education in speech pathology and audiology.* Washington, DC: Author.

Auer, J. J. (1959). *An introduction to research in speech.* New York: Harper & Row.

Binder, A. (1973). The statistical method. In B. Wolman (Ed.), *Handbook of general psychology* (pp. 49–66). Englewood Cliffs, NJ: Prentice-Hall.

Bloom, L. (1970). *Language development: Form and function in emerging grammars.* Cambridge, MA: MIT Press.

Castle, W. E., Newman, P. W., & Johnson, K. O. (1967). An investigation of membership attitudes toward publications of the American Speech and Hearing Association. *Asha, 9,* 287–296.

Chaplin, J. P., & Krawiec, T. S. (1968). *Systems and theories of psychology.* New York: Holt, Rinehart & Winston.

Chomsky, N. (1968). *Language and mind.* New York: Harcourt, Brace & World.

Davidson, P. O., & Costello, D. G. (Eds.). (1969). *N = 1: Experimental studies of single cases.* New York: Van Nostrand Reinhold.

Drew, C. J. (1976). *Introduction to designing research and evaluation.* St. Louis, MO: C. V. Mosby.

Duffy, J. R., Watt, J., & Duffy, R. J. (1981). Path analysis: A strategy for investigating multivariate causal relationships in communication disorders. *Journal of Speech and Hearing Research, 24,* 474–490.

Emerick, L. L., & Hatten, J. T. (1974). *Diagnosis and evaluation in speech pathology.* Englewood Cliffs, NJ: Prentice-Hall.

Fox, D. J. (1969). *The research process in education.* New York: Holt, Rinehart & Winston.

Giles, H., & Giles, J. A. (1976). Comments on "Speech fluency fluctuations during the menstrual cycle." *Journal of Speech and Hearing Research, 19,* 187–188.

Hersen, M., & Barlow, D. H. (1976). *Single case experimental designs: Strategies for studying behavior change.* New York: Pergamon.

Jerger, J. F. (1963). Viewpoint: Who is qualified to do research? *Journal of Speech and Hearing Research, 6,* 301.

Jerger, J. F. (1964). Viewpoint: More on "Who is qualified to do research?" *Journal of Speech and Hearing Research, 7,* 4–6.

Jerger, J. F. (Ed.). (1975). *Handbook of clinical impedance audiometry.* Dobbs Ferry, NY: American Electromedics Corporation

Kerlinger, F. (1973). *Foundations of behavioral research* (2nd ed.). New York: Holt, Rinehart & Winston.

Marx, M. (Ed.). (1963). *Theories in contemporary psychology.* New York: Macmillan.

Minifie, F. D., Hixon, T. J., & Williams, F. (Eds.). (1973). *Normal aspects of speech, hearing, and language.* Englewood Cliffs, NJ: Prentice-Hall.

Perkins, W. (1979). *Speech pathology: An applied behavioral science.* St. Louis, MO: Mosby.

Plutchik, R. (1974). *Foundations of experimental research* (2nd ed.). New York: Harper & Row.

Punch, J. (1983). Characteristics of ASHA members. *ASHA, 25* (1), 31.

Ringel, R. L. (1972). The clinician and the research: An artificial dichotomy. *Asha, 14,* 351–353.

Rummel, R. J. (1967). Understanding factor analysis. *Journal of Conflict Resolution, 11,* 444–480.

Seaton, W. H., Cosker, L., & Weinrod, H. (1981). Post-convention dissemination of papers presented at ASHA national conventions, 1967–1976: Stuttering, hearing aids, and alaryngeal speech. *Asha, 23,* 425–433.

Shearer, W. M. (1982). *Research procedures in speech, language, and hearing.* Baltimore, MD: Williams & Wilkins.

Sherman, D. (1960). Report to the membership. *Asha, 2,* 221–224.

Sidman, M. (1960). *Tactics of scientific research.* New York: Basic Books.

Silverman, E., & Zimmer, C, H. (1975). Speech fluency fluctuations during the menstrual cycle. *Journal of Speech and Hearing Research, 18,* 202–206.

Silverman, E., & Zimmer, C. H. (1976). Reply to Giles and Giles. *Journal of Speech and Hearing Research, 19,* 189–191.

Silverman, F. H. (1977). *Research design in speech pathology and audiology.* Englewood Cliffs, NJ: Prentice-Hall.

Skinner, B. F. (1953). *Science and human behavior.* New York: Macmillan.

Skinner, B. F. (1972). *Cumulative record* (3rd ed.). New York: Appleton-Century-Crofts.

Stevens, S. S. (1968). Measurement, statistics, and the schemapiric view. *Science, 161,* 849–856.

Wood, G. (1974). *Fundamentals of psychological research.* Boston, MA: Little, Brown.

Young, M. A. (1976). Application of regression analysis concepts to retrospective research in speech pathology. *Journal of Speech and Hearing Research, 19,* 5–18.

2
Types of Research in Speech Pathology and Audiology

Introduction

This chapter reviews the various types of research prevalent in the speech pathology and audiology literature. Classification of research into neat categories is difficult because of the number of different research strategies and because researchers do not always agree on the exact separation and overlap of various types of research. Therefore, our categorization will be arbitrary, as are those of other texts.[1] We hope that it will illustrate some common aspects of empirical research in behavioral science, some of the differences among various types of research, and the appropriateness of certain strategies for the study of different problems.

Common Steps in Empirical Research

Examination of articles in the behavioral science literature reveals some common steps taken in empirical research. These steps exemplify the nature of the scientific approach discussed more thoroughly in texts such as Kerlinger (1973) and Kaplan (1964). Consideration of this simplified outline may enable consumers to understand the general framework underlying empirical research and to realize that the different types of research to be discussed here are variations on a common theme of empirical inquiry.

[1] See for example, Isaac and Michael (1971); Kerlinger (1973); Levine and Elzey (1976).

The common steps in empirical research are:

Statement of a *problem* to be investigated.

Delineation of a *method* for investigation of the problem.

Presentation of the *results* of this investigation.

Drawing *conclusions* from the results about the problem.

We outline as follows how these steps are usually presented in a research article. Part II of this book considers each of these steps in greater detail and presents examples with critical comments.

Statement of the Problem

The researcher usually begins with the formulation of a general problem, a statement of purpose, a research question, or a hypothesis. In some cases, there may be a general statement followed by its breakdown into a number of specific subproblems or subpurposes. Whether researchers choose to present their topics with a statement of the problem, a purpose, a research question, or a hypothesis seems to be a matter of personal preference and, in fact, there is disagreement among researchers as to which of these linguistic vehicles is best for conveying the nature of the topic under investigation. We are not interested here in the polemics surrounding the choice of wording in presenting the topic to be investigated. We are more concerned that researchers provide a *clear and concise statement of what it is they are investigating.*

The problem statement should also contain some material on the meaningfulness or relevance of the topic under investigation by placing it in context. This is generally accomplished by establishing a *rationale* for the study through a review of the literature that has already been published on the particular topic to be investigated. This review may provide a historical background of the research to date and perhaps provide a summary or organization of the existing data so that the reader has an overview of what is known, what is not known, and what is equivocal concerning this general topic. Eventually, the review should culminate in a statement of the need for the particular study and a statement of the significance of the particular study.

Method of Investigation

After stating the research problem and providing its rationale by placing it in perspective relative to the existing literature, the researcher outlines a *strategy* for investigating the problem. This is accomplished through the description of the method of investigation. It is common to find the Method section of an article divided into three subsections: (1) subjects, (2) materials, and (3) procedures. Although there are variations on these subsections, the important questions we are concerned with are: *How was the study carried out? Did the method provide valid and reliable results?*

Subjects.   In this section of the research article, the reseacher describes the people (or animals) that were studied. A careful description is generally provided of the relevant characteristics of the subjects (e.g., number of subjects, age, sex, intelligence, type of speech or hearing disorder, etc.). The important point is how well the general population under consideration (e.g., stutterers or presbycuscis) is defined and how well the sample of subjects represents the population the researcher wishes to study.

Materials.   In this section, the researcher describes the various tests, instruments, apparatus, or training materials used and may also describe the situation or environment in which the study took place. Information about the calibration, reliability, and validity of tests or instruments used is also presented here.

Procedure.   In this section, the researcher describes how the *materials* were used to study the *subjects*.

Results of Investigation

Here, the researcher presents the results of the collection of data by means of the method of investigation just described. Tables and figures are often used to summarize and organize the data. Tables and figures are usually easier to understand than is a simple listing of all the individual or raw data. It is important for a researcher to present a specific breakdown of the results as they relate to the specific subcomponents of the problem presented at the beginning of the article.

Conclusions

After presenting the results, the researcher draws conclusions from them that reflect on the original statement of the problem. The conclusions are often cast in the form of a discussion of the results in relation to previous research, theoretical implications, practical implications, and suggestions for further research.

This simplified discussion of the manner in which the common steps in empirical research are reported in a journal article may give beginning readers the impression that research is a drab activity that follows a single pattern. It is difficult to understand the excitement and creativity inherent in the design and execution of an empirical study unless the student experiences it directly. In fact all researchers may not necessarily follow the orderly steps outlined above in doing their research; adjustments may be made to meet the needs of a researcher in a particular situation. Skinner (1959, p. 363) has captured some of the flavor of scientific creativity and excitement in his famous statement:

Here was a first principle not formally recognized by scientific methodologists: when you run onto something interesting, drop everything else and study it.

The common steps just outlined, then, are meant to illustrate the major components of the scientific method as reflected in the structure of most journal articles that report empirical research and should not be construed to be an inviolate set of rules for defining *the* scientific method.

We also want to point out that readers are likely to encounter some articles that do not report original empirical research data, but, instead, review the existing literature on a particular topic in speech pathology or audiology. These reviews are usually much more comprehensive and detailed then the literature review found in the introduction to a typical research article. They provide a historical perspective of trends in the development of thought about a particular topic and demonstrate how these trends may have shaped research approaches to these topics. Discussion of method and theory in historical research is beyond the scope of this book and readers are referred to Barzun and Graff (1970) for a general overview of historical research. A few brief points should be made about literature reviews as they relate to the commonalities of empirical research.

First, such reviews are important in synthesizing research developments to date, organizing our thinking regarding how past research has contributed to our present knowledge, and suggesting new avenues for exploration. Second, such devices are valuable in theory construction and in placing data into theoretical perspective. Third, such reviews are important sources of *critical* evaluation of the research literature. Finally, comprehensive reviews of the research literature also help to illuminate what Boring (1950) has referred to as the *zeitgeist* (German: "time spirit"), or the prevailing outlook that is characteristic of a particular period or generation. The zeitgist influences research trends along particular lines and may proscribe other directions, but it may also shift to generate new research trends. Baken (1975), for example, has noted such a zeitgeist shift in his discussion of a renewed interest in physiological studies of stuttering behavior. Physiological studies of the 1930s had not proven to be particularly fruitful, partially because of technological difficulties that have now been overcome for the most part by advances in electronics. But of even more importance in the renewal of interest in physiological research is what Baken called, "a retreat from the cortex." After reviewing the traditional stress on higher cortical functions in stuttering etiology as exemplified by cerebral dominance, semantic, Freudian psychodynamics, and non-Freudian psychologic theories, Baken highlighted the new emphasis on peripheral physiological events in the "domain of quantifiable observations" that opened new areas of etiological research and has implications for biofeedback and behavior modification treatments. Lane and Tranel (1971) provided another example in their review of the Lombard sign. They pointed out that although this discovery has important implications for four areas of scientific investigation, researchers have failed to appreciate these ramifications and, therefore, have incorrectly relegated Lombard's work only to the area of audiometry. This constrained view of the importance of the Lombard sign has resulted in a narrow channel of research efforts concerning this phenomenon.

The best way for students of speech pathology and audiology to appreciate the common steps in empirical research that we have discussed thus far is to read journal articles that report empirical research. Sustained experience in the reading of empirical research will enable the student to eventually assimilate the concept or process of moving from the formulation of a problem that can be attacked empirically to the drawing of conclusions based on empirical evidence. Many students report that the reading of literature reviews is as important as the reading of original empirical articles in developing an appreciation of the common steps in empirical research.

Variables in Empirical Research

Empirical research is concerned with the relationships among *variables*. Variables are measurable quantities that vary or change under different circumstances rather than remain constant. In geometry, for example, the radius and circumference of a circle are two variables: draw a large and a small circle and you can measure the different values of the radius and of the circumference of each circle. However, the formula that relates the radius and the circumference of a circle ($c = 2\pi r$) contains the term π (pi), which has a constant value of approximately 3.14159. Thus, π is a constant; it never varies regardless of the size of the circle. But the radius and the circumference are variables, or measurable quantities that may differ from one circle to the next. In behavioral science, the variables studied are often common measurable quantities such as stimulus characteristics (tone intensity or frequency), environmental conditions (background noise level), speech behavior (rate of speech or number of nonfluencies), language performance (mean length of utterance or number of embedded clauses found in a language sample), or hearing ability (speech reception threshold). Kerlinger (1973) has outlined three classifications of variables that are important for understanding the ways in which behavioral research attempts to understand the relationships among important variables.

Independent and Dependent Variables

Kerlinger's most important notion is the distinction between *independent* and *dependent* variables. Indeed, this concept forms the core of the material in this chapter and underlies everything discussed in the rest of the book. According to Kerlinger (1973, p. 35):

The most important and useful way to categorize variables is as independent and dependent. This categorization is highly useful because of its general applicability, simplicity, and special importance in conceptualizing and designing research and in communicating the results of research. An independent variable is the presumed cause of the dependent variable, the presumed effect. The independent variable is the antecedent; the dependent is the consequent.

Independent variables, then, can often be conceptualized as conditions that cause changes in behavior; dependent variables can be conceptualized as the behavior that is changed. For example, delayed auditory feedback (independent variable) may cause a change in speech rate (dependent variable). Masking noise (independent variable) may cause a change in auditory threshold (dependent variable). Kerlinger cautions us, however, on the use of "the touchy word 'cause' and related words" in discussing independent and dependent variables. One problem is the level of causation that we talk about: the variable that we manipulate may cause a change in a variable that is unknown to us, and the change of the unknown variable is what causes the change we observe in our dependent variable.

Another problem facing researchers in discussing cause-and-effect relations among variables will be seen in our discussion in this chapter of the distinctions between experimenal and descriptive research. Cause–effect relations are more logically inferred from the results of experiments than from the results of descriptive research because of the nature of the independent variables in these two kinds of research. In experimental research, the experimenter manipulates an independent variable (while holding all other potential independent variables constant) to examine what effect the manipulation of the independent variable has on the dependent variable. In descriptive research, however, it is not possible for the researcher to manipulate the independent variable to see what effect that manipulation will have on the dependent variable. Independent variables in descriptive research usually include things like subject classification (e.g., normal vs. language-delayed children) that the researcher cannot manipulate. The descriptive researcher may be able to compare a group of normal children with a group of language-delayed children on some dependent variable, but he or she cannot directly manipulate the subject classification of the children to observe the effect of the manipulation on their behavior. (Some authors have called such descriptive research "experiments of nature" because nature has manipulated the independent variable in determining the children's subject classification.) Thus, direct cause–effect relations are difficult to infer from the results of descriptive research.

Kerlinger (1973) has also pointed out that the distinction between independent and dependent variables is really a distinction that is based on our use of variables rather than a distinction that is based on some inherent property of a variable. We conceive of a certain variable as the antecedent that causes a change in another variable and, therefore, use that first variable as the independent variable and the second variable as the dependent variable. It is sometimes possible for researchers to conceive of a particular variable as being an independent variable in one situation and a dependent variable in another situation. For example, mean length of utterance is sometimes used (instead of chronological age) to classify children into groups that vary in degree of language development; mean length of utterance thereby becomes the measure of the values of the independent variable. In another study, however, a researcher may study the effect of manipulation of an independent variable on children's mean length of utterance; mean length of utterance thereby becomes the dependent variable. We must always look carefully at how a researcher employs the variables studied to determine the independent and dependent variables.

Kerlinger (1973) advocates thinking of independent and dependent variables in mathematical terms where X is an independent variable and Y is a dependent variable and we may specify the relationship between X and Y as a mathematical *function*. Jaeger and Bacon (1962, p. 6) state:

> . . . *if two variables are related in such a way that the value of one is determined whenever the other is specified, the one is said to be a function of the other.*

Thus, if we know the functional relationship of X and Y, we know how Y varies whenever X is varied. When we know the value of X, we can determine the value of Y from the functional relation of the two variables. In other words, if we know how the independent variable and the dependent variable are related and we know the value of the independent variable, we can determine the value of the dependent variable.

Functions can be demonstrated graphically by plotting the values of X and Y on the coordinate axes of a graph. Functions can also be demonstrated by writing an equation that shows how to calculate the value of Y for any value of X. The equation can be used to generate a line that connects all the plotted values of X and Y on the graph. The equation and the graph are just two different ways of displaying the same function—the equation with mathematical symbols and the graph with a line that connects the coordinate values of X and Y.

It is useful to exemplify this concept by examining the manner in which research results may often be presented in a graph. For example, the results of a reasearch study examining the relationship of two variables might look like the hypothetical data shown in Figure 2.1. The values of the independent variable are indicated on the *abscissa* (horizontal or X axis) and the values of the dependent variable are indicated on the *ordinate* (vertical or Y axis). The values of the independent variable increase from left to right on the abscissa and the values of the dependent variable increase from bottom to top on the ordinate. The dots indicate coordinate points of values of the dependent variable (Y) that were found for each value of the independent variable (X), and the line drawn to connect these dots graphically shows the

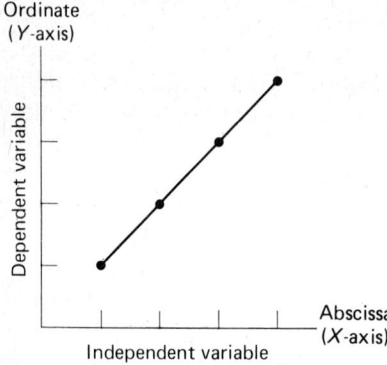

Ordinate
(Y-axis)

Dependent variable

Independent variable

Abscissa
(X-axis)

Figure 2.1 Hypothetical data illustrating a dependent variable that increases as a function of increases in the independent variable.

function relating the changes in the dependent variable to changes in the independent variable.

Figure 2.1 shows how the dependent variable varies as a function of changes in the independent variable in a graphic fashion. The function could also be shown with an equation relating the values of Y to the values of X. Because the function shown in Figure 2.1 is a straight line, a simple linear equation can be used to show the function:

$$Y = a + bX$$

This equation states that values of the dependent variable (Y) can be calculated by taking the value of the independent variable (X) and multiplying it by a value (b) and adding to it another value (a). The b term is the slope of the line that indicates how fast Y increases as X is increased. The a term is the value of Y at the point where the line intercepts the Y axis when the value of X is zero and is called the Y-intercept. The formula can be used to calculate the value of Y for any value of X and can also be used to generate the line drawn through the data points. The values of a and b are calculated from the actual X and Y data. The particular function shown in Figure 2.1 shows that Y increases as a function of increases in X. There are many other possible functions that can be seen in actual research data. For example, Y may decrease as a function of increases in X, in which case, the line would slope downward to the right rather than upward as in Figure 2.1. Or the data points may not fall along a straight line; they may show a curvilinear relationship between X and Y. In any case, the function is a mathematical or graphic way of depicting the relationship between the independent variable and the dependent variable by demonstrating how the dependent variable changes as a function of changes in the independent variable.

Active and Attribute Variables

A second notion about classifying variables that Kerlinger (1973) discussed is the distinction between *active* and *attribute* variables. A variable that can be *manipulated* is an active variable. Thus, the independent variable in an experiment is an active variable because the experimenter can manipulate it or change its value. For example, an experimenter can change the intensity of a tone presented to a listener by manipulating the hearing-level dial on an audiometer.

There are many independent variables, however, that cannot be manipulated by an experimenter. Variables such as subject characteristics cannot be manipulated. An experimenter cannot change things like a subject's age, sex, intelligence, type of speech disorder, degree of hearing loss, or previous history. Such variables have already existed for each subject—or have been "manipulated by nature." These variables are attributes of the subjects.

Some variables may be either active or attribute variables, depending on the circumstances of the research or on how the researcher uses the variable. Kerlinger (1973, pp. 38–39) uses the example of anxiety as a variable that may be either active or attribute. Anxiety may be thought of as an attribute of subjects—yet, anxiety could also be manipulated by inducing different degrees of anxiety in different subjects to see what effect the manipulation of anxiety has on some dependent variable. For example, anxiety could be raised in some subjects by telling them that the task they are about to undertake is a difficult one that will require great concentration, while telling other subjects not to worry about the task that they are about to complete because it is very easy.[2]

The important point is that the independent variable in an experiment is active—it can be manipulated in some way by an experimenter to see what effect it has on a dependent variable. However, the independent variable in descriptive research is an attribute—it cannot be manipulated by the researcher to see what effect it has on the dependent variable. In descriptive studies, the researcher must rely on comparisons of values of the dependent variable that correspond to some already existing value of an attribute independent variable.

Continuous and Categorical Variables

A third notion about classifying variables discussed by Kerlinger (1973) is the distinction between *continuous* and *categorical* variables. A continuous variable is one that may be measured along some continuum or dimension that reflects at least the rank ordering of values of the variable and possibly reflects even more refined measurement of the actual numerical values of the variable. The intensity of a tone, for example, can be measured along a numerical continuum from low to high values of sound pressure level. Stut-

---

[2]Kerlinger (1973, p. 39) points out, however: "Actually, we cannot assume that the measured (attribute) and the manipulated (active) 'anxieties' are the same. We may assume that both are 'anxiety' in a broad sense, but they are certainly not the same." Nevertheless, the example points out the principle that what may be an attribute variable in one situation may be an active variable in another.

tering frequency can vary from zero nonfluencies to a high number of nonfluencies.

Categorical variables, however, cannot be measured along a continuum. Instead, different values of the variable can only be categorized or named. For example, tones could be presented to a listener binaurally or monaurally. Subjects could be classified as "stutterers" or "nonstutterers" (although the degree of stuttering severity of the stutterers could be measured along some continuum from mild to servere). The ways in which we measure continous and categorical variables differ—more will be said about this in Chapter 5 when we discuss data organization and analysis. One immediate concern in this chapter is the way that continuous and categorical variables are displayed graphically. This is especially important in distinguishing between continuous and categorical independent variables. When graphing the change in a dependent variable as a function of changes in a continuous independent variable, it is common to use a line graph like the one in Figure 2.1. The line drawn through the data points in Figure 2.1 is an interpolation and is intended to demonstrate what the values of the dependent variable ought to be for intermediate values of the independent variable that were not actually used. However, when graphing the changes in a dependent variable as a function of changes in a categorical independent variable, it is customary to use a bar graph in which the height of the bar that is aligned at each categorical value of the independent variable on the X axis is meant to indicate the value of the dependent variable on the Y axis for that categorical value of the independent variable. Several examples of both types of graphs are seen in this and later chapters, but it may be useful to illustrate briefly the way in which a categorical independent variable is presented in a bar graph. Figure 2.2 shows the same hypothetical data that were illustrated in Figure 2.1, except that the four values of the independent variable are shown as four categories of a categorical variable rather than as four values on a continuous variable. The data in Figure 2.1 show a dependent variable that increases as the values of the independent variable increase along a continuum. The data in Figure 2.2 show the differences in the values of the dependent variable for four different categories of an independent variable. In general, throughout the rest of the book, we follow the convention of presenting data for a continuous independent variable with a line graph and data for a categorical independent variable with a bar graph.

Now that we have examined some common steps in empirical research and discussed the concept of variables in empirical research, we will look at some different types of research in speech pathology and audiology and discuss their similarities and differences. We outline various types of research by presenting a description of the general purpose and strategy of each type, giving an example of the application of each type to problems in the field of speech pathology and audiology and discussing some advantages and disadvantages of each.

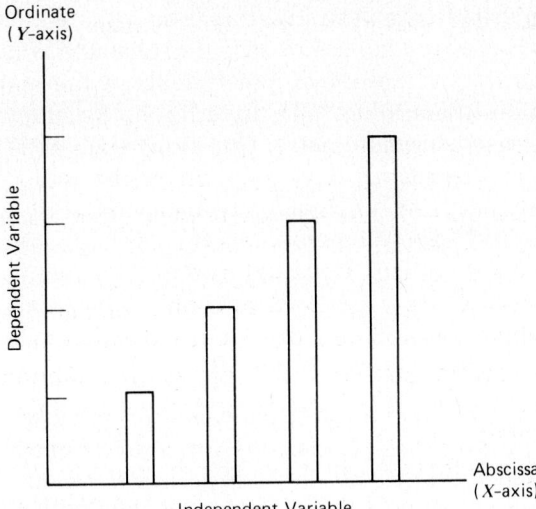

Figure 2.2 Hypothetical data illustrating differences in the values of the dependent variable for four different categories of an independent variable.

Experimental Research

Experimental research is the appropriate method for investigating cause-and-effect relations among variables. With regard to the investigation of cause and effect, Underwood and Shaughnessy (1975, p. 15) have stated:

> The critical strength of the experiment lies in the fact that when it is properly executed we learn about cause–effect relationships existing in nature. It is as near a foolproof technique for making these discoveries as has yet been devised. Those who have sought other approaches for determining cause–effect relationships in behavior have usually become discouraged.

The ability to make conclusions about cause–effect relationships among variables, then, is a hallmark of expermental research.

There are numerous different kinds of research problems in speech pathology and audiology that have been studied through the use of experimental research. Experiments have been carried out to examine the effects of therapy on the behavior of persons with speech or hearing disorders. The experimental question in such cases would be: Does therapy cause a change in behavior? In addition to such rather long-term therapy experiments, many experiments have examined more short-term cause–effect relationships in laboratories or clinics. For example, the research question, What effect does delayed auditory feedback have on speech behavior?, has been submitted to considerable experimental scrutiny over the years. Psychophysical experiments have been used to examine stimulus–response relationships to determine what effects certain changes in stimulus characteristics may have on people's responses. Psychophysical experiments of this nature have been especially common in audiology and underlie the development of most of the clinical tests used in audiometry. Questions such as What effect does change in pure-tone frequency have on auditory threshold? or What effect does presentation level of phonemically balanced (PB) words have on speech intelligibility? have been answered by psychophysical experiments.

In reality, there are so many potential uses of the experimental approach that it is difficult to classify all of its possible applications. As Kling and Riggs (1971, p. 3) have commented in attempting to define the experimental method in psychology:

> . . . contemporary methodology has become so highly specific that it is difficult to lay down general rules applicable to all experiments. However, a few characteristics of the experimental method may be mentioned.

The four characteristics of experimental research that Kling and Riggs listed (1971, p. 3) are: (1) experimenters start with some purpose, question, or hypothesis that allows them to know when to observe certain specific aspects of behavior; (2) experimenters can control the occurrence of events and, thus, observe changes in behavior when they are best prepared to make the observations; (3) because of this, experimenters (or others) can repeat these observations under the same conditions; and (4) because experimenters can control the conditions of observation, they can systematically manipulate certain conditions to measure the effects of these manipulations on behavior.

The experimenter, then, can manipulate an independent variable to study its effect on the dependent variable. But a change in an independent variable may be considered to cause a change in a dependent variable only if other potential independent variables have been controlled or held constant so that they will not be able to have a simultaneous effect on the dependent variable. Other potential independent variables are often called "extraneous" or "nuisance" variables becasue they may confuse the picture of a cause–effect relationship if left uncontrolled. Therefore, a major purpose of experimentation is to control potential extraneous variables while manipulating the independent variable of interest to the experimenter. We discuss several potential nuisance variables and how they may be controlled in Chapters 3 and 4. But, in this chapter, we are concerned mainly with the way in which the independent variable is manipulated as the basis for identifying different types of experiments.

Plutchik (1974) has outlined a classification of types of experiments that is based on the structure of the independent variables that are employed. Plutchik's classification is useful as a first step toward understanding experimental research and appreciating the strategies that an experimenter might employ to study the effects of manipulating an independent variable on some dependent variable. Not every experiment that you find in the literature falls into an exact niche in Plutchik's classification, but an understanding of the classification enables consumers of research to grasp the overall concept of how independent variables affect dependent variables and of how experimenters go about studying these effects. Plutchik's classification is based on the number of independent variables studied and on the number of manipulated values of the independent variable. Although it may seem trivial at first merely to count variables and their values, it eventually becomes apparent that the number of independent variables or the number of values of an independent variable can be critical in enabling an experimenter to determine the nature of the causes of changes in a given dependent variable.

Bivalent Experiments

The first type of experiment that Plutchik (1974) identified is the bivalent experiment in which the experimenter studies the effects of two values of one independent variable on the dependent variable. This type of experiment is called bivalent ("two values") because the independent variable is manipulated by the experimenter in a manner that allows for only two values of the independent variable to be presented to the subjects. In the case of a continuous independent variable, this means that the experimenter has selected only two of the many values that fall along the continuum of the independent variable to be the manipulated values of the independent variable. For example, an experimenter may wish to manipulate the intensity of tones presented to listeners and selects only two intensities to present to them: a "low" and a "high" intensity. In the case of a categorical independent variable, the researcher may select two of the many categories of the independent variable that are available. In some cases, the independent variable may be dichotomous and, therefore, only classifiable into two categories. For example, the experimenter may wish to study the effects of binaural vs. monaural listening. In any case, regardless of the potential number of values of the independent variable at the researcher's disposal, only two are employed in the bivalent experiment.

The study by Adams and Moore (1972) of the effects of masking noise on stuttering behavior is an example of a bivalent experiment. In this experiment, stutters spoke under two conditions: (1) in quiet and (2) when presented with a masking noise. The results of this bivalent experiment are illustrated in Figure 2.3, which shows that presentation of the masking noise caused a reduction in stuttering frequency relative to the quiet condition. A bar graph is used to display these results because the two conditions (quiet vs. noise) are categorical manipulations of the independent variable rather than manipulations that fall along a continuum of values of the independent variable.

In another example of a bivalent experiment, McClellan (1967) examined

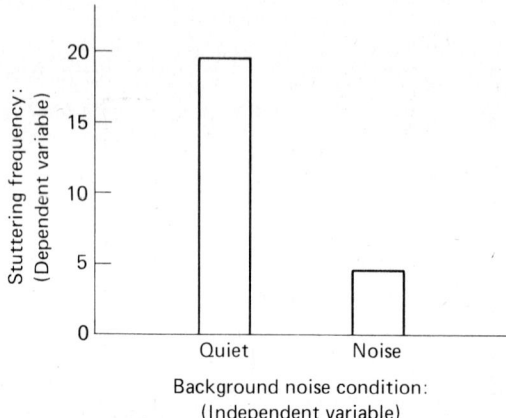

Figure 2.3 Results of a bivalent experiment, showing the effect of masking noise on stuttering frequency. (Drawn from the data of Adams and Moore, 1972.)

the effect of venting hearing-aid earmolds on speech discrimination in noise. Hearing-impaired subjects were given speech discrimination tests in a noisy background under two conditions: (1) while wearing hearing aid with an unvented earmold and (2) while wearing the same aid with a vented earmold. Figure 2.4 illustrates the results of this bivalent experiment. Inspection of Figure 2.4 reveals that the subjects showed better speech-discrimination scores when using the vented earmold than when using the unvented earmold. Again, the results of this bivalent experiment are presented with a bar graph because the independent variable was manipulated categorically (vented vs. unvented earmold) rather than along a continuum of values.

Other examples of bivalent experiments might include studies of the effect of therapy vs. no therapy on the articulation performance of articulation-impaired children, studies of the effect of binaural vs. monaural stimulation on speech perception, studies of the effect of fluency reinforcement vs. no reinforcement on stuttering, or studies of the effect of delayed vs. normal feedback on speech rate. All of these examples represent problems for which bivalent experiments could be valuable in examining the effects of these independent variables on these dependent variables because the independent variables can be dichotomized to form two values for manipulation.

Categorical independent variables very often form dichotomies that require the use of bivalent experiments. For example, Sherman (1954) considered the merits of playing speech backward vs. forward to listeners for scaling of voice quality, the rationale being that variables, like semantic content, that could bias the ratings would be removed with backward playing of the tapes. Backward vs. forward tape playback is a true dichotomy because there

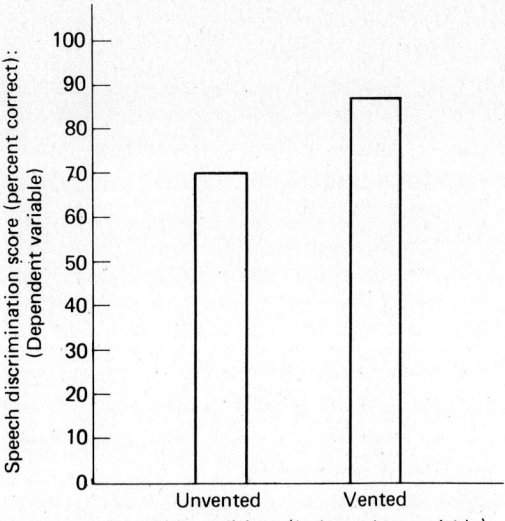

Figure 2.4 Results of a bivalent experiment, showing the effect of earmold venting on speech discrimination in noise. (Drawn from the data of McClellan, 1967.)

are only these two ways of presenting the stimuli. A truely dichotomous independent variable like this requires a bivalent experiment.

Some categorical independent variables comprise more than two categories. In that case, a researcher may select two of them to form a dichotomous independent variable, either because two of the categories are of more interest or because two of the categories do seem to be opposed in a dichotomous fashion. For example, we could conceive of binaural vs. monaural stimulation as a dichotomous independent variable because stimuli can be presented to either one ear or to both. However, we could also conceive of a more general categorical independent variable, mode of auditory stimulation, that includes values like monaural left, monaural right, true binaural (dichotic), pseudobinaural (diotic), and so on. We could then select various apparent dichotomies from the available categories such as left-ear vs. right-ear monaural stimulation, monaural vs. binaural, dichotic vs. diotic, and so on, to form the two values of a bivalent experiment. On the other hand, a researcher may decide to select more than two categories for manipulation and not do a simple bivalent experiment.

An experimenter may also take a continuous independent variable and use it to form a more-or-less artificial dichotomy in order to conduct a bivalent experiment. For example, the experimenter might study the effect of the presence vs. the absence of reinforcement on nonfluencies. Amount of reinforcement could be conceptualized as a continuous independent variable that could be artificially dichotomized into values of zero vs. a large amount, or "present" vs. "absent." In a sense, this is what happened in the Adams and Moore (1972) study of the effects of noise on stuttering. Noise intensity is a continuous independent variable that Adams and Moore artificially dichotomized into "quiet" and "noise," or presence vs. absence of noise.

Although bivalent experiments are valuable in examining the effects of categorical independent variables (especially those that reflect true dichotomies), Plutchik (1974) has indicated that they are limited in scope and may even lead to erroneous conclusions when the independent variable is continuous. Bivalent experiments are limited in scope because they do not always encompass as much of the potential range of values of the continuous independent variable as may be possible. In other words, presenting only two values of a continuous independent variable may not give as clear a picture of the function relating it to a dependent variable as presenting a larger number of values of the independent variable might. Bivalent experiments can lead to erroneous conclusions when the function being studied is not linear. Discussion of the next type of experiment in Plutchik's classification will help to clarify these two problems.

Multivalent Experiments

The second type of experiment that Plutchik (1974) identified is the multivalent experiment in which the experimenter studies the effects of several values of the independent variable on the dependent variable. This type of experiment is called multivalent ("many values") because the independent variable is manipulated in a manner that allows for at least three (and usually more) values of the independent variable to be presented to the subjects. When the independent variable is continuous, a multivalent experiment is more appropriate than a bivalent experiment for two reasons.

First, the multivalent experiment gives a broader picture of the relationship between the independent and dependent variables than the bivalent experiment does because the experimenter samples the range of possible values of the independent variable more completely. If the dependent variable changes linearly as a function of changes in the independent variable (i.e., the graph slopes upward or downward in a straight-line fashion), then the bivalent experiment would show a pattern of results similar to the multivalent experiment. The results of the bivalent experiment, however, would be limited in scope, and the multivalent experiment would broaden the picture of the functional relationship between the independent and dependent variables.

A second, and more serious, problem occurs when the function takes the form of a curve rather than a straight line on the graph relating changes in the dependent variable to manipulations of the independent variable. At least three values of the independent variable must be employed to identify a curvilinear function because at least three coordinate points on a graph must be used to plot a curve. Because a bivalent experiment examines only two values of the independent variable, its resultant graph cannot reveal the shape of a curvilinear function. A multivalent experiment must be performed to reveal a curvilinear function. We now examine some examples from the research literature to demonstrate the appropriateness of multivalent experiments for studying the effects of a continuous independent variable on a dependent variable.

In the previous section, the study by Adams and Moore (1972) on the effects of noise on stuttering was presented as an example of a bivalent experiment. Although this study showed that stuttering frequency decreased from the quiet to the noise condition, it was somewhat limited in scope because it could not show how stuttering frequency changed as a function of increases in the intensity of noise. Adams and Hutchinson (1974) hypothesized, as a logical extension of the Adams and Moore study, that increases in the intensity of masking noise might cause decreases in stuttering frequency. To test this hypothesis, the authors conducted a multivalent experiment in which the masking noise was varied from quiet to 10, 50, and 90 dB above threshold. The results of this study are illustrated in Figure 2.5, which plots stuttering frequency as a function of masking noise intensity. Inspection of Figure 2.5 reveals systematic decreases in stuttering frequency from the quiet condition to the noise conditions. Also, stuttering frequency decreased in a roughly linear fashion as masking noise was progressively increased in intensity from 10 to 90 dB above threshold. This multivalent experiment broadens the picture of the relation between stuttering and masking noise by showing the functional dependence of stuttering frequency on increases in the masking noise intensity.

An example of a multivalent experiment that demonstrates a curvilinear

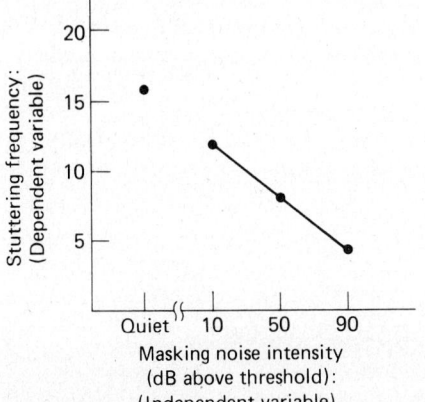

Figure 2.5   Results of a multivalent experiment, showing the effect of masking noise intensity on stuttering frequency. (Drawn from the data of Adams and Hutchinson, 1974.)

relationship is the commonly seen performance-intensity function. It dem-onstrates how word recognition varies as a function of the intensity at which words are presented to the listener. For normal-hearing persons listening to PB words, this curve rises rather sharply as presentation level is increased from 0 to about 50 dB sound pressure level (SPL) and then it flattens out at a ceiling of about 95 to 100% correct as intensity is further increased to about 100 dB SPL. Figure 2.6 depicts a typical performance-intensity function for normal-hearing persons listening to PB words. The dependent variable is performance (percent of words correctly recognized) and the independent variable is the intensity of presentation level of the words. As we can see in Figure 2.6, performance rises steeply from the lowest presentation level to about 50 dB SPL and then the curve flattens out from about 50 dB to 100 dB SPL.

Clearly, a multivalent experiment is necessary to discover the shape of this function. If a bivalent experiment were performed using the values of the independent variable indicated at points *A* and *B* on Figure 2.6, the function would seem to rise sharply, but there would be no indication of the cur-vilinearity of the relationship. If a bivalent experiment were performed using the values of the independent variable indicated at points *B* and *C* on Figure 2.6, the conclusion would be that presentation level had no effect on perfor-mance! Thus, a bivalent experiment would not be appropriate for examining the effect of presentation intensity level on word recognition because the

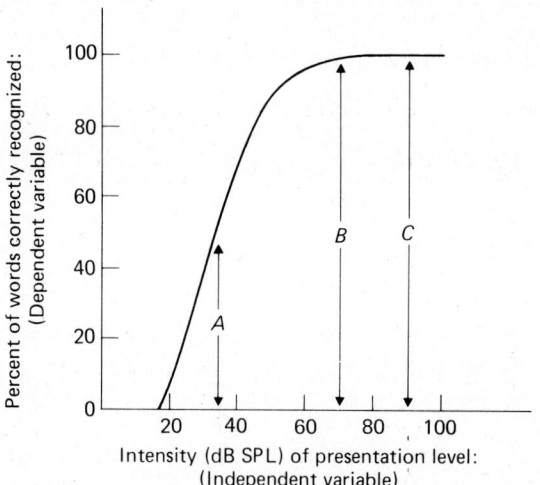

Figure 2.6   Results of a multivalent experiment, showing the effect of presentation-intensity level on recognition of monosyllabic PB words. *A* and *B* or *B* and *C* indicate possible outcomes of bivalent ex-periments. (Adapted from data of Hirsh et al., 1952.)

dependent variable changes as a curvilinear function of changes in the independent variable.

In summary, a multivalent experiment is more appropriate than a bivalent experiment in the case of a continuously manipulable independent variable. Consumers of research should be cautious in drawing conclusions from bivalent experiments unless the independent variable can be dichotomized. When the independent variable can be manipulated along some continuum of values for presentation to the subjects, bivalent experiments suffer from two disadvantages. First, the picture of the functional relation of the dependent to the independent variable is limited in scope. Plutchik (1974) cautions that this limitation may force readers to overgeneralize to the effects of other possible values of the independent variable. Second, when the function is curvilinear, a bivalent experiment could lead to incorrect conclusions because at least three values of the independent variable (and preferably more) are necessary to determine the shape of the curve. These disadvantages can be overcome by conducting a multivalent experiment in which several values of the independent variable are manipulated or presented to the subjects. The multivalent experiment, then, is a much more comprehensive type of experiment for studying the functional dependence of one variable on another variable, especially when examining nonlinear functions.

Parametric Experiments

The third type of experiment Plutchik (1974) described is the *parametric* experiment in which the researcher studies the simultaneous effects of more than one independent variable on the dependent variable. It is called a parametric experiment because the second independent variable is referred to as the parameter.[3] The main effect of one independent variable on the dependent variable can be examined at the same time that the main effect of another independent variable on the dependent variable is studied. In addition, the *interaction* of the two independent variables in causing changes in the dependent variable can also be determined.

An example of a parametric experiment is the study by Erber (1971) of the simultaneous effects of distance (independent variable) and syllabic pattern of words (parameter) on visual recognition of speech through lipreading by deaf children (dependent variable). The results of this experiment are illustrated in Figure 2.7. Inspection of the figure reveals that recognition of words by lipreading decreased as the talker moved farther away from the receiver and that this function held true for three types of words differing in syllabic pattern. Also demonstrated was the fact that at any given distance, spondees

---

[3]This is a special use of the term parameter, a word that has several uses. In mathematics, parameter means a variable quantity that may be arbitrarily held constant or changed to generate a family of curves. In statistics, parameter means a variable population characteristic, and this statistical use of the word will be explained in more detail in Chapter 5.

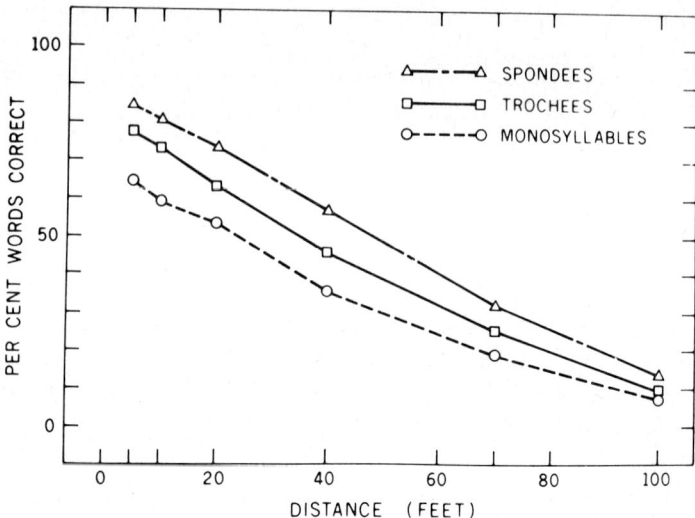

Figure 2.7 Results of a parametric experiment, showing the main effects of distance of talker from receiver and syllabic pattern of words on recognition of words by lipreading. (From Erber, 1971, p. 852.)

were easiest to recognize by lipreading, trochees were somewhat more difficult, and monosyllables were most difficult. Therefore, there were two main effects operating on lipreading recognition: distance of talker from receiver and syllabic pattern of words spoken.

In a parametric experiment on time-compressed speech, Beasley, Schwimmer, and Rintelmann (1972) examined the simultaneous effects of presentation intensity and amount of time compression on the intelligibility of speech with normal adults. Figure 2.8 shows the main effects of the independent variable (presentation intensity measured in sensation level) and the parameter (percent time compression of the speech) on the dependent variable (speech intelligibility measured in percent correct). Inspection of Figure 2.8 reveals two things: (1) intelligibility increased as presentation intensity increased and (2) for each presentation level, intelligibility generally decreased as time compression was increased from 0 to 70%. Thus, the main effects of two independent variables on the dependent variable were explored.

So far, we have discussed only the *main effects* of the independent variable and the parameter on the dependent variable. The main effects of each of these independent variables and parameters could also be studied if the experimenters each performed two different multivalent experiments to examine the effects of each of their independent variables on their dependent variables. For example, Erber could have studied the effect of distance on lipreading and then done a second experiment to study the effect of syllabic pattern on lipreading. Beasley et al. could have studied the effect of pre-

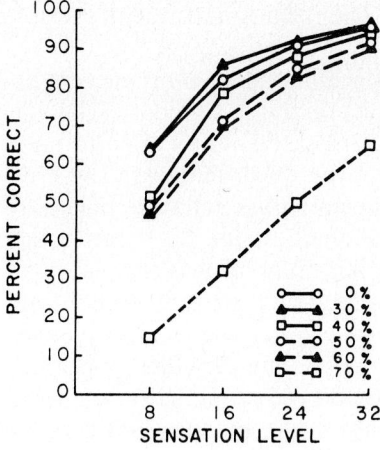

Figure 2.8 Results of a parametric experiment, showing the main effects of presentation intensity and percent time compression on speech intelligibility. (From Beasley, Schwimmer, and Rintelmann, 1972, p. 343.)

sentation level on speech intelligibility and then done a second experiment on the effect of time compression on speech intelligibility. So far, the experimenters have improved efficiency by studying the two main effects in the same experiment rather than performing a different experiment for each main effect. But the most important advantage of performing a parametric experiment rather than two multivalent (or bivalent if both independent variables are categorical) experiments is that the *interaction* of the two independent variables in causing changes in the dependent variable can be examined.

An interaction effect is a *joint* or *simultaneous* or *mutual* effect of the two (or more) independent variables on the dependent variable. We say that an interaction effect occurs when the independent variable affects the dependent variable in different ways for different levels of the parameter. An interaction effect can only be seen when two (or more) independent variables are studied *simultaneously* in a parametric experiment. An interaction effect cannot be seen when two separate multivalent experiments have been completed, even if the two independent variables employed in the two experiments would have interacted in a parametric experiment.

An interaction effect occurs when the function relating changes in the dependent variable to changes in the independent variable is not the same shape for all values of the parameter. For example, the dependent variable may *increase* as a function of increases in the independent variable for one value of the parameter, but the dependent variable might show *no change* as a function of increases in the independent variable for another value of the parameter. In fact, the dependent variable may increase with increases in the independent variable for one value of the parameter and *decrease* with increases in the independent variable for another value of the parameter. Whenever the shape of the function relating changes in the dependent variable to changes in the independent variable has a different form for different values of the parameter, an interaction between the independent variable and the parameter is said to occur.

An example of a parametric experiment that illustrates an interaction between two independent variables in their effect on the dependent variable is seen in the study by Shriner and Daniloff (1970) of the ability of children to reassemble syllables that were segmented by the experimenters. The children were presented with meaningful and meaningless syllables that were recorded with silent intervals between the phonemes, and they were asked to reassemble the syllables. The interphonemic interval was the independent variable and was manipulated over a range from 50 to 400 msec. Meaningfulness of the syllables was the parameter and assumed two values: meaningful and meaningless. Thus, the independent variable was multivalent and the parameter was bivalent. (Note: because a parametric experiment employs two or more independent variables, any independent variable used in a parametric experiment is either bivalent or multivalent.) The dependent variable was reassembly performance measured in percent correct. Figure 2.9 shows the effects of interphonemic interval and meaningfulness of the syllables on reassembly performance for all of the children who were studied. Inspection of Figure 2.9 reveals that meaningful syllables were more often reassembled correctly than meaningless syllables. In addition, there was a general trend for better reassembly performance when the interphonemic interval was shorter and poorer reassembly performance when the interphonemic interval was longer.

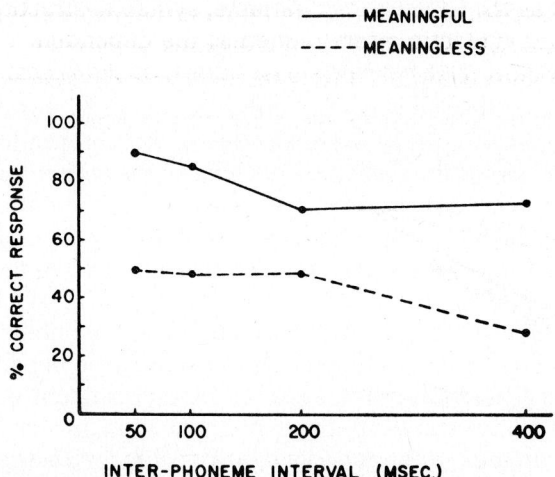

Figure 2.9 Results of a parametric experiment, showing the main and interaction effects of interphonemic interval and syllable meaningfulness on children's syllable-reassembly performance. (From Shriner and Daniloff, 1970, p. 542.)

However, there was a significant interaction between interphonemic interval and meaningfulness in determining the changes in reassembly performance. In other words, there was an interaction between the independent variable and the parameter in causing the changes in the dependent variable. For the meaningful syllables, there was a decrease in the children's performance as the interphonemic interval increased from 50 to 200 msec, but their reassembly scores remained about the same from 200 to 400 msec. This pattern of results was reversed for the meaningless syllables. As the interphonemic interval increased from 50 to 200 msec, there was no change in reassembly performance, but as interphonemic interval increased from 200 to 400 msec, reassembly performance decreased. Thus, the function relating performance on the dependent variable to manipulation of the independent variable was not the same for the two levels of the parameter. In other words, there was an interaction between interphonemic interval and meaningfulness of the syllables in their mutual effect on the dependent variable of reassembly performance.

Another example of a parametric experiment with an interaction between two independent variables is seen in the study of Panagos and Prelock (1982) concerning the effects of phonological and syntactical constraints on sentence productions of language-disordered children. The children were presented with sentences that varied in both phonological structure (simple vs. complex) and in syntactical structure (center embedded, right embedded, and unembedded), and they were asked to repeat each sentence. The dependent variable was the number of syntactic errors made by the children in repeating each sentence. Figure 2.10 shows the results with phonological structure plotted as the independent variable, syntactic structure plotted as the parameter, and syntactic errors plotted as the dependent variable.

Inspection of Figure 2.10 reveals a main effect of phonological structure

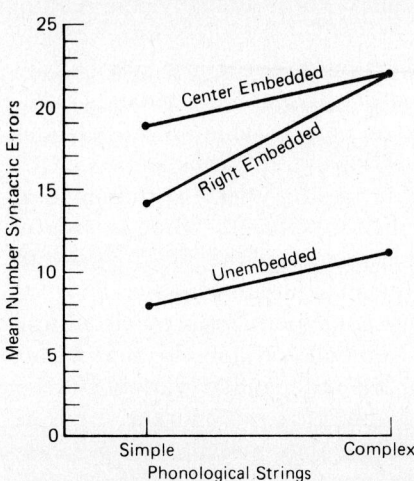

Figure 2.10 Results of a parametric experiment, showing the main and interaction effects of phonological constraints and syntactic constraints on children's syntactic errors. (From Panagos and Prelock, 1982, p. 174.)

(more errors on complex than on simple structures) and a main effect of syntactic structures (generally more errors on center embedded than on right embedded structures and more errors on right embedded than on unembedded structures). In addition, an interaction between phonological and syntactic structures is seen in the figure. The increase in number of errors from simple to complex phonological structures was greater for right embedded sentences than for either center embedded or unembedded sentences. In fact, the increase was so sharp that the right embedded/complex mean equaled the center embedded/complex mean, even though there was a large difference between the center embedded and right embedded means for simple phonological structures. The more rapid acceleration of the right embedded line in the figure shows this interaction graphically. As a general rule of thumb, when the lines on a graph, like those in Figure 2.10, are roughly parallel, there is no interaction between the independent variables. But when the lines deviate grossly from parallel, there is an interaction between the independent variables. Parallel lines on the graph indicate that the functions relating the changes in the dependent variable to the independent variable are the same for each level of the parameter. Lines that are not parallel indicate that the functions relating the changes in the dependent variable to the independent variable are not the same for each level of the parameter.

Consumers of research should also be aware of the fact that experiments are often conducted that employ more than one dependent variable. In such a case, the effects of the independent variable on the different dependent variables are examined. In the bivalent experiment by Adams and Moore (1972) discussed earlier, the researchers actually studied more than just the effects of noise masking on stuttering frequency. They examined the effects of noise on four dependent variables: stuttering frequency, palmar sweat anxiety, vocal intensity, and reading time. In the multivalent experiment cited earlier, Adams and Hutchinson (1974) examined the effects of noise on three dependent variables: stuttering frequency, vocal intensity, and reading time.

To summarize Plutchik's (1974) classification, experiments may be categorized as bivalent, multivalent, or parametric. Bivalent experiments examine the effects of two values of one independent variable on a dependent variable and are appropriate when the independent variable can be dichtomized. These experiments are inappropriate for studying independent variables that can be continuously manipulated, especially when examining nonlinear functions. Multivalent experiments examine the effects of several values of one independent variable on the dependent variable. They are more comprehensive and accurate than bivalent experiments in determining functional relationships when the independent variable is continuous. When there is the possibility of more than one independent variable having an effect on the dependent variable, the parametric experiment is appropriate for simultaneously manipulating an independent variable and a parameter to study their combined effects on the dependent variable. Any of these types of experiments could employ more than one dependent variable.

Descriptive Research

Descriptive research is employed to examine group differences, developmental trends, or relationships among variables that can be measured by the researcher. Research of this type provides an empirical picture of what was observed at one time or of observed changes over a period of time, without manipulation of independent variables by the researcher. In descriptive research, researchers are essentially passive observers who try to be as unobtrusive as possible so that their presence (or the presence of their measuring instruments or techniques) cause a minimum of alteration of the naturalness of the phenomena under investigation. As pointed out earlier in this chapter, experimental research involves manipulation of an active independent variable to see its effect on a dependent variable, whereas descriptive research involves the observation of relations between attribute independent variables and dependent variables. Descriptive research is an important endeavor in the behavioral sciences and constitutes a large portion of the research found in the speech pathology and audiology literature. There are, however, some common misunderstandings of descriptive research that should be discussed.

First, descriptive research does not lead to the formulation of cause-and-effect statements. The description of differences between groups or of relationships among variables does not provide sufficient grounds for establishing *causal* relations. The discovery of cause and effect falls within the purview of experimental research, and the experimenter's ability to make things happen under controlled conditions is simply not possible in descriptive research. It is, therefore, difficult to draw conclusions from descriptive research about cause–effect relations because many factors beyond the control of the researcher may confound the results.

Second, statements such as the foregoing have led some people to disparage descriptive research as an inferior method. It is not an inferior method. There are situations in which descriptive research is more appropriate and situations in which experimental research is more appropriate. Descriptive research is more appropriate in a situation in which the researcher is interested in behaviors as they occur naturally without the interference of an experimenter. In other situations, when the researcher wishes to manipulate conditions to study cause–effect relations, experimental research is more appropriate.

There are, however, situations in which experimental research is desired, but ethical concerns such as the regard for protection of human subjects preclude the use of certain experimental techniques. For example, it would be unethical to conduct an experiment that would produce a conductive hearing loss in humans in order to study the effects of middle ear pathology on auditory perception or academic achievement. Therefore, researchers must rely on descriptive studies of children with and without middle ear pathology. Such descriptive research is not equal to experiments in determining cause–effect relationships, but it must be relied on as the best available compromise because of the ethical concern that forbids experimental studies of the effects of pathology on humans. The problems inherent in such a situation have led to much controversy concerning descriptive research such as investigations of the relations between middle ear pathology and auditory perception (Ventry, 1980). A recent exchange of letters in the *Journal of Speech and Hearing Disorders* between Ayukawa and Rudmin (1983) and Karsh and Brandes (1983) illustrates the dilemma facing researchers who must substitute a descriptive study for an experiment that is impossible to conduct.

Another example concerns research on the etiology of stuttering. It has been hypothesized that various conditions in the child's speaking environment may be responsible for the onset of stuttering. But it would be unethical to manipulate systematically environmental conditions in an attempt to cause stuttering in children. Therefore, much research concerned with environmental factors related to the onset of stuttering has focused on descriptions of stuttering and nonstuttering children around the time of typical onset.

In summary, when observation of natural phenomena is necessary to solve a particular problem, descriptive research is appropriate. When the researcher wishes to examine cause-and-effect relations by manipulating variables, experimental research is appropriate. There may be situations in which experimental research is desirable but impossible. When descriptive research is substituted for experimental research in such a situation, the ensuing investigation is unable to determine the kind of direct cause-and-effect links that the experiment might have found.

Before discussing the different types of descriptive research, it is worth commenting on the various terms that are used to describe independent and dependent variables in descriptive research. As stated previously, experimental independent variables are active and can be manipulated by the experimenter to examine their effects on dependent variables. The independent variables of descriptive research, however, are attribute variables that cannot be manipulated.

In certain kinds of descriptive research, subjects can be *classified* according to certain variables and comparisons can be made between the classifications with regard to some *criterion* variable. The terms *classification variable* and *criterion variable* are analogous, respectively, to the terms *independent variable* and *dependent variable*. For example, aphasics might be compared with persons without aphasia on some measure of linguistic performance. In such a case, the classification variable would be language status (aphasic vs. nonapahsic) and linguistic performance would be the criterion variable.

In certain other kinds of descriptive research, subjects of one classification are measured on a number of criterion variables to determine the relationships among these variables and the ability to predict one variable from another. In such a case, one of the variables can be designated the *predictor variable* and the other can be designated the *predicted variable*. Again, the terms *predictor variable* and *predicted variable* are analogous to the terms *independent variable* and *dependent variable*. The real difference between the two sets of terms lies in the ability of the researcher to manipulate the independent variable.

It might help consumers of research to differentiate experimental and descriptive research if they would examine the manipulability of the variables used in a research study. If the independent variable can be manipulated to see its effect on the dependent variable, then the study is experimental. If the subjects are classified according to some nonmanipulable dimension and compared on some criterion, or if relationships are examined between nonmanipulable predictor and predicted variables, then the research is descriptive. It should be pointed out to consumers that many authors use the terms independent and dependent variables for *both* experimental and descriptive research, so an analysis of the manipulability of variables is often necessary to determine whether or not a given research study is experimental or descriptive. As will be seen later, much research in speech pathology and audiology is a *combination* of experimental and descriptive research.

Many different types of descriptive research can be found in the literature and those outlined below illustrate some of the common approaches found in speech pathology and audiology. Four different types of descriptive research will be considered: (1) *comparative*, (2) *developmental*, (3) *correlational*, and (4) *survey* research.

Comparative Research

Comparative research is designed to measure the behavior of two or more types of subjects at one point in time in order to draw conclusions about the similarities or differences between them.

For example, Shriner, Holloway, and Daniloff (1969) were interested in the syntactic performances of children with and without articulatory defects. They asked 30 children with severe articulation problems and 30 children with normal articulation to tell stories about pictures of children engaged in various activities, and they derived six measures of each child's syntactic use from their responses: length-complexity index (LCI), four subcategories of LCI, and mean length of response (MLR). Children with normal articulation performed better than did those with articulation defects on LCI, two subcategories of LCI that involve elaboration of noun phrases and verb phrases in sentences, and MLR.

The LCI scores of the two groups of children are illustrated in Figure 2.11. Inspection of Figure 2.11 shows that the children with normal articulation had higher LCI scores than did the children with impaired articulation. It also reveals that comparative research that examimes dichotomous groups is analogous to a bivalent experiment, but it involves the selection of subjects from dichotomous classifications rather than manipulation of a dichoto-

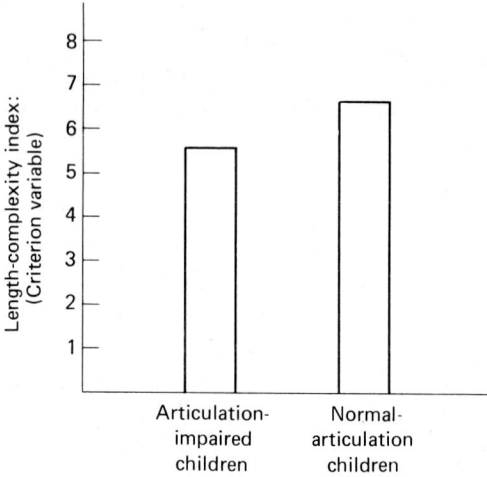

Figure 2.11   Results of a bivalent comparison of the length-complexity index (LCI) scores of children with normal and impaired articulation. (Drawn from data of Shriner et al., 1969.)

mous independent variable. Comparative research studies may also be found that are analogous to multivalent and parametric experiments.

A comparative research study analogous to a multivalent experiment would involve comparison of three or more groups of subjects who could be classified along some continuum. For example, Brannon (1968) compared linguistic word-class usage in samples of the spoken language of normal-hearing, hearing-impaired, and deaf children. The children were classified along the continuum of hearing status from normal to hearing impaired to deaf, and linguistic word-class usage was the criterion variable on which they were compared.

To illustrate the analogy between this comparative study and a multi-valent experiment, Brannon's data on the average number of words per subject found in the speech samples of the three groups are shown in Figure 2.12. The similarity between Figure 2.12 and Figure 2.5 illustrates the analogy between a multivalent comparison and a multivalent experiment. The graph relating the criterion variable to the classification variable can be evaluated in much the same manner as the graph relating the dependent variable to the independent variable in experimental research. The major difference between the multivalent comparison and the multivalent experiment concerns the ability to manipulate the independent variable in the experiment vs. the need to select already existing members of the classifications in the descriptive comparison. It would not have been possible to produce hearing impairment in the children and then study the effects of this impairment on word-class usage.

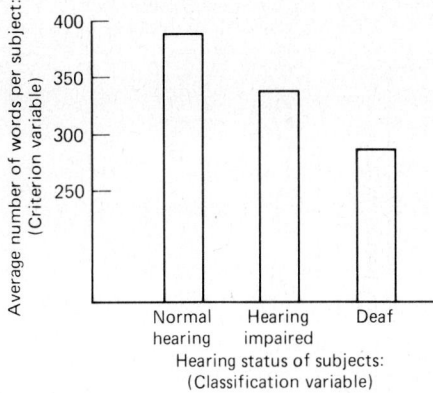

Figure 2.12 Results of a multivalent comparison of number of words per subject produced by three groups of subjects differing in hearing status. (Drawn from data of Brannon, 1968.)

There is one minor difference between Brannon's (1968) results, as illustrated in Figure 2.12, and the results of Adams and Hutchinson (1974), illustrated in Figure 2.5. A bar graph was used instead of a line graph to illustrate Brannon's data. This was done because the three levels of the independent variable were three categorical values of hearing status rather than numbers on a numerical continuum to indicate degrees of severity of hearing loss. The line graph was used for the Adams and Hutchinson data in Figure 2.5 because their independent variable was continuous rather than categorical. The categories in Brannon's data do, however, represent an approximation, at least, to a multivalent ordering of categories along a continuum of degree of hearing-loss severity. This graphical convention should not be construed as a reflection of a difference between experimental and descriptive independent variables, but, rather, as reflecting a difference between categorical and continuous independent variables.

A comparative study that is analogous to a parametric experiment would involve comparisons of groups that differ simultaneously with respect to two or more classification variables. Parasnis (1983) provides such an example in her descriptive comparison of performance on several dependent variables of deaf students who differed with regard to early manual communication exposure and sex. The first classification (independent) variable—early manual communication exposure—included two levels: delayed sign language (a group of congenitally deaf children of hearing parents who learned to sign between the ages of 6 and 12 years) and native American Sign Language (ASL) signers (a group of congenitally deaf children of deaf parents who had learned to sign from birth). The second classification (independent) variable—sex—had two levels: male and female. Figure 2.13 shows the mean performances of each of the four groups for the dependent variable of speechreading without sound. Inspection of Figure 2.13 reveals that the delayed sign language students outperformed the native ASL students and that the females outperformed the males in each of these groups. In other words, there was a main effect of early manual communication experience

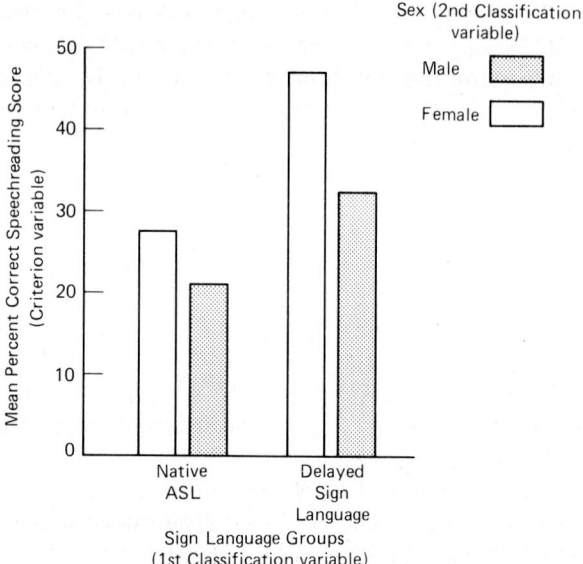

Figure 2.13 Results of a parametric comparison of speechreading scores of male and female deaf students who were native sign language (ASL) users or delayed sign language users. (Drawn from data of Parasnis, 1983.)

and a main effect of sex. No interactions were found between sex and early manual communication exposure for any of the dependent variables.

Comparative research, then, involves the examination of differences and similarities among existing variables or subject classifications that are of interest to the researcher. This type of research has the advantage of allowing researchers to study variables that could not be manipulated experimentally. Sometimes these experiments are called "experiments of nature" because subjects belong to the classifications as a result of the vagaries of nature. These experiments may also be referred to as "natural-group" research studies for the same reason.

These are two disadvantages of comparative research that should be mentioned. First, it is difficult to draw conclusions about the causes of criterion-variable differences that may be found. This difficulty in attributing causation is due to the possibility that other variables may concurrently operate with the classification variable to influence the criterion variable. The lack of experimental control in the descriptive approach makes it difficult to preclude such a possibility.

Second, Young (1976)[4] criticized the use of group-difference data for gen-

---

[4]Young uses the term "retrospective" to describe what we call comparative research, and our use of the term retrospective later in this chapter has a more restricted meaning than the one Young implied.

erating knowledge about the performance of different groups of subjects on various criterion measures. He suggested some correlational plans as better methods of assessing the performance of differently classified subjects on various criterion measures. The use of such correlational plans is considered later in this chapter.

Developmental Research

A developmental research study is designed to measure changes over time in the behavior or characteristics of subjects, usually with reference to aging or maturation of the subjects. The independent or classification variable in developmental research is maturation (e.g., physical or intellectual growth) and is usually indicated by measurements of chronological or mental age or by some index of maturation (e.g., mean length of response as an index of language maturity). Researchers, for example, have been interested in studying the form and function of emerging grammars as children develop language (Bloom, 1970) or in changes in hearing thresholds as adults progress through old age (Bergman, 1971). Three different developmental plans may be encountered in the literature: *cross-sectional, longitudinal,* and *semilongitudinal.*

A *cross-sectional* plan of observation involves the selection of subjects from various age groups and observing differences between the behaviors or characteristics of the different groups. For example, Lodge and Leach (1975) examined idiomatic comprehension of adults and six-, nine-, and 12-year old children. Sentences that could be interpreted idiomatically or literally were read to 20 subjects in each age group and they were asked to choose pictures closest in meaning to each sentence. More idiomatic comprehension was found for older subjects than younger ones, whereas all subjects performed at about the same level in literal comprehension. The authors concluded that literal meaning was acquired first by children and followed by acquisition of idiomatic meaning.

Figure 2.14 shows a portion of the data that Lodge and Leach presented in their article and is included here only to illustrate how developmental data are often presented in a journal article. The data in Figure 2.14 illustrate the conclusion that comprehension of literal meaning appeared to be acquired before comprehension of idiomatic meaning. The data for literal meaning show only a small increase in performance from six to nine years and a similar performance for the three upper age groups, whereas those for idiomatic comprehension indicate a pronounced increase in performance as a function of increasing age. In developmental research, then, some criterion variable is plotted as a function of age. This function is similar to the functions seen earlier in experimental and comparative research, with age acting as the independent or classification variable.

A weakness of cross-sectional studies is that observations of differences *between* subjects of different ages are made in order to generalize about developmental changes that would occur *within* subjects with the passage of

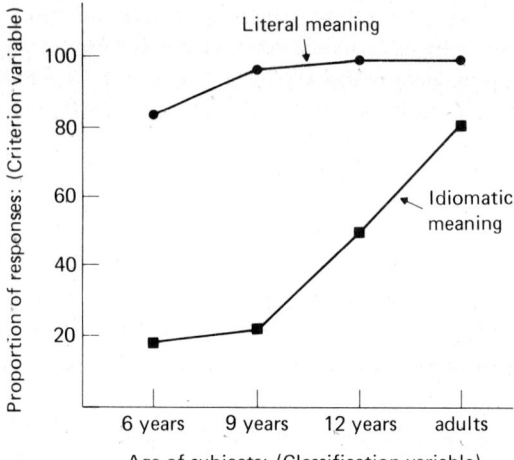

Figure 2.14 Illustration of the results of a cross-sectional developmental study of two dependent variables (comprehension of literal and of idiomatic meaning). Correct literal and idiomatic responses are plotted as a function of age. (Adapted from the data of Lodge and Leach, 1975.)

time. Only the next developmental plan can make direct observations of how subjects actually develop as they age and mature.

A *longitudinal* plan of observation involves following subjects as they mature or age and observing changes with the passage of time in the behaviors or characteristics of each subject. For example, Bloom (1970) followed three children for 18 months and sampled their language to study the form and function of emerging grammars in their utterances. Longitudinal studies have the advantage of directly showing how subjects mature or develop certain characteristics or behaviors while the subjects are actually aging.

Longitudinal studies, however, have the disadvantage of being expensvie and time consuming, and they suffer from problems of subject attrition. Subjects may die, move to new locations that are inaccessible to the investigator, or lose interest in participating in the study before it is completed. Often, as a result of the expense, the time demands on the researcher, and the time demands on the subjects, only a small number of subjects can be included in a longitudinal study. Also, if the study is conceived as spanning a wide age range, it would be years before the study were completed and published, and, quite possibly, the investigator could die or lose interest before the study was finished. Cross-sectional investigations are often substituted for longitudinal plans because they are less costly, less time consuming, and suffer less from attrition.

A logical compromise to minimize the weaknesses and maximize the strengths of cross-sectional and longitudinal studies is the *semilongitudinal* plan of observation. This plan involves dividing the total age span to be studied into several overlapping age spans, selecting subjects whose ages are at the lower edge of each new age span, and following them until they reach the upper age of the span. Wilder and Baken (1974), for example, were interested in observing respiratory parameters underlying infant crying behavior with a technique called impedance pneumography to record thoracic and abdominal movements. Ten infants entered the study at ages ranging from 2 to 161 days, and each was observed over a period of four months. Rather than making one observation of infants of different ages or waiting for infants to be born and then following them for a year, a semilongitudinal approach was adopted that allowed Wilder and Baker to make observations between *and* within subjects over a period of time in a more efficient manner.

Correlational Research

A correlational research study is designed to study the relationships among two or more variables by examining the degree to which changes in one variable correspond with or can be predicted from variations in another. Details of the statistical procedure called correlation and regression analysis will be discussed in Chapter 5, but the logical framework of correlational research should be considered along with the other types of descriptive research. Correlational research may range from a simple problem in which only two variables are studied to complex research in which the interrelation of a large number of variables is considered.

There are two basic questions asked in correlational research. First, how closely related are the variables? This question is answered by examining the performance of a group of subjects on the variables. The appropriate correlation coefficient is computed to indicate the strength of the relationship with regard to how much variation the two share in common. The correlation also indicates the direction of the relationship. A positive correlation indicates that increases in one variable are associated with increases in the other, whereas a negative correlation indicates that increases in one variable are associated with decreases in the other. A zero correlation indicates that the two variables are unrelated.

The concept of the correlation between variables can also be depicted visually on a graph called the "scatterplot" or "scattergram," which will be discussed in more detail in Chapters 5 and 8. The scattergram will be mentioned here only to illustrate correlational research. Briefly, the scattergram shows the pairs of scores on the two variables that were attained by each subject. The graph is a plot of the functional relationship between the two variables and is similar to the functions plotted for the data of experimental, comparative, and developmental research.

An example of a study of the correlation between two variables can be seen in the work of Shipp and Hollien (1969) on perception of age by listening to a person's voice. Listeners made judgments of the age of talkers by listening to recorded samples of their voices. The researchers then correlated the perceived ages with the actual ages of the talkers. Figure 2.15 shows the scatterplot and the correlation coefficient for the two variables of perceived age and actual age of the talkers. Perceived age is indicated on the ordinate and actual age is indicated on the abscissa of the graph. Each dot represents the intersection of the perceived age and the actual age of each of the 175 talkers. The correlation is strong and positive ($r = +.88$), indicating that perceived age and actual age are closely related to each other. If all the dots had fallen along the line drawn on the graph, the correlation would have been perfect ($r = +1.0$).

The second question that can be asked in correlational research is how well can performance on one variable be predicted from knowledge of performance on the other for a typical subject? This question is answered by completing a regression analysis that develops an equation for predicting the expected score (with a margin of error for the prediction) on one variable from knowledge of a subject's score on the other variable.

In the regression problem, one variable (or set of variables) is designated as

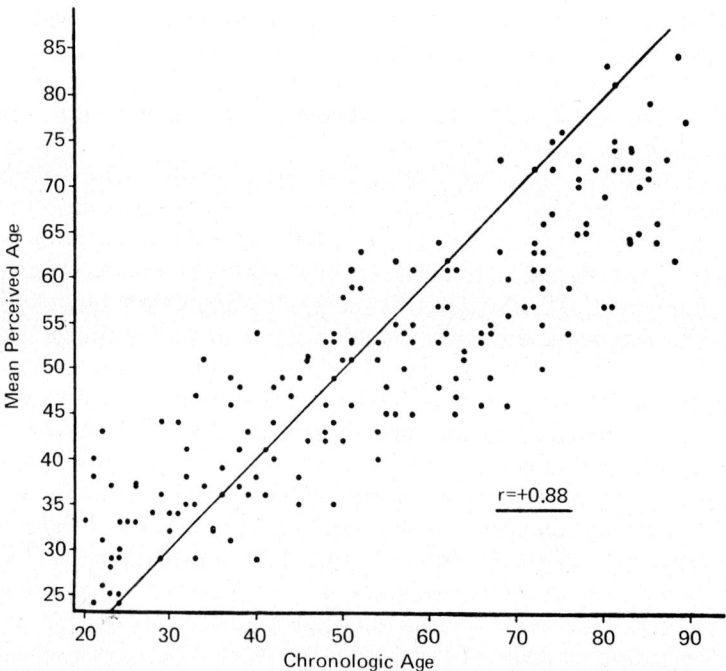

Figure 2.15   Scatterplot depicting the relationship between perceived age and chronological age of 175 talkers. Perceived age was judged by subjects listening to voice recordings of the talkers. (From Shipp and Hollien, 1969, p. 707.)

the predictor and another variable (or set of variables) is designated as the predicted variable. As mentioned previously, some researchers designate the predictor and predicted variables as independent and dependent variables, respectively. The terms predictor and predicted variables may provide a more accurate description of the nature of the variables studied in correlational research than do the terms independent and dependent variables. In correlational research, an independent variable is not manipulated to examine its effect on a dependent variable. Rather, two variables are measured and then one is used to try to predict the other one. Consumers should be aware, however, that they may encounter the terms independent and dependent variables used interchangably with the terms predictor and predicted variables in correlational studies.

An example of such a prediction problem is found in the task of the college admissions office in predicting how well an applicant should do in college, given the applicant's high school background and performance on standardized tests. Variables such as high school grade-point average, college board aptitude and achievement test scores, and interview ratings are designated as predictor variables, and college grade-point average is designated as the predicted variable. The admissions office has correlated the predictor and predicted variables of college students from previous years and developed a regression equation for predicting college grade-point average from high school grade-point average, college board scores, and interview rating. This equation can then be applied to a new applicant's record to predict the expected college grade-point average to help in deciding whether or not to admit the applicant.

Carhart and Porter (1971) provide an example of multiple regression analysis in their study of the predictive relation between pure-tone thresholds and speech reception threshold (SRT) with six groups of patients classified according to audiometric configuration. A separate regression analysis was performed for each subject group: patients with flat, gradual, marked high-tone, rising, trough-shaped, and atypical pure-tone configurations. Predictor variables were pure-tone thresholds at 250, 500, 1000, 2000, and 4000 Hz; the predicted variable was SRT measured with spondees. Pure-tone threshold at 1000 Hz emerged as the most important predictor variable for all groups except those subjects with marked high-tone loss, for them, 500 Hz was the best single predictor of SRT. Combinations of frequencies in the multiple prediction equations were also studied, and a noticeable, although not dramatic, improvement in prediction of SRT was achieved by adding a second frequency to the equation; adding a third frequency did not significantly improve the prediction. Also, the second frequency that most improved the prediction differed for various categories of audiometric configuration. The authors summarized the best combinations of predictor variables for each audiometric configuration and suggested an optimal combination for use if separation of patients by audiometric configurations could not be accomplished.

Jordan (1960) provides an example in speech pathology with his study of the relationship between children's performance on articulation tests and listener ratings of articulation defectiveness. The Templin-Darley articulation test was administered to 150 children, and a sample of each child's connected speech was played to 36 listeners for rating the severity of their articulation defectiveness. A multiple-regression analysis was then performed, using various measures from the articulation tests as predictor variables to predict scaled severity of articulation defectiveness (predicted variable). Jordan found that the number of defective single sounds, the proportion of misarticulations that were omissions, and consistency of misarticulations were the most important predictors of scaled severity of misarticulations.

A number of rather complicated extensions of correlation and regression plans have been developed over the years but discussion of all of these is beyond the scope of this book. Interested readers might wish to consult Monge and Capella (1980) or Kerlinger and Pedhazur (1973), but they should be aware that both a good understanding of mathematics and considerable preparation in statistics are necessary for a full appreciation of advanced correlation and regression analysis. We have only scratched the surface here, but we hope that readers have captured some of the flavor of the correlational plan.

One advantage of correlational research has already been pointed out in referring to Young's (1976) criticism of comparative research. Correlational research could be used to estimate the amount of variation in a criterion measure that could be accounted for on the basis of knowledge of group classification rather than simply looking at average differences in a criterion measure between two groups of subjects. Correlational research can be a most powerful tool for learning what aspects of human behavior share common properties. If a strong relationship exists between two variables, then a researcher can predict what one variable will be like if he or she knows the value of the other. But there are also disadvantages. Correlation does not imply causation, and many people have seemed to miss this fact in applying cause-and-effect statements to correlational data. In addition, correlational studies suffer from problems in the interpretation of the meaning of correlation coefficients. Two variables may be significantly correlated, but this may occur because both variables are correlated with a third variable that may be unknown to the researcher. Knowledge of the third variable may be crucial to understanding the true nature of the correlation between the original two variables. For these and other more technical reasons, it may be difficult to assess the theoretical or practical implications of a correlation. Sometimes correlational studies employ a shotgun approach in attempting to intercorrelate many variables and a large number of significant but fairly small correlation coefficients are found that make it difficult to assess the meaning of the complex interrelation of the variables.

Survey Research

A survey research study is designed to provide a detailed inspection of the prevalence of conditions, practices, or attitudes in a given environment by asking people about them rather than observing them directly. The instruments used in survey research include questionnaires, interviews, and, sometimes, a combination of the two. From a practical point of view, questionnaires are generally more appropriate for collecting relatively restricted information from a wide range of persons, whereas interviews are generally more appropriate for gathering more detailed information from a more restricted sample. When a balance of depth of information and breadth of respondents is desired, a combination of the two methods may be appropriate. For example, a relatively restricted or superficial questionnaire may be administered to a large number of people and a follow-up interview of a sample of these persons may be conducted.

Surveys do not usually encompass the entire population of interest for a number of practical reasons. For example, the population may be enormous and may be widely distributed geographically so that the time and expense necessary to study the entire population would be prohibitive. Therefore, a sample is usually drawn from the population for study, and inferences are made concerning the population from the study of the sample. Such surveys are often called sample surveys, and problems often arise in determining how well the data of the sample survey can be applied to make a generalization about the entire population.

A particular problem with the use of questionnaires should be mentioned. Regardless of whether a questionnaire is sent to the whole population or to a sample of the population, not all the questionnaires are returned, so the ones that are returned may not be an unbiased representation of the population. Interviews and questionnaires both may suffer from problems in determining the accuracy and the veracity of respondents' answers to various questions.

The American Speech-Language-Hearing Association regularly uses questionnaires to study such things as salaries or personal and professional characteristics of its members and reports these findings periodically in *Asha*. For example, Curlee (1976) recently presented questionnaire results concerning professional and personal characteristics such as employment setting, job tasks, sex, age, years of professional experience, academic training, and certification status of responding members. A recent follow-up survey by Fein (1984) presents an update of some of the variables surveyed by Curlee (1976) and illustrates the kind of periodic survey consumers are likely to encounter in *Asha*.

Martin and Pennington (1971) provide another example of a questionnaire study in their analysis of trends in audiometric practice. Questionnaires were sent to 500 persons randomly selected from the roll of ASHA-certified audiologists and 342 usable forms were returned. Results concerning the use of various procedures in pure-tone and speech audiometry were analyzed, and trends were noted in the degree of adoption of certain procedures.

Johnson & Associates (1959) provide an example of an in-depth interview study with their investigations of parental diagnoses of the onset of stuttering in children. Extensive interviews were conducted with parents who had judged their children as stutterers and parents who regarded their children as normal speakers, and it was found that sound repetitions were the speech characteristic reported as the basis of most of the judgments of stuttering. In most other respects, the interview data indicated that the stuttering and nonstuttering children were alike. In audiology, Harford and Dodds (1966) used interviewing to follow up on clinical tests in their evaluation of the success of users of CROS hearing aids. Patients were questioned several months after the hearing aids were recommended to gather information about hearing-aid purchases, use, and satisfaction of the wearers.

Case Study and Retrospective Research

Two variations of descriptive research encountered in the literature merit discussion. Therefore, some special considerations in the design of case studies and retrospective research are discussed here, with comments on the limitations of these approaches.

Retrospective research is designed to examine data already on file before the formulation of the research problem. A clinic may have kept routine records of patients with a particular disorder and a researcher may review these records to study important independent and dependent variables. Or a researcher may look back at data collected in a previous research study to reexamine old data or to examine some aspect of the data that had not been previously examined.

Some authors (e.g., Plutchik, 1974; Young, 1976) have used the term "retrospective" to describe what we have called comparative research in this chapter, but we believe that a distinction should be made between the two plans of observation. In comparative research, the investigator has control over the selection of subjects and the administration of criterion-variable measures. In retrospective research, however, the investigator depends on subject classifications and criterion-variable measurements that were performed at a different time and possibly by a different person. Thus, there arises the danger in retrospective research that the investigator may not know the reliability and validity of these file data. For example, audiograms in patients' files may have been obtained by a new and unpracticed graduate student who committed procedural errors; the equipment may have been out of calibration on the day of testing; or shortcuts in measurement method may have been taken to save time on a busy day.

Such shortcomings may be overcome to ensure reliable and valid measures in the files if the researcher was responsible for all of the measurements in the first place or is absolutely certain of the conditions under which the data were collected. This could be documented by keeping careful records of calibration and measurement methods. Otherwise, the records used in retrospective research may provide the researcher with incorrect or inaccurate information that, in turn, will be passed on to the profession. Retrospective research, then, should be conducted when the researcher has had administrative control over the collection of the data and when it would be very difficult to collect new data because of financial or other administrative considerations. In the Carhart and Porter (1971) study cited above (and discussed in greater detail in Chapter 7), retrospective analysis of file data was employed and the authors carefully detailed the conditions under which the data were gathered to justify the use of retrospection.

The Carhart and Porter (1971) study illustrates the use of clinical files as the source of previously gathered data in a retrospective study. An alternative source of data for retrospective analysis can be the data of previous research studies. Using old research data may, in fact, be a better approach then using clinical file data because it is probable that old research data would have been collected under more rigorous and standardized conditions than old clinical file data. An example of the use of old research data in retrospective research can be seen in the study of Colburn and Mysak (1982) of developmental disfluency and emerging grammar in young children. Audiotapes of their subjects were available from a previous study of normal language development (Bloom, 1970) and Colburn and Mysak did a retrospective analysis of the development of disfluencies in these longitudinal data. An extra advantage of the retrospective approach in this study is that the subjects proved to have followed a normal course in development of language and fluency over the subsequent ten years between the original data collection and the retrospective analysis, thus allowing the researchers to specify long-term subject characteristics.

Case study research is designed to examine in depth specific individuals to illustrate important principles that might be overlooked in examining group data. Several specific reasons for performing case studies are apparent. First, case studies may be used to evaluate phenomena that may occur rarely but that can provide important information. For example, Jerger, Weikers, Sharbrough, & Jerger (1969) attempted to learn more about central auditory processes by examining in great deatil the auditory abilities of a young man with bilateral temporal lobe lesions. Schiff-Myers (1983) studied the development of personal pronouns from reversal to correct usage in a highly imitative child with otherwise normally developing language and none of the other behavioral characteristics of autism. Second, the case study approach may aid in the development of insights in the use of certain clinical or research techniques. Webster and Brutten (1972), for instance, used sound motion pictures of a stutterer to measure the course and frequency of several different stuttering behaviors and found two divergent categories of behavior that they felt would have been masked by a more traditional molar analysis of stuttering. Zimmermann and Rettaliata (1981) presented a detailed kinematic analysis of articulatory gestures of an adventitiously deaf speaker to examine physiological correlates of intelligibility deficit and the role of auditory information in speech production. Third, case studies have proven valuable in examining exceptions to generally accepted rules. Chaiklin and Stassen (1968) presented a case in which the fitting of a hearing aid to the indicated ear was not a correct decision and the patient actually preferred to wear the aid in the other ear. Fourth, important case studies have also appeared in the literature to alert the profession to phenomena that have been previously overlooked in clinical practice. Ventry, Chaiklin, and Boyle (1961), for example, first described the condition of collapse of the ear canal during audiometry, and this case report led to numerous research studies on ear canal collapse.

Case studies have their weaknesses in addition to their benefits. Because they are limited in the number of subjects or situations studied, they may allow little generalization. Thus, case studies may need to be combined with follow-up studies of larger numbers of cases that exhibit the same phenomenon. Also, case studies may be contaminated by subjective biases on the part of the investigator. The excitement often generated by dramatic or atypical cases may cause the investigator or the subject to react in a manner that may not be characteristic of typical cases.

Nevertheless, retrospective and case study research are sometimes the only methods available for studying some phenomena. This may happen when few cases are available for study or when financial or administrative considerations preclude the use of other types of research. As long as caution is exerted in the interpretation of retrospective and case study data, they may provide the profession with important information.

Combined Experimental–Descriptive Research

There are numerous articles in speech pathology and audiology that are combinations of experimental and descriptive research. Because of the prevalence and importance of these investigations in the literature, they merit some discussion on their own. These articles generally summarize the investigation of the effects of manipulation of one or more independent variables on the performance of subjects who have been selected from groups that differ on the basis of classification variables such as age, sex, or pathology. The effect of the experimental manipulation on the dependent variable for one group is compared with the effect of the experimental manipulation for the other group. The research is partly descriptive because the experimenter cannot directly manipulate the classification of subjects, that is, the experimenter cannot cause a disorder or accelerate maturation or change the sex of a subject. Therefore, the experimenter has to select subjects who fall into preexisting classifications of age, sex, or pathology.

An example of a combined experimental–descriptive investigation is the study by Lahey (1974) on the effects of prosody and syntactic markers on children's comprehension of sentences. She systematically manipulated prosody and syntactic markers in recording three different types of sentences and presented these recordings to four- and five-year-old children. The effects of these manipulations on the comprehension of the sentences of both groups of subjects were examined. The experimental aspect of the study was the researcher's ability to manipulate prosody and syntactic markers in the recordings to study the effects of these manipulations on sentence comprehension. The study was also partly descriptive because Lahey selected subjects from different age groups to examine the development of comprehension in four- and five-year-olds with a cross-sectional plan of observation. In other words, the effects of the experimental manipulations on the four-year-olds were compared with the effects on the five-year-olds.

In another example, Hochberg and Waltzman (1972) studied the effects of presenting pulsed vs. continuous pure tones on the auditory thresholds of persons with and without tinnitus. The study was partly experimental because the researchers could manipulate the manner in which the stimuli were presented to subjects and examine the effect of this manipulation on thresholds. The study was also partly descriptive because they compared the effect that the presentation mode had on listeners with tinnitus with the effect it had on persons without tinnitus. Because they could not manipulate the status of the subjects with regard to tinnitus, they selected subjects who were classified as either having or not having tinnitus.

Examination of some illustrative data from combined experimental–descriptive studies may aid consumers in recognizing this important combination of research strategies in the literature. Pashek and Brookshire (1982) studied auditory comprehension of high-level and low-level adult aphasics. In one of their experiments, they examined the effect of paragraph presentation rate (normal speech rate vs. slow speech rate) on the auditory comprehension of the two groups of subjects. Figure 2.16 shows the effect of rate of paragraph presentation on the responses of the two subject groups. Inspection of Figure 2.16 reveals that both groups of aphasics made more correct

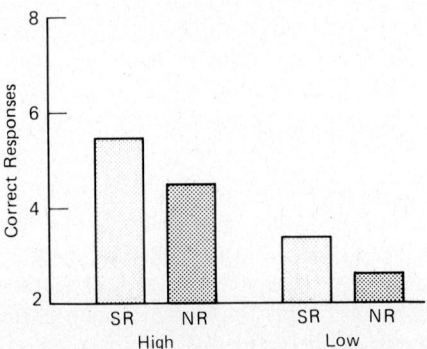

Figure 2.16 Results of a combined experimental–descriptive study of the effects of speech rate on auditory comprehension of high-level and low-level aphasics. (From Pashek and Brookshire, 1982, p. 380.)

responses when the rate of the speech that they listened to was slower than normal. In other words, there was a main effect of rate. There was also a main effect for subject groups because the high-level subjects always did better than the low-level subjects. Because both groups of aphasics showed the same main effect of rate, there was no interaction between rate and subject group.

In another example of a combined experimental–descriptive study, Cohen and Keith (1976) studied the effects of noise on the word-recognition performance of normal hearing subjects, subjects with flat cochlear hearing loss, and subjects with high-frequency cochlear hearing loss. Word recognition was tested while subjects selected from the three classifications were in a quiet background and while exposed to two different background noise levels. Figure 2.17 presents some of their results and shows how word recognition changed as noise was increased from the quiet condition to signal-to-noise ratios of −4 dB and −12 dB. Inspection of Fig. 2.17 reveals that increased noise levels reduced word-recognition scores but that the amount of reduction was different for each of the three groups of subjects. The high-frequency-loss group showed the greatest reduction, the normal group showed the least reduction, and the flat-loss group was in between these two groups. Also, there was an interaction between subject classification and the independent variable in determining the dependent variable. The manipulation of the independent variable had a different effect on the dependent variable for subjects in the different classifications. Because combined experimental–descriptive research is both common and important in speech pathology and audiology research, subsequent portions of this book devote considerable attention to the evaluation of this type of research.

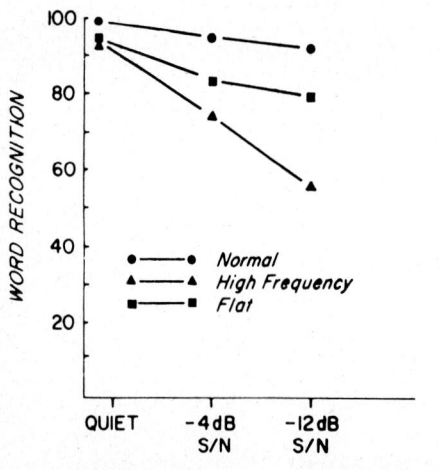

Figure 2.17 Results of a combined experimental–descriptive study of the effects of noise on word recognition of subjects with normal hearing, flat hearing loss, and high-frequency hearing loss. (From Cohen and Keith, 1976, p. 51.)

Summary

This chapter has provided a brief overview of experimental and descriptive empirical research. An outline of some common steps in empirical research illustrated the similarities among the various types of research. The discussion of the differences among these research approaches emphasized the appropriateness of certain strategies for the study of different kinds of research problems. Plutchik's (1974) model of bivalent, multivalent, and parametric experiments was employed to illustrate the investigation of the effect of manipulation of an independent variable on a dependent variable. Investigations employing nonmanipulable independent variables such as comparative, developmental, and correlational studies were considered in the discussion of descriptive research. The next three chapters of Part I will be concerned with some fundamental concepts of research design and data analysis that are integral parts of experimental and descriptive research strategies.

Study Questions

1. Read the following articles: Lloyd, L. L., & Doherty, J. E. (1983). The influence of production mode on the recall of signs in normal adult subjects. *Journal of Speech and Hearing Research, 26,* 595–600.
   Seider, R. A., Gladstein, K. L., & Kidd, K. K. (1983). Recovery and persistence of stuttering among relatives of stutterers. *Journal of Speech and Hearing Disorders, 48,* 402–409.Robinson, D. O., & Allen, D. V. (1984). Racial differences in tympanometric results. *Journal of Speech and Hearing Disorders, 49,* 140–144.
   Write a brief abstract of each article that outlines the four common steps in reporting empirical research: problem, method, results, and conclusions. Identify the type of research in each article.

2. Read the following article: Abbs, J. H., Folkins, J. W., & Sivarajan, M. (1976). Motor impairment following blockade of the infraorbital nerve: Implications for the use of anesthetization techniques in speech research. *Journal of Speech and Hearing Research, 19,* 19–35.
   (a) Identify the various dependent variables that were measured before and after anesthesia.
   (b) What differences were observed as a result of the anesthetization?

3. Read the following article: Robbins, J., Fisher, H. B., Blom, E. C., & Singer, M. I. (1984). A comparative acoustic study of normal, esophageal, and tracheoesophageal speech production. *Journal of Speech and Hearing Disorders, 49,* 202–210.
   (a) What three groups of subjects were compared (i.e., what was the classification variable)?
   (b) What were the criterion variables used to compare them?
   (c) What differences were found among the three groups?

4. Read the following article: Schwartz, A. H., & Goldman, R. (1974). Variables influencing performance on speech sound discrimination tests. *Journal of Speech and Hearing Research, 17,* 25–32.
   (a) What types of research are combined in the article?
   (b) Identify the manipulated independent variables, the classification variable, and the dependent variable. Pay close attention to Figure 1 on page 29 of the article in your attempt to identify the variables.

5. Read the following article: Quigley, S. P., Wilbur, R. B., & Montanelli, D. S. (1974). Question formation in the language of deaf students. *Journal of Speech and Hearing Research, 17,* 699–713.
   (a) What types of descriptive research are combined in this study?
   (b) Identify the independent and dependent variables.

6. Read the following article: Guitar, B. (1976). Pretreatment factors associated with the outcome of stuttering therapy. *Journal of Speech and Hearing Research, 19,* 590–600.
   (a) What were the predictor and predicted variables in this correlational study?
   (b) Which group of variables would you identify as independent? Which group as dependent?

References

Adams, M. R., & Hutchinson, J. (1974). The effects of three levels of auditory masking on selected vocal characteristics and the frequency of disfluency of adult stutterers. *Journal of Speech and Hearing Research, 17,* 682–688.

Adams, M. R., & Moore, W. H. (1972). The effects of auditory masking on the anxiety level, frequency of dysfluency, and selected vocal characteristics of stutterers. *Journal of Speech and Hearing Research, 15,* 572–578.

Ayukawa, H., & Rudmin, F. (1983). Does early middle ear pathology affect auditory perception skills and learning? Comment on Brandes and Ehinger (1981). *Journal of Speech and Hearing Disorders, 48,* 222–223.

Baken, R. J. (1975). Overview of the conference. In L. M. Webster & L. C. Furst (Eds.), *Vocal tract dynamics and disfluency* (pp. 1–9). New York: Speech and Hearing Institute.

Barzun, J., & Graff, H. F. (1970). *The modern researcher.* New York: Harcourt, Brace & World.

Beasley, D. S., Schwimmer, S., & Rintelmann, W. F. (1972). Intelligibility of time-compressed CNC monosyllables. *Journal of Speech and Hearing Research, 15,* 340–350.

Bergman, M. (1971). Hearing and aging. *Audiology, 10,* 164–171.

Bloom, L. (1970). *Language development: Form and function in emerging grammars.* Cambridge, MA: MIT Press.

Boring, E. G. (1950). *A history of experimental psychology.* New York: Appleton-Century-Crofts.

Brannon, J. B. (1968). Linguistic word classes in the spoken language of normal, hard-of-hearing, and deaf children. *Journal of Speech and Hearing Research, 11,* 279–287.

Carhart, R., & Porter, L. S. (1971). Audiometric configuration and prediction of threshold for spondees. *Journal of Speech and Hearing Research, 14,* 486–495.

Chaiklin, J. B., & Stassen, R. A. (1968). Distorted perception of speech in hearing aid consultation. *Journal of Speech and Hearing Disorders, 33,* 270–274.

Cohen, R. L., & Keith, R. W. (1976). Use of low-pass noise in word-recognition testing. *Journal of Speech and Hearing Research, 19,* 48–54.

Colburn, N., & Mysak, E. D. (1982). Developmental disfluency and emerging grammar: I. Disfluency characteristics in early syntactic utterances. *Journal of Speech and Hearing Research, 25,* 414–420.

Curlee, R. F. (1976). Characteristics of ASHA members employed full time during 1973. *Asha, 18,* 68–76.

Erber, N. P. (1971). Effects of distance on the visual perception of speech. *Journal of Speech and Hearing Research, 14,* 848–857.

Fein, D. J. (1984). Findings from the 1983 ASHA omnibus survey *Asha 26*(4), 45–48.

Harford, E., & Dodds, E. (1966). The clinical application of CROS. *Archives of Otolaryngology, 83,* 455–464.

Hirsh, I. J., Davis, H., Silverman, S. R., Reynolds, E. G., Eldert, E., & Benson, R. W. (1952). Development of materials for speech audiometry. *Journal of Speech and Hearing Disorders, 17,* 321–337.

Hochberg, I., & Waltzman, S. (1972). Comparison of pulsed and continuous tone thresholds in patients with tinnitus. *Audiology, 11,* 337–342.

Isaac, S., & Michael, W. B. (1971). *Handbook in research and evaluation.* San Diego, CA: Edits.

Jaeger, C. G., & Bacon, H. M. (1962). *Introductory college mathematics.* New York: Harper & Row.

Jerger, J., Weikers, N. J., Sharbrough, F. W., & Jerger, S. (1969). Bilateral lesions of the temporal lobe. *Acta Otolaryngologica* (Supplementum 258).

Johnson, W., & Associates. (1959). *The onset of stuttering.* Minneapolis: University of Minnesota Press.

Jordan, E. (1960). Articulation test measures and listener ratings of articulation defectiveness. *Journal of Speech and Hearing Research, 3,* 303–319.

Kaplan, A. (1964). *The conduct of inquiry.* Scranton, PA: Chandler.

Karsh, D. E., & Brandes, P. (1983). Response to Ayukawa and Rudmin. *Journal of Speech and Hearing Disorders, 48,* 223–224.

Kerlinger, F. (1973). *Foundations of behavioral research.* New York: Holt, Rinehart & Winston.

Kerlinger, F., & Pedhazur, E. J. (1973). *Multiple regression in behavioral research.* New York: Holt, Rinehart & Winston.

Kling, J. W., & Riggs, L. A. (Eds.). (1971). *Woodworth and Schlossberg's experimental psychology.* New York: Holt, Rinehart & Winston.

Lahey, M. (1974). Use of prosody and syntactic markers in children's comprehension of spoken sentences. *Journal of Speech and Hearing Research, 17,* 656–668.

Lane, H., & Tranel, B. (1971). The Lombard sign and the role of hearing in speech. *Journal of Speech and Hearing Research, 14*, 677–709.

Levine, S., & Elzey, F. F. (1976). *A programmed introduction to research*. Belmont, CA: Wadsworth.

Lodge, D. N., & Leach, E. A. (1975). Children's acquisition of idioms in the English language. *Journal of Speech and Hearing Research, 18*, 521–529.

Martin, F. N., & Pennington, C. D. (1971). Current trends in audiometric practice. *Asha, 13*, 671–677.

McClellan, M. E. (1967). Aided speech discrimination in noise with vented and unvented earmolds. *Journal of Auditory Research, 7*, 93–99.

Monge, P. R., & Cappella, J. N. (1980). *Multivariate techniques in human communication research*. New York: Academic Press.

Panagos, J. M., & Prelock, P. A. (1982). Phonological constraints on the sentence productions of language-disordered children. *Journal of Speech and Hearing Research, 25*, 171–177.

Parasnis, I. (1983). Effects of parental deafness and early exposure to manual communication on the cognitive skills, English language skill, and field independence of young deaf adults. *Journal of Speech and Hearing Research, 26*, 588–594.

Pashek, G. V., & Brookshire, R. H. (1982). Effects of rate of speech and linguistic stress on auditory paragraph comprehension of aphasic individuals *Journal of Speech and Hearing Research, 25*, 377–383.

Plutchik, R. (1974). *Foundations of experimental research*. (2nd ed.). New York: Harper & Row.

Schiff-Myers, N. B. (1983). From pronoun reversals to correct pronoun usage: A case study of a normally developing child. *Journal of Speech and Hearing Disorders, 48*, 394–402.

Sherman, D. (1954). The merits of backward playing of connected speech in the scaling of voice quality disorders. *Journal of Speech and Hearing Disorders, 19*, 312–321.

Shipp, T., & Hollien, H. (1969). Perception of the aging male voice. *Journal of Speech and Hearing Research, 12*, 703–710.

Shriner, T. H., & Daniloff, R. G. (1970). Reassembly of segmented CVC syllables by children. *Journal of Speech and Hearing Research, 13*, 537–547.

Shriner, T. H., Holloway, M. S., & Daniloff, R. G. (1969). The relationship between articulatory deficits and syntax in speech defective children. *Journal of Speech and Hearing Research, 12*, 319–325.

Skinner, B. F. (1959). A case history in the scientific method. In S. Koch (Ed.), *Psychology: A study of a science* (Vol. 2, pp. 359–379). New York: McGraw-Hill.

Underwood, B. J., & Shaughnessy, J. J. (1975). *Experimentation in psychology*. New York: Wiley.

Ventry, I. M. (1980). Effects of conductive hearing loss: Fact or fiction. *Journal of Speech and Hearing Disorders, 45*, 143–156.

Ventry, I. M., Chaiklin, J. B., & Boyle, W. F. (1961). Collapse of the ear canal during audiometry. *Archives of Otolaryngology, 73*, 727–731.

Webster, L. M., & Brutten, G. (1972). An audiovisual behavioral analysis of the stuttering moment. *Behavior Therapy, 3*, 555–560.

Wilder, C. N., & Baken, R. J. (1974). Respiratory patterns in infant cry. *Human Communication, 3*, 18–34.

Young, M. A. (1976). Application of regression analysis concepts to retrospective research in speech pathology. *Journal of Speech and Hearing Research, 19*, 5–18.

Zimmermann, G., & Rettaliata, P. (1981). Articulatory patterns of an adventitiously deaf speaker: Implications for the role of auditory information in speech production. *Journal of Speech and Hearing Research, 24*, 169–178.

3
Criteria for Evaluating Research Designs

Introduction

The purpose of this chapter is to review: (1) the meaning and purpose of research design, (2) the criteria of internal and external validity (which determine the efficacy of research designs), (3) some factors which jeopardize internal and external validity, and (4) the reliability and validity of measurements and tests that may be used in research designs.

Much of the material in this chapter is based on the survey of research designs in educational psychology research by Campbell and Stanley (1966) entitled *Experimental and Quasi-experimental Designs for Research*. Their classification of research designs and of the factors that threaten the internal and external validity of these designs has had a strong impact on research in psychology and education. The popularity of their classification is evident in the many textbooks on educational and psychological research that have adopted it (e.g., Drew, 1980; Isaac & Michael, 1971; Levine & Elzey, 1976).

The Campbell and Stanley classification comprises experimental and quasi-experimental designs commonly used in educational psychology, especially in research on teaching. Because we are dealing with research in speech pathology and audiology that includes some other designs and that excludes some of the designs they used, some modification of their classification is necessary. Our discussion, however, is mainly based on their system, and we wish to express our debt to them for the influence that their work has had in shaping our thinking about the evaluation of research designs.

Meaning and Purpose of Research Design

Many textbooks on research (e.g., Kerlinger, 1973; Plutchik, 1974) state that research design has two main purposes. The first purpose is to solve the research problem. This means the development of an experimental or descriptive strategy for obtaining empirical data that will answer the question or test the hypothesis posited in the problem statement. The second purpose of research design is to eliminate (or at least minimize) contamination of the results by extraneous or nuisance variables. This means the arrangement of the experimental or descriptive strategy in a manner that will provide as clear an explanation as possible of the empirical data without having to worry about many competing explanations that could arise because of contamination of the results by extraneous influences.[1]

These two general purposes of research design are common to both experimental and descriptive research, but some specific objectives are different for these two types of research. In experimental research, the first design objective is to manipulate the independent variable in order to answer the question: What effect does this have on the dependent variable? The second design objective is to arrange the experiment so that extraneous variables are controlled and, therefore, cannot have a confounding effect on the dependent variable. In descriptive research, the first objective is to select the variables for observation in order to answer questions such as: What are the dimensions or differences or relationships found in the natural phenomena? The second objective is to make these observations in a systematic and unobtrusive fashion so that the dimensions, differences, or relationships of the criterion variables are not confounded by extraneous variables.

We have merely rephrased the general purposes of research design into specific objectives to fit the descriptive and experimental models. The main point is that both types of research should be designed to: (1) answer the research question empirically and (2) reduce or eliminate contamination of the answer by extraneous variables.

Kerlinger (1973, pp. 300–301) has indicated that it may be tempting to omit the first purpose (because it is so obvious) and concentrate on the second. But he points out that this is a dangerous delimitation because research design could then degenerate into a "sterile technical exercise" in which one may lose sight of the importance of uniting the research questions, the empirical evidence, and the conclusions of the study. The research

---

[1]Technically, the second objective of research design is to control variance, according to Kerlinger (1973, pp. 306–313). He indicates that the research design should be used to maximize the systematic variance associated with the variables that the researcher manipulates or selects for observation, to minimize error or random variance, and to control extraneous variance that might arise from the influence of extraneous variables on the dependent or criterion variables. Because a technical discussion of variance is beyond the scope of this introductory book, we will eschew the term "variance" in our discussion and try to explain research design with less technical language. Those readers who prefer a more technical discussion after reading this chapter are referred to Kerlinger's text.

question or problem, then, should be a common unifying element in the design of research.

The next two sections of this chapter will be concerned with the two major criteria of internal and external validity formulated by Campbell and Stanley (1966) for evaluation of the efficacy of research designs and with the factors that jeopardize internal and external validity. These criteria were intended to be used for the evaluation of experimental designs in which the independent variable could be manipulated easily and extraneous variables well controlled as well as for quasi-experimental designs in which the independent variable could not be manipulated easily and the extraneous variables could not be well controlled. The latter designs were compromise attempts to approximate experiments in which certain demands of the research situation would not allow for the easy manipulation of the independent variable and control of extraneous variables. These criteria are easily applied to experimental research in speech pathology and audiology. Much of the material concerning the validity criteria and factors that jeopardize them also can be made relevant to the evaluation of descriptive research.

Campbell and Stanley (1966, p. 5) stated that internal validity concerns the question: "Did in fact the experimental treatments make a difference in this specific experimental instance?" If an experiment has internal validity, the experimenter can assert with confidence that the manipulation of the independent variable (experimental treatment) caused the change in the dependent variable and competing explanations that could have arisen from lack of control of extraneous variables are eliminated, at least within the confines of the specific experiment. If, indeed, a study has internal validity, the next concern is the degree to which the results of the experiment can be generalized. External validity according to Campbell and Stanley (1966, p. 5) "asks the question of generalizability: To what populations, settings, treatment variables, and measurement variables can this effect be generalized?"

Campbell and Stanley have formulated a list of 12 factors, of which eight jeopardize the internal validity and four jeopardize the external validity of experiments. An examination of the degree to which an experimental design minimizes these 12 factors indicates the degree to which the experiment has internal and external validity in demonstrating the effect of the independent variable on the dependent variable.

Although some of the jeopardizing factors cited by Campbell and Stanley are mainly relevant to the effect of manipulating an independent variable in an experiment, many of their factors are also relevant to descriptive studies of nonmanipulable independent variables. In evaluating descriptive research a question of internal validity can be asked: Did, in fact, the descriptive study adequately measure the dimensions, differences, and relationships without contamination of these measures by extraneous variables? Many of the factors that jeopardize the internal validity of an experiment could jeopardize the internal validity of a descriptive study, and it is important that they be minimized. If, indeed, a descriptive study has internal validity, the next concern is the degree to which the results of the descriptive study can be generalized, and this is the question of external validity.

In other words, for both experimental and descriptive research, internal validity indicates the degree to which the design has accomplished what it intended to accomplish within the confines of the specific investigation, and external validity indicates the degree to which the results of the study can be generalized.

In summarizing these important criteria, Campbell and Stanley (1966, p. 5) have stated:

> Both types of criteria are obviously important, even though they are frequently at odds in that features increasing one may jeopardize the other. While internal validity is the sine qua non, and while the question of external validity, like the question of inductive inference, is never completely answerable, the selection of designs strong in both types of validity is obviously our ideal.

Internal Validity and Factors that Affect It

A major consideration in the evaluation of any research, be it experimental or descriptive, is whether the researcher has controlled or accounted for the variety of factors that could have a significant effect on the validity of the data collected. In experimental research, the experimenter (and the reader) need to be certain that the change in the dependent variable was, in fact, caused by the experimental treatment and *not* by factors that can mimic the effect of the treatment. That is, the experimenter needs to eliminate alternative explanations that might account for the treatment effect. The fewer the alternative explanations, the greater the internal validity of the experiment. In descriptive studies, the researcher is faced with the very same problem. The researcher (and reader) must ensure that extraneous influences have not contaminated or confounded the results that show differences or relationships. The importance of internal validity is identical in both types of research; the difference lies in the experimenter's greater ability to minimize the influence of the extraneous variables. It is to the factors that can affect internal validity in both experimental and descriptive studies that we now turn.

History

The first factor that can have an effect on internal validity is *history*. History, in an experimental context, is defined as events occurring between the first and second (or more) measurements in *addition* to the experimental variable. In other words: Has some event occurred to a subject or group of subjects between measurements to confound the effect of the experimental variable or treatment? In such an instance, the experimenter cannot determine whether the result was a function of the extraneous events alone, the extraneous events interacting with the experimental treatment, or the experimental treatment alone. History has essentially the same meaning in descriptive research.

Several examples should help clarify the impact that history can have on validity. Assume that an experimenter is evaluating a particular therapy approach for a group of young children who stutter. Unbeknownst to the experimenter, several of the subjects are receiving therapy in their local schools. The experimenter evaluates fluency before and after treatment and concludes that the particular treatment produced increased fluency. The conclusion is suspect because an equally plausible explanation for the improved fluency is that the therapy received in school rather than the experimental treatment accounted for the decreased stuttering or, even more likely, the two treatment approaches (one in school, the other given by the experimenter) interacted to produce the observed result.

Another illustration can be drawn from descriptive audiologic research. With hearing screening programs used in schools, it is common practice to evaluate the efficiency of a hearing screening test by comparing the results of such a test with the results obtained on the "standard" measure, that is, the measure against which the screening test is being compared. In this case, the standard measure is usually threshold audiometry. History can have a profound influence on the judged efficiency of the screening procedure if a significant amount of time elapses between the administration of the threshold test and the administration of the screening test. The reason is simply that the status of the child's hearing may have changed as a result, for instance, of a middle ear infection occurring or resolving during the interval between the screening test and the threshold test. The wise researcher deals with the problem by reducing the interval between tests as much as is feasible to eliminate middle ear history from affecting the evaluation of efficiency of the screening test.

Some types of descriptive research and some types of experimental designs are more prone to the contaminating effects of history than others. Longitudinal studies, for example, are subject to greater history effects than cross-sectional studies; therapy studies are generally more prone to the effects of history than laboratory studies when, in the latter instance, experimental isolation is more or less guaranteed; long-term studies are more likely to be contaminated by history effects than are studies in which data are collected over a short time span. A research design that is especially susceptible to history effects is the one-group pretest–posttest design. In this design, one group of subjects is evaluated prior to treatment (pretest), is given the treatment, and is then evaluated subsequently (posttest) to determine if treatment had an effect. In such cases, the longer the interval between the pretest and the posttest, the greater the likelihood that history will serve to contaminate the results. Even if the interval is relatively short, say one day, external events may still serve to confound the data.

Recapitulation. External events, not under the researcher's control, can produce effects that confound or confuse experimental data making it difficult, if not impossible, to attribute an effect to an experimental treatment. The greater the interval between treatments, the greater can be the effect of history. History effects can contaminate both descriptive and experimental research. Thus, the careful evaluator of research should pay particular attention to whether or not the experimenter has taken into account the possible effects of history on the data.

Maturation

The effect of maturation is similar to the effect associated with history. History refers to events that occur outside the experimental setting and, thus, outside the control of the experimenter. Maturation, on the other hand, refers to changes in subjects themselves that cannot be controlled by the experimenter, changes that may cause effects that are attributed, incorrectly, to the experimental treatment. Examples of maturational factors are age changes, changes in biological or psychological processes that take place over time, and the like. It is important to understand that maturation, in this context, need not be a long-term process. That is, even within a single experimental session, short-term changes in motivation, interest, attention, and so forth, can serve to contaminate the data and to confound the effects of the experimental treatment.

Obviously, maturation effects can play an important role in longitudinal studies, long-term therapy research, and in other kinds of descriptive research that require extensive time for completion. Take, for example, a language-stimulation program designed to improve expressive language in young children. The program might be introduced to two-year-old children whose language performance is evaluated prior to the initiation of the program. Then, the effects of the treatment program might be evaluated when the group of children reaches three years of age. Because of changes that occur in language performance (pretest at two years vs. posttest at three years), the experimenter concludes that the language stimulation program was successful in enhancing language development for young children. It is hardly likely, although not impossible, that such a study would appear in print because it is obvious that maturational processes—neurological, physiological, psychological—could have had an equal or greater role in producing changes in language performance than the language intervention program itself. Furthermore, the interaction between maturational factors and the experimental treatment could have produced the improved performance rather than either maturational processes or the treatment operating singly.

Maturation has served to confuse certain types of research in speech pathology and audiology or, at the very least, has made these kinds of research difficult to perform. A good illustration deals with the efficacy of early therapy for stroke patients. There is still controversy over whether early therapeutic intervention for aphasic patients produces benefits over and above what might be expected merely as the result of spontaneous recovery. The major difficulty confronting the researcher is to isolate or eliminate the effects of maturation (spontaneous recovery) so that changes in language performance can be attributed solely to the therapy program.

Laboratory experimental research is not immune to the effects of maturation. Lengthy experimental sessions, for instance, may produce boredom, fatigue, and inattention. Hunger pangs may affect a subject's responsivity if an experimental session goes through the lunch hour. Retesting the same subject after the subject has consumed a satisfactory lunch may produce response behavior affected by drowsiness. As a result, performance could be differentially affected, and the results contaminated.

The critical evaluator of research should not only be aware of the possible confounding effects of maturation but should also be alert to the ways in which the researcher has tried to minimize these effects. First, it is almost impossible to account for the effects of maturation in single-group pretest–posttest designs. The only way to do this is to know for certain that maturation cannot or does not have an effect on the *dependent* variable. This knowledge is difficult to come by. In the illustration used earlier dealing with a hypothetical language-intervention program, the researcher cannot know that maturational processes will not affect language performance (dependent variable). In fact, the good researcher knows that it is just the reverse, that is, that maturation will probably have a significant effect on language performance. To deal with this problem, the researcher might assign the subjects, at random, to an experimental group that receives the language-stimulation program, or to a control group that does not receive the stimulation treatment. The basic assumption in this approach is that if the subjects are assigned randomly, then maturation effects will be about the same for both the experimental and control groups and that any differential performance at the conclusion of the intervention program is due primarily to the program itself. Note that although random assignment deals with long-term maturation, the reader must still evaluate how the experimenter dealt with short-term maturation factors intrinsic to the test situation, that is, fatigue, boredom, and so on.

Maturation effects intrinsic to an experimental or test session can have a dramatic impact on both descriptive and experimental research. If the experimenter has failed to take into account such factors as fatigue, learning, and boredom, these factors can serve to contaminate the data. Several important procedures are available to the researcher and, again, the critical evaluator must determine if the experimenter has employed these or other procedures to control for maturational influences. One simple method, if feasible, is to keep experimental sessions (or test or therapy sessions) relatively short. Rather than having a four-hour test session, two sessions of two hours each or four sessions of one hour each can be employed. This helps to elimintate short-term fatigue, boredom, and inattention as contaminating factors in each session.

Still another approach, one that is often used in research, is to *randomize* or *counterbalance* conditions. To explain, let us take an example of a study of pure-tone threshold sensitivity in which seven or eight frequencies are tested. Rather than use one test order for all subjects, say measuring thresholds in octave intervals and always starting at 125 Hz, the experimenter can randomize frequency presentations so that any order, learning, or fatigue effects on pure-tone sensitivity are distributed equally over all subjects. For some subjects, then, 125 Hz may be tested first, then 4000 Hz, then 1000 Hz, and so on, with the same test order never or infrequently repeated for other subjects. A similar example can be used to illustrate counterbalancing. Let us assume that we are interested in the effect of a particular treatment on pure-tone sensitivity at 1000 Hz and 4000 Hz. Half the subjects could be tested at 1000 Hz first and 4000 Hz second, whereas the other half would have the reverse order. The assumption is that fatigue, practice, and other short-term maturation effects, if they exist at all, are distributed equally for all conditions and subjects. Incidentally, mention should be made of the fact that in some experiments the investigator wishes to study the effects of order rather than controlling or eliminating order effects. That is, the experimenter might want to know if order *AB* produces a different result from that produced by order *BA* on the dependent variable. In a sense, order becomes an independent variable.

Recapitulation.   Maturation influences can easily serve to confound the results of descriptive or experimental research. With respect to subjects, physiological, neurological, and psychological maturation can mimic the effects of treatment. Maturation effects are most pronounced for longitudinal studies or for studies in which significant amounts of time elapse between experimental treatments or between pretest and posttest sessions. Single-group pretest–posttest designs are most vulnerable to maturational factors. Random assignment of subjects to experimental and control groups is a valuable way of minimizing the effects of maturation. In addition to long-term maturation, short-term maturation effects such as fatigue, practice, and motivation can influence a given experimental session. Randomizing or counterbalancing conditions can reduce or eliminate maturation effects. The critical reader must determine if such methods have been used by the researcher to minimize maturational influences.

Testing or Test-Practice Effects

A third factor that can affect internal validity is the effect that merely taking a test may have on scores achieved later on subsequent administrations of the same test. This effect may be due to the practice afforded by the first test, familiarity with the test items or format, reduction of test anxiety, and so on. By their very nature, pretest–posttest designs are especially vulnerable to test-sensitizing effects or test-practice effects. As a simple illustration, take the measurement of speech discrimination in the audiology clinic. Let us assume that the investigator wishes to determine if a hearing aid will improve speech discrimination. The subject is tested for the first time with a standard discrimination test without a hearing aid and then retested while wearing a hearing aid. The subject's score improves significantly and the investigator concludes that the hearing aid is beneficial. An equally plausible alternative hypothesis, however, is that the improvement in discrimination is simply a function of testing or practice with the discrimination test and that a similar improvement might have been observed if the subject had been merely retested without the hearing aid. It may also be, of course, that a portion of the change was due to practice effects and another portion was due to the hearing aid. Obviously, in these circumstances, it would be extremely difficult to know which was which. Any time tests are used to establish pretreatment baseline data, the reader must ask whether posttreatment changes are due to treatment effects, testing effects, or a combination of the two. It is important to emphasize that both experimental and descriptive research are subject to the influences of pretests on posttests.

Brief mention should be given here to *reactive* vs. *nonreactive* measures. Huck, Cormier, and Bounds (1974), among others, have noted that tests, inventories, and rating scales are referred to as *reactive* measures. They are reactive because they may change the phenomenon that the researcher is investigating. Huck et al. (1974, p. 235) emphasize that

> *any measure is reactive if it has the potential for modifying the variables under study, if it may focus attention on the experiment, if it is not part of the normal environment, or if it exercises the process under study.*

As Campbell and Stanley (1966, p. 9) point out, ". . . the more novel and motivating the test device, the more reactive one can expect it to be." Videotapes and tape recordings may also be reactive measures. As a result, special care must be taken by the investigator to reduce the reactive effects of these recording devices.

A *nonreactive* measure, on the other hand, does not change what is being measured. Isaac and Michael (1971) put nonreactive measures into three categories: (1) *physical traces*—for instance, examining the condition of library books on speech pathology to determine their actual use rather than giving students in speech pathology a questionnaire on book usage; (2) *archives and records*—such as clinic folders, attendance records, and school grades; and (3) *unobtrusive observation*—in which the subject may not know that a particular behavior is being observed.[2] Although Isaac and Michael emphasize that nonreactive measures are not impervious to sampling biases and other kinds of distortion, Campbell and Stanley (1966) urge the use of such measures whenever possible.

---

[2]For the interested reader, unobtrusive measures are discussed at length by Webb, Campbell, Schwartz, & Sechrest (1966).

Recapitulation.   Because testing is a frequent component of research studies in speech pathology and audiology, it is incumbent on the careful reader of such research to evaluate the effects of testing on the outcomes reported. Pretests can affect posttest results, and tests themselves may cause behavior to change in a manner unanticipated by the investigator. Nonreactive measures should be used whenever they are consistent with the investigator's goals but, at the very least, both reader and researcher must be aware of the effect of testing on the behavior to be measured.

Instrumentation

Campbell and Stanley (1966, p. 5) define the instrumentation threat to internal validity as one "in which changes in the calibration of a measuring instrument or changes in the observers or scorers used may produce changes in the obtained measurements." It should be clear from the discussion that follows that this threat to validity transcends types of research in speech pathology and audiology. Instrumentation effects can be a threat to the internal validity of any research studies.

The most obvious instrumentation threat to the validity of studies in speech and hearing is faulty, inadequate, or changing calibration of the equipment employed in the research. Because all students in speech pathology and audiology are taught about the importance of calibration in their clinical work, there is no need to belabor the point here. Appropriate calibration and ongoing monitoring of calibration are absolutely essential ingredients in the collection of valid data, whether the data are for research purposes or for clinical purposes.

How does the reader of a research article determine whether the equipment was calibrated or maintained in calibration throughout the duration of the study? In many instances, the researcher provides a detailed description of the equipment employed and the calibration techniques utilized. Provided that the reader has some knowledge of instrumentation and calibration procedures, the adequacy of the instrumental array can be assessed by a careful reading of the method section. Often, however, only sketchy information is available on the instrumentation used and the calibration procedures employed. Because journal space is at a premium, editors have a tendency to prune procedures to a bare minimum. As a result, we may run across such statements as, "the equipment was calibrated and remained in calibration throughout the study" or "calibration checks were conducted periodically during the course of the investigation." Here the reader must rely on the integrity and honesty of the investigator.

Although it is readily apparent that mechanical and electrical instruments can be sources of error that pose threats to validity, it may be less obvious that such devices as rating scales, questionnaires, attitude inventories, and standardized intelligence tests are also instruments and that their use or misuse can have a profound influence on the adequacy of the data collected in either experimental or descriptive research. A poor pencil-and-paper test, one that has not been standardized, one that has poor reliability, or one that was standardized on a sample different from that under investigation can have serious consequences for internal validity. For speech pathology and other behavioral disciplines as well, considerable attention and research effort have been given to the development and evaluation of rating scales. These efforts have been made in recognition of the need to develop valid and reliable rating scale instruments to reduce the chances that the rating scale itself would pose an instrumentation threat to validity. Because tests are so widely used in research in speech and hearing, the last part of this chapter deals with the validity and reliability of tests and measurements per se.

The next instrumentation threat is posed by the investigator or the observers employed by the investigator to collect data. When human beings are used as judges, there is ample opportunity for their judgments to be confounded by their biases in rating samples of behavior of different subjects or of subjects participating in various conditions. For example, judges' standards may change from one experimental session to another, raters may be influenced by knowledge of the purpose of the investigation, or observers may make judgments based partially on their expectations about the behavior of subjects in different groups (e.g., stutterers vs. nonstutterers).

Rosenthal (1966) has written extensively about the problems of human observers as measuring instruments and, in fact, some researchers call the validity threat posed by biased human observations the "Rosenthal effect." Rosenthal categorized experimenter effects on research results on the basis of whether or not the experimenter effect actually changes the subjects' behavior. The first class of experimenter effect does not actually affect the subjects' performance but does affect the research results. This class of experimenter effect includes error or bias in the experimenter's observation of behavior, unintentional error in mathematical calculation or interpretation of responses, and intentional fabrication of data. As an example of observer bias, consider what might happen if judges were asked to rate the hypernasality in speech samples taken from children with cleft palates before and after pharyngeal flap surgery. Observers might expect less hypernasality after surgery and thereby unconsciously rate the post-surgery tape recordings with lower hypernasality ratings. The second class of experimenter effect includes those factors that actually may change the behavior of the subjects during the study. For example, Rosenthal's research has shown that bisocial attributes of experimenters (e.g., sex, bodily activity, etc.) or psychosocial attributes of experimenters (e.g., friendliness, encouragement, anxiety, hostility, authoritarianism, etc.) may influence the way subjects behave in an experiment.

Rosenthal's research has demonstrated, then, that both experimenter expectancies and attributes can influence the outcome of research results by either directly changing the subjects' behavior or by affecting the manner in which the experimenter measures their behavior. Rosenthal has outlined several approaches to the control of experimenter artifacts, including replicating experiments with different observers, training observers to apply uniform criteria in their judgments, and the use of "blind" experiments, in which observers do not know the treatment condition or group assignment of the subjects whose behavior they are measuring.

The final instrumentation threat to internal validity is the test environment. We will see later how test environment may threaten external validity as well. With respect to internal validity, poor test environment can have a dramatic effect on the adequacy of the data obtained. Without question, the internal validity of audiologic data obtained in both school and industrial settings has often been compromised by the poor quality of the test environment. Research data collected in a speech clinician's office or in a classroom setting may be contaminated by distractions, noise, interruptions, and the like. The researcher must describe the test environment and the critical consumer must determine if the test environment has posed an instrumentation threat to internal validity.

Recapitulation. Instrumentation effects can sorely compromise internal validity. Confounding effects can occur as a result of poor calibration of mechanical and electrical apparatus, as a result of the use of poorly standardized tests or rating scales, and as a result of bias operating on human observers, raters, or judges. Neither experimental nor descriptive research is immune to the threats posed by instrumentation effects.

Statistical Regression

Statistical regression is a phenomenon in which subjects who are selected on the basis of atypically low or high scores change on a subsequent test so that their scores are now somewhat better (in the case of the low scorer) or somewhat poorer (in the case of the high scorer) than they were originally. The investigator may conclude that the treatment produced the change when, in reality, the scores have simply moved or regressed toward a more typical, mean score, that is, the scores have become less atypical. This occurs primarily because of measurement errors associated with the test instrument used in selecting and evaluating the subjects. The more deviant or atypical the score, the larger the error of measurement it probably contains (Campbell & Stanley, 1966). Regression effects may occur in either experimental or descriptive research if groups selected on the basis of extremely atypical scores are retested.

To illustrate, let us say that an experimenter is interested in assessing the value of an articulation-therapy program in a school setting. After screening all the children with an articulation screening test, the experimenter selects for study those 10 children who performed the poorest on the test, that is, had the lowest scores. The therapy program is initiated for the children and a month later, the children are retested. An improvement is noted and the experimenter concludes that the therapy program is a success. The conclusion may be unwarranted, in that the changes noted could have been caused by the extreme, atypical performance (scores) becoming less atypical (regressing toward the mean). If no intervention had been provided, the retest scores might still have shown an improvement comparable to that shown with the therapy program.

To give another example, a group of hearing-impaired people might be evaluated and chosen to participate in a counseling study on the basis of their high scores on the Hearing Handicap Scale (HHS). In this case, a high score represents considerable handicap and a low score represents little handicap. A counseling program is initiated and after four counseling sessions, the subjects are retested with the HHS. The investigator finds that after counseling the scores are lower than they were before counseling and concludes, again erroneously, that the counseling program was successful in reducing self-assessed hearing handicap. An equally plausible explanation is that the improved scores simply represent statistical regression and that the atypical scores would have become more typical scores even without counseling. It should be emphasized that statistical regression is not always a concomitant of extreme scores. As Campbell and Stanley (1966) pointed out, if a group selected for independent reasons turns out to have extreme scores, there is less likelihood that the data will be contaminated by regression effects.

Recapitulation. Statistical regression occurs when subjects are selected because of their extreme scores. Because research in speech pathology and audiology often involves the use of subjects who give atypical scores or who can give extreme scores, it is important for the critical reader to determine if changes in performance are a result of a treatment or the result of regression toward the typical or mean scores. Random selection of subjects and random assignment to treatment and no-treatment groups help reduce the threat to internal validity posed by statistical regression effects.

Differential Selection of Subjects

The selection of subjects to form experimental and control groups in experimental research or to form comparison groups in descriptive research can affect internal validity if subject selection is not done properly. In experimental research, internal validity may be threatened because differences between subjects in the experimental and control groups may account for the treatment effects rather than the treatment itself. In most experimental research, one important requirement is that the subjects should be equal, on important dimensions, prior to experimental treatment or manipulation. The experimenter attempts to ensure equality by random assignment of subjects to experimental and control groups. The absence of equality prior to treatment poses a subject-selection threat to the internal validity of experimental research.

To further explain, let us use an example dealing with an experimental study of articulation therapy. Assume that a researcher wishes to conduct an experiment to evaluate the effectiveness of a new method of articulation therapy with young children. The researcher selects a sample of children with articulation defects and assigns subjects *randomly* to one of three groups: (1) a no-treatment group, (2) a standard-treatment group, and (3) a new-treatment group. Through random assignment, the researcher attempts to reduce the effects of any pretreatment differences among subjects by distributing these differences randomly among the three groups. In this way, the effects of differences between experimental and control subjects on treatment outcomes are minimized and differential selection of subjects poses little threat to internal validity.

In descriptive research, especially in comparative descriptive research, groups are chosen on the basis of some preexisting condition that the researcher wishes to investigate. A subject-selection threat to internal validity arises, however, when the subjects are also different on dimensions (e.g., socioeconomic status or intelligence) other than the preexisting condition. The differences between subjects on these extraneous variables could account for group differences on the criterion (dependent) variable just as easily as the preexisting condition on which the subjects were initially selected.

A second example involving articulation-impaired children can be used to illustrate the subject-selection threat to the internal validity of descriptive comparative research. In this instance, the researcher might wish to determine, for example, if there are personality differences between children with normal articulation and children with impaired articulation. The preexisting condition—adequacy of articulation—provides the basis for group composition. The important point to recognize is that the subjects are *not equal* to begin with. In fact, this type of study would not be possible if the two groups were equal prior to the administration of the personality tests.

The two groups of subjects (normal vs. articulation-impaired children) are given a battery of personality tests and the researcher might find that the two groups differ on certain personality dimensions. The differential-selection threat to internal validity arises because the two groups of subjects may have been quite different on certain important extraneous variables in addition to the difference in adequacy of articulation. Suppose that all the normal speakers were from upper middle-income families, whereas the articulation-impaired speakers were from lower income families. Or suppose that all of the normal speakers were much more intelligent than the articulation-impaired speakers. The extraneous variables of intelligence or socioeconomic status could account for any personality difference between the groups as easily as could the difference in articulation.

A basic problem in descriptive research, then, is that systematic differences between comparison groups must be minimized with the exception of the classification variable under study. Unless this is done, the threat to internal validity is substantial. It is clear that a number of subject variables need to be controlled if group differences are to be meaningful. It is also important to note that any preexisting condition that forms the primary basis of group composition needs to be spelled out clearly by the investigator and needs to be substantiated by the research literature. That is, there should be no overlap between groups on the variable that presumably distinguishes the groups from one another. As an example, let us assume that an investigator wishes to explore the differences between individuals with conductive hearing loss and subjects with sensorineural hearing loss on a new site-of-lesion diagnostic test. It is imperative that the subject selection criteria assure that the groups are indeed different regarding type of hearing loss. There cannot be subjects with conductive hearing loss in the sensorineural group or vice versa. Any subjects with a mixed hearing loss would have to form a third comparison group. The consumer of research should evaluate carefully the adequacy of the criteria used to establish the comparison groups, and the researcher has a responsibility to justify these criteria to consumers.

Recapitulation.   The differential selection of subjects is an important threat to internal validity because so many research studies in speech pathology and audiology deal with experimental treatment of different groups or with descriptive comparisons of different groups. Many of these studies may stand or fall not only on the adequacy of the criteria used to select subjects for the groups that are compared but also on the researcher's ability to deal with other subject variables that may confound the results if left uncontrolled. As a consequence, the critical evaluator of research must give careful attention to the jeopardizing effects of subject selection procedures.

Mortality

Mortality simply refers to the differential loss of subjects between experimental and control groups or between other comparison groups. Mortality can threaten the internal validity of both experimental and descriptive studies. This occurs because the subjects who are lost or who drop out or who fail to complete the research procedure may be quite different in important respects from those subjects who continue to participate in the study. It is difficult, if not impossible, for the investigator to know how the dropouts may differ from those subjects who remain.

A brief example should suffice to clarify the effects of mortality in a descriptive study. Let us assume that we are interested in investigating personality differences between subjects who are successful hearing-aid users and subjects who are not. Two groups of 20 subjects each are formed by using carefully defined selection criteria. Subjects are asked to participate in two test sessions, one devoted to audiologic tests, the other to personality tests. All of the subjects report for the initial test session but eight subjects—two from the successful group (10%) and six from the unsuccessful group (30%)—fail to report for the second test session. Repeated attempts to solicit the cooperation of the subjects are not fruitful, so, data are reported for the subjects who did participate in both sessions. The question facing us is whether the personality data for the unsuccessful hearing-aid-users group have been compromised by the 30% mortality for that group. Unfortunately, we simply cannot determine if the six subjects who dropped out have personality characteristics that caused them not to participate and that are different from the personality characteristics of the unsuccessful users who continued to participate in the study.

Mortality in an experimental study may differentially affect experimental and control-group composition by posttest time to such a degree that meaningful and valid comparison of posttest scores is impossible. It might be possible, for example, that subjects who dropped out were the ones who might have benefited the least (or the most!) from the experimental treatment. Because these possibilities remain unknown to the experimenter, the only ways to account for them would be to find all the dropouts or to replicate the entire study with a new sample.

Follow-up studies are especially prone to the problems of mortality. In speech and hearing, we are often interested in the long-term success of our therapy programs. Is the stuttering adult still reasonably fluent six months after the termination of therapy? Was our voice therapy program successful, in the long run, in ameliorating the vocal pathology in the group of children who received our therapy program? This type of research is among the most difficult to do and the problem of experimental mortality is at the core of the difficulty. If we cannot locate or follow all, or a significant majority of, the subjects, then there is no way of determining if the subjects who cannot be followed are different on any number of dimensions from the subjects who can be located. The investigator might simply choose to reevaluate those subjects that can be located, but the data will hardly be representative.

Recapitulation. Both experimental and descriptive research may suffer from mortality in which subjects, for whatever reason, fail to complete the research protocol. The differential mortality of subjects can affect both within-group and between-group comparisons and raise substantial threats to internal validity. Follow-up studies are especially vulnerable to mortality effects. The careful reader of such studies must determine if the investigator has dealt adequately with the issue of mortality.

The Hawthorne Effect

Although Campbell and Stanley (1966) do not specifically cite the Hawthorne effect as a threat to internal validity, many other texts (e.g., Drew, 1980) consider it to be an internal validity problem. (Campbell and Stanley describe a similar problem with external validity, called reactive arrangement, which will be treated later in this chapter.) The Hawthorne effect refers to changes in a subject's behavior that occur simply because the subject knows that he or she is participating in a research study. The increased attention that the subject receives, the change in routine, the experimental setting itself may all act to cause a performance change that may mimic or accompany the change attributed to the independent variable alone. This effect was first noticed in studies of worker performance at a Hawthorne, Illinois, Western Electric Company telephone-assembly plant in the 1920s; hence, the name, Hawthorne effect.

Drew (1980) indicates that the Hawthorne effect is especially important in group comparisons when one group receives special attention that the other group does not receive. Drew cautioned against the assumption that experimental research using experimental and control groups may be immune to the Hawthorne effect when the control group does nothing during the course of the experiment. For this reason, experiments often have a control group do something (e.g., receive an old therapy treatment while the experimental group receives a new treatment) or use a do-nothing control group and a do-something control group in a three-group experiment. Drew states that it is difficult, if not impossible, to control the Hawthorne effect by removing it from the experimental group, so researchers have tried to control it by applying an added Hawthorne effect to a control group by paying special attention to its members. The group that receives the nonexperimental treatment is often called a placebo group or is said to receive a placebo treatment. This term is derived from drug studies where one group receives the active drug, a second group receives no drug, and a third group receives an inert drug (e.g., a sugar pill) called a placebo drug. Such an experiment allows the researcher to separate the effect of the drug from the effect of the subjects' perception that a treatment would help them.

Parsons (1974) completed an exhaustive reanalysis of the Hawthorne research and concluded that the key elements of the Hawthorne effect are feedback to subjects about their performance and reinforcement of performance. Parsons (1974, p. 930) concluded by defining the Hawthorne effect as ". . . the confounding that occurs if experimenters fail to realize how the consequences of subjects' performance affect what subjects do." In other words, the Hawthorne effect is not just the simple problem of subjects' awareness that they are participating in a research study but is related to how they perceive the consequences of their behavior during the course of the research. Drew has suggested that the Hawthorne effect is most potent immediately after subjects' routines are disrupted and that the influence of the Hawthorne effect may be reduced as subjects become more acclimated to the research situation. For this reason, many researchers begin experimental sessions or test administrations with a brief period of acclimation to establish rapport.

Recapitulation.   Subjects participating in research may show changes in behavior that are a function of their knowledge of experimental participation rather than a function of the treatment. The Hawthorne effect poses a threat to internal validity because it can serve as an alternative explanation to the treatment effect. The control of the Hawthorne effect is best accomplished by ensuring comparability of treatment between groups in their knowledge of the nature of experimental treatments.

Interaction of Factors

The final threat to internal validity deals with the possible interaction effects among two or more of the previously described jeopardizing factors. Although these factors have been treated singly in this discussion, there is little question that they can interact with one another to cause an effect greater than each operating independently and, more important, greater than the experimental effect under investigation. As noted earlier, each of the jeopardizing factors or a combination of factors may also interact with the experimental variable to produce an effect that can be mistaken for the experimental effect alone. Oftentimes, however, it is the interaction between subject selection and some other factor, especially maturation, that confounds the interpretation of the data.

One example may suffice. Let us say that we have an experimental group composed of second graders with articulation problems on whom we wish to assess the efficacy of an experimental articulation therapy program. We use third-grade children with articulation problems as the control group. The therapy program is initiated, significantly greater gains are noted for the experimental group than are noted for the control group; we conclude that our experimental therapy program is a success. Note, however, that maturational influences may be operating differentially for the two groups so that more rapid maturation and development and change in articulatory proficiency have occurred for the younger children. Thus, the effect of the experimental therapy program could be in large part due to subject-selection–maturation-interactions rather than to the program itself. The picture is further clouded if a history threat has also occurred so that a significant portion, or perhaps any portion, of the experimental group is receiving speech therapy outside school. Instrumentation can interact with maturation and history if the articulation test used to evaluate performance has low reliability, especially for second-grade children. The major point is that the factors that can jeopardize internal validity can act singly or in concert to produce changes in performance or behavior that can be mistaken for the effect of the experimental treatment.

Recapitulation.   Interaction effects among the various jeopardizing factors can magnify the threat that each might post individually. If the interaction effects are significant, a reasonable interpretation of the results of the research becomes virtually impossible.

External Validity and Factors that Affect It

As noted earlier in this chapter, external validity, as defined by Campbell and Stanley (1966), simply refers to the generalizability of the data, that is, the extent to which the results of a research study can be generalized to other subjects, other settings, other measurements, and other treatments. Each of these four ways of generalizing results will be considered in this section. Four threats to external validity that were identified by Campbell and Stanley (1966) are outlined here. Each of these four threats provides an example of a problem in generalizing in one of these four ways: to other subjects, settings, measurements, or treatments.

Bracht and Glass (1968) have extended Campbell and Stanley's (1966) discussion of external validity to include 12 threats to generalization that they classified under the rubrics of population validity and ecological validity. Population validity factors concern the populations of subjects to which results can be generalized. Ecological validity factors concern the environments to which results can be generalized (i.e., settings, measures, treatments). Consideration of all 12 factors is beyond the scope of this chapter, and we have chosen to review the four Campbell and Stanley threats as examples of threats to each of the main areas of generalization: subjects, settings, measures, and treatments. Interested readers are referred to the Bracht and Glass (1968) article for a fuller treatment of external validity.

It should also be pointed out that threats to external validity are qualitatively different from threats to internal validity. Serious threats to internal validity render results meaningless and uninterpretable and preclude the drawing of valid conclusions about the relations among the variables studied. Threats to external validity, however, only *limit* the degree to which internally valid results can be generalized. No single research study is expected to have wide-ranging generalizability to many different kinds of subjects, settings, measures, or treatments. Generalizations grow from cumulative research centered on a given topic. Researchers build a case for generalization from comparison of the results of many studies. Also, efforts to control threats to internal validity often reduce external validity by introducing greater specificity to the population and environment of the research design. Therefore, the accumulation of several internally valid research studies is necessary to overcome limitations to external validity.

Subject Selection

The first threat to external validity presents a problem in generalizing to other subjects. This threat concerns the degree to which the subjects chosen for the study are representative of the population to which the researcher wishes to generalize. If there are important differences between the two (and these differences may not always be apparent to the experimenter), then meaningful generalizations will be limited. We have emphasized earlier the importance of subject selection to internal validity. It should be clear that subject selection procedures can pose an equally important threat to external validity, especially because subject selection may interact with the experimental variable to produce positive results only for certain types of subjects and not for others. Subject selection bias may also jeopardize the external validity of descriptive research because a difference or a relationship may hold true only for certain types of subjects and not for others.

The number of examples that could be cited here is limitless. Several brief ones should suffice to illustrate the point. Spriestersbach, Moll, and Morris (1964) pointed out the danger of failing to recognize that the "cleft palate population" contains various pertinent subgroups that may be identified by variables such as age, cleft type, or speech characteristics. Generalization from research with cleft palate subjects should be limited, therefore, to the specific subgroups that are studied. Elliott (1982) has pointed out the difficulties that arise in attempts to generalize from data concerning the effects of noise on speech perception of normal-hearing young adults to the effects of noise on speech perception of normal-hearing children, normal-hearing older adults, normal-hearing individuals with speech or learning disorders, and hearing-impaired persons of all ages. Brookshire (1983, p. 342) has discussed the problems of generalization of results of experiments with aphasics and stated:

> In any experiment, the population to which experimental findings can be generalized is determined by the characteristics of the subjects who participate in the experiment. In order for the results of an experiment to be generalizable to a given population, the sample of subjects which participates in the experiment must be representative of the population. That is, the sample must resemble the population with regard to those variables which are likely to affect the relationship between the independent and dependent variable(s).

Brookshire further stated that investigators should report both the relevant variables used to select subjects and the characteristics of the subjects on these variables in order to make legitimate generalizations to a specific population. He discussed 18 specific subject characteristics (e.g., age, severity of aphasia, handedness, visual acuity, time post onset, etc.) that could be relevant in specifying an intended target population of aphasics for generalization.

The important point is that generalization should be limited to subjects who have characteristics in common with the subjects studied. In other words, the subjects must be representative of the population to which the researcher wishes to generalize and the relevant characteristics of the subjects that determine their degree of representativeness should be specified in the article to allow readers to evaluate the generality of results to other subjects.

Recapitulation. Subject selection is critical to both internal and external validity. With respect to the latter, the type of subject used has considerable impact on the generalizations that can be drawn about the population at large. Extensions of the data are possible when the investigator is certain that classes of nonsampled people would perform in essentially the same manner as those used in the research.

Reactive or Interactive Effects of Pretesting

The second threat to external validity presents a problem in generalizing to other measures. This threat concerns the degree to which a reactive pretest may interact with an independent variable in determining the subjects' performance on the dependent variable. In other words, subjects who are exposed to a reactive pretest may react to an experimental treatment in a way that is different from people who have not been exposed to the pretest. The effect of the treatment may be demonstrated only for subjects who were tested just prior to treatment and not for the population at large who might receive the treatment without the specific pretest.

To illustrate the point, assume that an investigator wishes to study the attitudes of parents toward children with a significant physical handicap such as cerebral palsy. Parents would first be pretested on their attitudes toward handicapped children and then shown a 10-minute film depicting the children at play. Following the film, each parent is asked to complete a posttest attitude questionnaire. The basic question regarding external validity is whether the attitudes of the parents in the study can be generalized to parents who have not been pretested before the film because the pretest may have sensitized them for an attitude shift during the film. Of course, there are design strategies that can circumvent this problem so that generalizations could be made.

Let us take another example. Suppose a researcher is interested in assessing a particular aspect of stuttering therapy designed to reduce a stutterer's fear of speaking situations. The pretest involves an interview in which various measures of speaking fear are taken. The therapy program is initiated and following its completion, the subject is again required to answer questions about fear or to demonstrate his or her mastery of fear. The experimenter notes a significant decrease in fear of speaking situations and concludes that the program is successful. Although it may be true for the subjects in the experiment, it may very well be that the therapy program would not be successful or would be less successful if administered to individuals who have not had the pretest experience. In this example, external validity is in jeopardy because of the interaction of the pretest and the experimental treatment.

Recapitulation. The effect of pretesting may limit the generalizations that can be made to people who have not been pretested. Preexperimental activity may sensitize the subject to the experimental variable or condition so as to enhance the experimental effect only for those people subject to the preexperimental activity. Fortunately, there are research designs (see Chapter 4) that minimize this threat to external validity.

Reactive Arrangements

The third threat to external validity presents a problem in generalizing to other settings. This threat concerns the degree to which the setting of the research is reactive or interacts with the independent variable in determining the subjects' performance on the dependent variable. Campbell and Stanley (1966, p. 6) note that the "reactive effects of experimental arrangements" are such that they ". . . would preclude generalization about the effect of the experimental variable upon persons being exposed to it in non-experimental settings." In essence, it is the Hawthorne effect operating as a threat to external validity. A child is taken from the classroom to the speech clinician's office to be given an experimental language stimulation program. Is the effect of that language stimulation program specific to the experimental setting of the clinician's office or can the language stimulation program be equally effective in the normal classroom environment? How does the experimental arrangement interact with the treatment to produce the observed effect? If there is an interaction (and it cannot be ruled out easily), then the treatment effects cannot be generalized to people who have not experienced the experimental arrangement. In the aforementioned example, the experimental language stimulation program might be modified so that it could be administered in the classroom and its effect there directly evaluated. If the treatment program is designed specifically to be administered by the speech clinician working in an office and no claims are made about the efficacy of the program in the classroom, then the experimenter would be justified in generalizing the treatment to all similar "experimental arrangements," that is, *limiting* the generalization to similar settings rather than trying to extend it to a large variety of settings without sufficient evidence.

Reactive arrangements may also operate to jeopardize the external validity of descriptive research. If the measuring situation were reactive, subjects might behave in a different fashion than would other similar subjects in nonreactive situations. For example, subjects might be more candid in completing an anonymous questionnaire than they would normally be in discussing their speech problems with a friend; on the other hand, they might be less candid in an interview with a professional then they would be in talking to a friend. Generalization about their expressed opinions, therefore, would be somewhat limited by the reactive arrangements of the survey.

Recapitulation.   A treatment effect can interact with an experimental arrangement so that generalizations about the treatment effect in a nonexperimental arrangement are not justified. In such a case, generalization is limited to similar settings, but the results would still be important if a large number of similar settings exist in the real world. Reactive arrangements could also limit generalizations from descriptive research.

Multiple-Treatment Interference

The fourth threat to external validity presents a problem in generalizing to other treatments. This threat concerns the degree to which various parts of a multiple treatment interact with each other in determining subjects' performance on the dependent variable. This effect is likely to occur when more than one experimental treatment is administered to the same subjects or when a treatment consists of a carefully sequenced set of steps. The threat to external validity lies in the fact that the results of a multiple-treatment study can only be generalized to people who would receive the same sequence and number of treatments.

An example might be a study in which fluency is reinforced and nonfluency is punished during a conditioning segment of an experiment on stuttering. It would be difficult to ferret out the individual effects of the punishment and the reinforcement in examining any reduction in nonfluency because of the multiple-treatment effect. Separate studies would be needed of the individual effects of punishment of nonfluency, reinforcement of fluency, and the combined punishment of nonfluency and reinforcement of fluency. In other words, the treatment must be representative of the kind of treatment to which the results can be generalized.

Recapitulation.   If a series of experimental treatments is administered to a subject, generalizations about the effects of the multiple treatments can be made only to others who experience the same multiple treatments.

Reliability and Validity of Tests and Measurements

Much of the research in speech pathology and audiology involves the use of tests and measurements. In fact, the variety of tests is nothing short of bewildering. Tests range from the simple pencil-and-paper test to the sophisticated measurement of a physiologic phenomenon, from the well-standardized test available commercially to the test developed for a specific research purpose, from questionnaires to rating scales, and so on. It is well beyond the purview of this text to discuss the intricacies of test development and evaluation. Further, we assume the reader has been exposed to tests through diagnostics or testing courses. However, because tests and measurements are such an integral part of research in speech and hearing, we will review here two fundamental aspects of tests and measurements, aspects important to the judicious consumption of research and to the evaluation of tests used in research. These aspects are *reliability* and *validity*.

Reliability of Tests and Measurements

Reliability means precision of measurement (Kerlinger, 1973; Thorndike & Hagen, 1977) and can be assessed by examining the consistency or stability of a test or measure. A reliable measure provides precise results that can be expected to remain reasonably stable if the measurement procedure is repeated with the same subject. An unreliable measure, however, would not provide precise results and could be expected to fluctuate more or be unstable if the measurement procedure were repeated with the same subject. Actually, reliability is not an all-or-none phenomenon: different measures have different degrees of reliability.

There are many factors that can influence the reliability of a measure. Thorndike and Hagen (1977, p. 74), for example, have identified three important general classes of reasons for inconsistency in a test or measure. First, the person under test may actually change from day to day. The person may be more rested or more motivated on the second testing day and thereby score higher on the second administration of a test than on the first administration. Second, the task may be different in two forms of the same measure or in the different parts of one measure. Task-item comparability in various parts or forms of a measure is important to ensure reliability. Third, many measures provide a limited sample of behavior and small samples of behavior may not provide dependable characterizations of behavior over the long run.

Thorndike and Hagen (1977) described three approaches to evaluation of the reliability of a test or measurement. The first approach involves performing a complete repetition of the exact same test or measurement and comparing the results of the two administrations. This approach is referred to as *test-retest* reliability. Second, they suggest administration of a *parallel* or *equivalent form* of the test or measurement and an examination of the consistency of the results across the two parallel forms. Their third suggestion is to subdivide the test or measure into two equivalent parts and to examine the consistency of the results of the two halves of the test. This type of reliability check is called assessment of *split-half* reliability, or *odd-even* reliability if the odd items of a test are compared to the even items of a test in dividing the test into two halves. There are advantages and disadvantages to each of these methods of checking reliability and readers who are interested in further pursuit of these matters are urged to consult Chapter 3 "Qualities Desired in Any Measurement Procedure" of the Thorndike and Hagen (1977) book for a more detailed discussion of reliability assessment than is possible within the scope of this book.

There are basically two statistical procedures for quantifying reliability when reliability data have been gathered by one of the methods above (Thorndike and Hagen, 1977). The first procedure is to examine the variability found with repeated measures. If the measurement could be repeated a number of times with a single individual and the distribution of these repeated measurements were examined, the researcher could compute their standard deviation to describe their variability. This standard deviation of the repeated measurements is called the *standard error of measurement*. Rarely, however, do we encounter situations in which it is practical to gather an extended set of repeated measurements with all of the individuals to be measured. Therefore, statisticians have developed methods for estimating the standard error of measurement in situations in which an individual can be tested only once. These estimates of the standard error of measurement give an indication of the variability that might be expected in the score of any individual if the measurement were to be repeated a number of times. If the standard error of measurement were large, then greater variability would be expected with repeated measurement and the test or measure would be considered to be less precise or reliable. If the standard error of measurement were small, then less variability would be expected with repeated measurement and the test or measure would be considered to be more precise or reliable.

The second statistical procedure for quantifying reliability, which is more commonly found in the research literature, involves the computation of reliability coefficients for repeated measurements or for split-half comparisons. If reliable measurements were made on a group of persons, someone with a high score on the first measurement (or in one-half of the test) would be expected to maintain a high score on subsequent measurement attempts (or on the other half of the test), and persons with low scores would be expected to maintain low scores. If two sets (or two halves) of the measurement were available for the same group of individuals, then a correlation coefficient showing the relationship between the two sets of measurements could be computed. If the individuals who scored high on the first measurement also scored high on the second and those who achieved low scores on the first also scored low on the second, then this correlation coefficient (which could be called a reliability coefficient) would be high. If there were instability in the measurement, however, such that individuals' scores changed from the first to the second measurement to such an extent that each individual did not maintain the same relative place in the two distributions of measurements, the relability coefficient would be very low. The nature of correlation coefficients and the interpretation of their directions and magnitudes will be explained in more detail in Chapter 5.

A measurement, then, can be said to be reliable if it is precise or consistent. In such a case, the standard error of measurement would be low and the reliability coefficient would be high. Some good examples of reliability studies of various tests and measures can be found in the speech pathology and audiology literature. For instance: Chaiklin, Ventry, and Barrett (1961) have reported on the reliability of conditioned galvanic skin response (GSR) audiometry with adults; Fujiki and Brinton (1983) have reported on the reliability of elicited imitation procedures in language assessment; and Chermak, Pederson, and Bendel (1984) has reported on equivalent forms and split-half reliability of the NU-CHIPS test.

It should be borne in mind that although these concepts of reliability and its assessment are generally known to apply to standardized tests and measures (e.g., tests of intelligence, language usage, and articulation that are available commercially), many people fail to realize that they also apply to measurements made by researchers who develop their own measuring material. Readers who are often aware of the reliability of commercial material may not stop to ask about the reliability of a test or measure developed by a researcher to suit a particular investigation. Researchers who develop their own measuring material have as much responsibility as a commercial producer to justify its use by examining its reliability. This is not always easy to do. Usually, commercial measures have been previously standardized on a large sample of subjects and, therefore, reliability data are readily available in the test manual. But when researchers develop new material for use in measurement, they must spend extra time examining its reliability by means of the methods described above, before reporting on the use of these measurements in the research design.

Validity of Tests and Measurements

The validity of a test or measure can be defined as the degree to which it measures what it purports to measure (Kerlinger, 1973; Thorndike & Hagen, 1977). Whereas reliability means consistency or precision of measurement, validity means truth or correctness or reality of measurement. A reliable measure may be quite repeatable or precise, but it may not be true or correct. For example, a scale in a butcher shop may consistently and precisely weigh the meat put on it at a half-pound over the true or correct weight. Such a scale would be reliable, but not valid, and customers of this shop would consistently and repeatedly pay the price of an extra half-pound for all of the meat they purchased. Reliability, then, does not ensure validity, but it is a necessary prerequisite for validity. That is to say, to be valid, a measure must first be reliable. Once reliability has been established, then the validity of a measure can be assessed.

As Kerlinger (1973, pp. 456–457) has pointed out, if the measure in question is a physical one (e.g., measuring the sound pressure level of a pure tone), there is usually little difficulty in determining its validity. Physical measures generally present a more or less direct analogue of the property that the researcher wishes to measure. The validity of behavioral or cognitive measures, however, is often more difficult to determine. In some cases, it may be so difficult to measure directly certain human behaviors or characteristics that researchers may have to resort to indirect measures to make inferences about them. This has often occurred, for instance, in language research when data concerning linguistic performance have been used to make inferences about linguistic competence or language-processing strategies. The validity of such indirect measures may be difficult or even impossible to establish.

There are basically three ways to establish the validity of a test or measure (Kerlinger, 1973; Thorndike & Hagen, 1977). First, the *content validity* may be established by logical examination of the content of test items to see how well they sample the behavior or characteristics to be measured. The various parts of the test or measure should be representative of the behaviors or characteristics that the test is supposed to measure. This is usually determined by first describing all of the behaviors or characteristics to be measured and then checking the test or measure to see how well it samples these behaviors or characteristics. Suppose, for example, that researchers wanted to test the language performance of a group of children. First, the researchers would have to outline all of the behaviors that would constitute those aspects of language performance they wished to sample (e.g., use of past and future tense of certain verbs or comprehension of grammatical relation between subject and object). Then they would have to determine how well their test or measure sampled this universe of possible behaviors.

Content validation, then, is basically a subjective procedure for logically or rationally evaluating the items on a test to see how well they reflect what the tester wishes to measure. This analysis is usually done by the researcher or by a panel of judges assembled by the researcher for this task. As such, the analysis is not a strictly empirical measure of validity, but more a rational one, and it may be subject to error arising from the particular biases of the judges. There are many situations, however, in which content validity is the only type of validity that can be established.

Second, the *criterion validity* of a test or measure may be established by empirical examination of how well the test or measure correlates with some outside validating criterion. The degree to which the test or measure correlates with a known indicator of the behavior or characteristic it is supposed to measure gives an indication of its criterion validity. There are two types of criterion validity that differ from one another only with respect to the time of administration of the outside criterion.

The first is *concurrent validity*. Concurrent validity is assessed when a test or measure and an outside validating criterion are administered at the same time. It might be important, for example, to develop a test that is less time consuming, cumbersome, and expensive than an existing one. The concurrent validity of the shorter version would be established by examining how well it correlates with the longer version. Concurrent validity may also be important in determining how well a test or measure is related to some concomitant occurrence in the real world outside the testing situation. A good example of this can be found in Jordan's study (1960) of the relationship between various measures taken from the Templin-Darley articulation tests and the listeners' judgments of the defectiveness of children's articulation. The listeners' judgments were used as an outside validating criterion and correlated with the children's scores on the articulation tests. Another example can be found in Dever's study (1972) of the validity of a morphology test when compared to the occurrence of morphemes in the free speech of mentally retarded children.

The second type of criterion validity is *predictive validity*. Predictive validity is assessed when a test or measure is used to predict some future behavior. In such a case, the test or measure is administered first, time elapses, and then the criterion measure is administered. For example, college admissions officers may use college board scores to predict how well high school students might be expected to do in college. A therapy study may involve the use of certain pretherapy measures to predict how much patients might be expected to improve during the course of therapy. Guitar (1976) presents such a study on the validity of certain pretherapy measures for predicting the outcome of stuttering therapy. In each case, the future outcome is the outside validating criterion for determining the validity of the earlier test. In Chapter 2, we described regression analysis in the use of correlational research plans in descriptive research. Readers will recognize this as the method for quantifying the degree of either concurrent or predictive criterion validity.

The greatest difficulty in determining criterion validity lies in the selection of an appropriate outside validating criterion. There may be none in existence or it may be very difficult to measure one. The outside criterion itself needs to be valid and reliable and available for measurement. Many tests and measures have never been subjected to examination of their criterion validity simply because no suitable outside criteria are available for measurement.

A third approach to measuring validity is to establish the *construct validity* of a test or measure by means of both empirical and rational examination of the degree to which the test or measure reflects some theoretical construct or explanation of the behavior or characteristic to be measured. Kerlinger (1973, p. 461) calls construct validity "one of the most significant advances of modern measurement theory and practice" because it brings both empirical and theoretical considerations together in examining *why* a test is valid. As we emphasized in Chapter 1, a theory is an explanation of empirical knowledge of some phenomenon. If such an explanation exists, then the results of a test or measure should confirm the theory if the test is valid *and* the theory is correct.

Construct validity could be established in several different ways. For instance, a theory might predict that a particular behavior should increase with age. The test or measure could be administered to persons of different ages, and if the measured behaviors were found to increase with age, the construct validity of the measure with respect to the age aspect of the theory would be established. The theory might also predict that different kinds of subjects (e g., pathological vs. normal) should score in certain ways. If empirical testing with the measure confirmed this, then the measure would have construct validity with respect to that aspect of the theory. The theory might also state that certain experimental manipulations should affect the test or measure; for example, drug administrations should reduce scores, whereas reinforcement should increase scores on the test or measure. If experiments were carried out that confirmed these effects, the test or measure would have construct validity with respect to this aspect of the theory. Factor analysis, a statistical technique for reducing a large number of tests or variables to a smaller number of clusters of common tests or variables that identify common traits, might also be used to establish construct validity. This would involve the determination of how much the test or measure shares in common with other tests known to fit certain theoretical constructs. Also, the internal consistency of the test or measure might be assessed by item analysis, a statistical technique for correlating each item in the test with the overall test score to see if each item measures the construct as well as the overall test or measure does. Muma (1984) recently discussed several aspects of construct validity in his analysis of problems with the Clinical Evaluation of Language Functions (CELF); Schiavetti, Metz, and Sitler (1981) reported an experiment that examined the construct validity of scaled measures of speech intelligibility in reference to Stevens' (1975) psychophysical constructs regarding prothetic and metathetic continua.

The greatest problem in establishing construct validity lies in the validity or the correctness of the theoretical constructs used to predict test performance. This is analogous to the problem finding a suitable outside validating criterion in predictive and concurrent validity. As Thorndike and Hagen (1977) have pointed out, the construct validity of a test or measure is borne out if measurements agree with the theoretical prediction, but if the prediction is not verified, it may be the result of an invalid measure or an incorrect theory or both. A variety of sources are available to those interested in test validity and reliability, test development and standardization, and similar topics (American Psychological Association, 1974; Buros, 1972; Cronbach, 1970; Thorndike & Hagen, 1977; Weiner & Hoock, 1973). The reader is urged to consult these sources.

An excellent review of the reliability and validity of language and articulation tests was published by McCauley and Swisher (1984). They applied 10 psychometric criteria to 30 currently used articulation and language tests for preschool children and found many of the tests lacking in specificity regarding the 10 criteria. The criteria included aspects of test construction such as description of the normative sample, sample size, evidence of test–retest reliability, information about criterion validity, and so on. Their results were not particularly encouraging and they concluded:

> . . . the reviewed tests failed to provide compelling evidence that they can reliably and validly be used to provide information concerning the existence of language or articulation impairment. These findings suggest important limitations on the use of such tests that must be considered by investigators and by speech-language clinicians. (McCauley & Swisher, 1984, pp. 40–41)

McCauley and Swisher suggested that test authors and publishers should be encouraged to gather empirical evidence of test reliability and validity as an integral part of test development and that test users can wield considerable influence as consumers by evaluating the adequacy of tests before purchasing them.

Summary

This chapter has identified the factors that can affect the validity of both experimental and descriptive research. Two types of validity were described. If a research study is internally valid, extraneous factors that could account for the results reported have been controlled or accounted for. The extraneous factors discussed were history, maturation, testing, instrumentation, statistical regression, subject selection, mortality, the Hawthorne effect, and interactions among the various factors. The careful evaluator of research must pay particular attention to the way the researcher has tried to ensure internal validity. External validity refers to the researcher's ability to generalize results to other subjects, settings, measures, or treatments. Four factors that can affect external validity were discussed: subject selection, interactive pretesting, reactive arrangements, and multiple-treatment interference. The last section considered briefly the reliability and validity of tests and measures.

Study Questions

1. Define internal and external validity and explain why these concepts are important to consumers of research.

2. Discuss the reasons for the following points made by Campbell and Stanley (1966):
   (a) efforts to increase internal validity may jeopardize external validity and vice versa;
   (b) internal validity is the sine qua non of research; and
   (c) the question of external validity can never be completely answered.

3. Read the following article: Brookshire, R. H. (1983). Subject description and the generality of results in experiments with aphasic adults. *Journal of Speech and Hearing Disorders, 48,* 342–346. What subject characteristics did Brookshire suggest should be reported in experiments with aphasics in order to determine the population to which results can be generalized?

4. Read the following article: McCauley, R. J., & Swisher, L. (1984). Psychometric review of language and articulation tests for preschool children. *Journal of Speech and Hearing Disorders, 49,* 34–42.
   (a) What were the 10 criteria suggested for reviewing the language and articulation tests?
   (b) Identify the consequences described if each criterion is unmet.

5. Read the following article: Arndt, W. B. (1977). A psychometric evaluation of the Northwestern Syntax Screening Test. *Journal of Speech and Hearing Disorders, 42,* 316–319. What issues of test validity did Arndt raise in his critique of the Northwestern Syntax Screening Test?

6. Read the following article: Kirk, S. A., & Kirk, W. D. (1978). Uses and abuses of the ITPA. *Journal of Speech and Hearing Disorders, 43,* 58–75.
   (a) What three criteria did the Kirks present for evaluating research dealing with the ITPA?
   (b) What issues of validity are addressed in these criteria?

7. Read the following article: Spekman, N. J., & Roth, F. P. (1984). Clinical Evaluation of Language Functions (CELF) diagnostic battery: An analysis and critique. *Journal of Speech and Hearing Disorders, 49,* 97–100.

   What questions did Spekman and Roth raise about the reliability and validity of the CELF?

8. Read the following articles: Goldsmith, H. (1983). Some comments on "Articulatory dynamics of fluent utterances of stutterers and nonstutterers." *Journal of Speech and Hearing Research, 26,* 319–320. Zimmermann, G. N. (1983). In agreement with Goldsmith. *Journal of Speech and Hearing Research, 26,* 320.

   What issues regarding internal and external validity in research comparing stutterers and nonstutterers were discussed by Goldsmith and by Zimmermann?

9. Read the following article: Andrews, G., & Harvey, R. (1981). Regression to the mean in pretreatment measures of stuttering. *Journal of Speech and Hearing Disorders, 46,* 204–207.

   Summarize Andrews and Harvey's findings regarding regression to the mean in stuttering measures and identify their implications for the design of stuttering therapy experiments.

References

American Psychological Association. (1974). *Standards for educational and psychological tests.* Washington, DC: Author.

Bracht, G. H., & Glass, G. V. (1968). The external validity of experiments. *American Educational Research Journal, 5,* 437–474.

Brookshire, R. H. (1983). Subject description and generality of results in experiments with aphasic adults. *Journal of Speech and Hearing Disorders, 48,* 342–346.

Buros, O. K. (1972). *The seventh mental measurements yearbook.* Highland Park, NJ: Gryphon Press.

Campbell, D. T., & Stanley, J. C. (1966). *Experimental and quasi-experimental designs for research.* Chicago, IL: Rand McNally.

Chaiklin, J. B., Ventry, I. M., & Barrett, L. S. (1961). Reliability of conditioned GSR pure-tone audiometry with adult males. *Journal of Speech and Hearing Research, 4,* 269–280.

Chermak, G. D., Pederson, C. M., & Bendel, R. B. (1984). Equivalent forms and split-half reliability of the NU-CHIPS administered in noise. *Journal of Speech and Hearing Disorders, 49,* 196–201.

Cronbach, L. J. (1970). *Essentials of psychological testing* (3rd ed.). New York: Harper & Row.

Dever, R. B. (1972). A comparison of the results of a revised version of Berko's test of morphology with the free speech of mentally retarded children. *Journal of Speech and Hearing Research, 15,* 169–178.

Drew, C. J. (1980). *Introduction to designing and conducting research* (2nd ed.). St. Louis, MO: C. V. Mosby.

Elliott, L. L. (1982). Effects of noise on perception of speech by children and certain handicapped individuals. *Sound and Vibration, 16*(12), 10–14.

Fujiki, M., & Brinton, B. (1983). Sampling reliability in elicited imitation. *Journal of Speech and Hearing Disorders, 48,* 85–89.

Guitar, B. (1976). Pretreatment factors associated with the outcome of stuttering therapy. *Journal of Speech and Hearing Research, 19,* 590–600.

Huck, S. W., Cormier, W. H., & Bounds, W. G. (1974). *Reading statistics and research.* New York: Harper & Row.

Isaac, S., & Michael, W. B. (1971). *Handbook in research and evaluation.* San Diego, CA: Edits.

Jordan, E. (1960). Articulation test measures and listener ratings of articulation defectiveness. *Journal of Speech and Hearing Research, 3,* 303–319.

Kerlinger, F. (1973). *Foundations of behavioral research* (2nd ed.). New York: Holt, Rinehart & Winston.

Levine, S., & Elzey, F. F. (1976). *A programmed introduction to research.* Belmont, CA: Wadsworth.

McCauley, R. J., & Swisher, L. (1984). Psychometric review of language and articulation tests for preschool children. *Journal of Speech and Hearing Disorders, 49,* 34–42.

Muma, J. R. (1984). Semel and Wiig's CELF: Construct validity? *Journal of Speech and Hearing Disorders, 49,* 101–104.

Parsons, H. M. (1974). What happened at Hawthorne? *Science, 183,* 922–932.

Plutchik, R. (1974). *Foundations of experimental research* (2nd ed.). New York: Harper & Row.

Rosenthal, R. (1966). *Experimenter effects in behavioral research.* New York: Appleton-Century-Crofts.

Schiavetti, N., Metz, D. E., & Sitler, R. W. (1981). Construct validity of direct magnitude estimation and interval scaling of speech intelligibility: Evidence from a study of the hearing impaired. *Journal of Speech and Hearing Research, 24,* 441–445.

Spriestersbach, D. C., Moll, K. L., & Morris, H. L. (1964). Heterogeneity of the "cleft palate population" and research designs. *Cleft Palate Journal, 1,* 210–216.

Stevens, S. S. (1975). *Psychophysics.* New York: Wiley.

Thorndike, R. L., & Hagen, E. P. (1977). *Measurement and evaluation in psychology and education* (4th ed.). New York: Wiley.

Webb, E. J., Campbell, D. T., Schwartz, R. D., & Sechrest, L. (1966). *Unobtrusive measures: Nonreactive research in the social sciences.* Chicago, IL: Rand McNally.

Weiner, P. S., & Hoock, W. C. (1973). The standardization of tests: Criteria and criticism. *Journal of Speech and Hearing Research, 16,* 616–626.

4

Evaluation of Research Designs

Introduction

This chapter reviews some research designs that may be applied in speech pathology and audiology and examines their internal and external validity in light of the jeopardizing factors that were discussed in Chapter 3. The number of possible research designs that could be discussed is large; different texts cover different number of designs, selecting those that may be more common in their areas of interest or those that may best exemplify the major advantages and disadvantages of various design strategies. As Kerlinger (1973) has pointed out, theoretically, at least, there are as many designs as there are hypotheses to be tested. Therefore, rather than attempt to present an exhaustive taxonomy of descriptive and experimental research designs, we have limited our discussion to a general discussion of some basic types of designs and to a specific discussion of some designs that are commonly used to study the effectiveness of therapy. The former discussion is intended to introduce the student to some general considerations in the design of research that have broad applicability to many descriptive and experimental studies. The latter discussion is meant to serve as an example of how many of these general principles can be applied to the analysis of research designs in a specific area. We have selected the latter group because many students have expressed interest in studying the design of therapy experiments and because much has been written about the validity of these designs (e.g., Campbell & Stanley, 1966; Huck, Cormier, & Bounds, 1974).

General Research Design Considerations

This section will be concerned with some general principles important for the consumer's understanding of the design of experimental and descriptive research. Specific examples of many of these principles are included in the excerpts from the literature that are presented in Chapter 7.

Experimental design is concerned with the manipulation of the independent variable and with the measurement of its effect on the dependent variable. Descriptive research design is concerned with the classification of subjects and with the application of measurement procedures to subjects in order to assess group differences, developmental trends, or relationships among variables. Experimental and descriptive research designs are often classified as *between-subjects, within-subjects,* or *mixed* (both between-subjects and within-subjects) designs.

In between-subjects designs, different groups of subjects are compared to each other. Within-subjects designs involve the comparison of the same group of subjects in different situations. Mixed designs include both types of comparison in the same study. Some problems are well suited to between-subjects designs, whereas other problems are more logically attacked through within-subjects designs. In some cases, a combination of the two in a mixed design is necessary in order to study the problem appropriately. The selection of an appropriate design is dependent, to a large extent, on a clear understanding of the research problem and a logical analysis of the alternative means for studying the problem.

Between-Subjects Designs

In between-subjects research designs, the performances of separate groups of subjects are measured and comparisons are made between the groups. In experimental between-subjects designs, different groups of subjects are exposed to different treatments or levels of the independent variable. In descriptive between-subjects designs, different groups of subjects are compared with each other with regard to their performance on some criterion variable. We will first discuss some issues in between-subjects experimental designs and then consider some points concerning between-subjects descriptive research designs.

In between-subjects experimental designs, the independent variable or experimental treatment is applied to one group of subjects (experimental group) but not applied to another group of subjects (control group). The difference between the performance of the two groups is taken as an index of the effect of the independent variable on the dependent variable. This would be the case, for example, in a therapy experiment in which the experimental group is given therapy and the control group is not given therapy. The two groups are then compared on some dependent variable that is usually some measure of performance improvement.

Ferguson (1976, p. 212) has summarized the process of designing a be-tween-subjects experiment:

> In developing the design for an experiment, the investigator must (1) select the values or categories of the independent variable, or variables, to be compared; (2) select the subjects for the experiment; (3) apply rules or procedures whereby subjects are assigned to the particular values or categories of the independent variable; (4) specify the observations or measurements to be made on each subject.

Between-subjects experimental designs may be bivalent, in which case one experimental group is compared to one control group to study the effect of the presence vs. the absence of the experimental treatment (independent variable). These designs may also be multivalent, in which case each of several experimental groups is exposed to a different value of the indepen-dent variable and the control group receives no treatment. Finally, between-subjects designs may be parametric, in which case several groups could receive different values of the different independent variables in different combinations and could also be compared with a control group that receives no treatment.

A major consideration in the evaluaton of the design of between-subjects experiments is the equivalence of the experimental and control groups. The subject-selection threat to internal validity (and its interaction with other threats) must be controlled in between-subjects designs. Otherwise, differ-ences in the relative performances of the experimental and control groups might be attributable to subject-selection differences between groups in ad-dition to, or instead of, the effects of the experimental treatment. Re-searchers, then, must attempt to ensure that subjects in the experimental and control groups are equivalent in all respects except for the varied distribu-tion of the independent variable to these groups. There are basically two techniques for attempting to equate experimental and control groups for between-subjects experimental designs: *randomization* and *matching*.

Randomization is usually considered the better of these two techniques and will be discussed first. Christensen (1977, p. 124), in commenting on the importance of randomization as a technique for equating groups, stated:

> Randomization is the most important and basic of all the control methods. It provides a control not only for known sources of variation but also for unknown sources of variation. In fact, it is the only technique for controlling unknown sources of variation.

Randomization means the assignment of subjects to experimental and con-trol groups on a random basis. Random, in this sense, does not mean that subjects are assigned in a haphazard fashion. Rather, randomization is a technique for group assignment that ensures each subject has an equal prob-ability of being assigned either to the experimental group or to the control group. Christensen (1977, p. 127) summarized the objective of randomization in dealing with extraneous variables in experimental and control groups:

> *Random assignment produces control by virtue of the fact that the variables to be controlled are distributed in approximately the same manner in all groups (ideally the distribution would be exactly the same). Since the distribution is approximately equal in all groups, the influence of the extraneous variables is held constant because they cannot exert any differential influence on the dependent variable.*

With a random assignment of subjects to experimental and control groups, extraneous variables, (e.g., age, sex, intelligence, and socioeconomic status), which could effect the subjects' performance on the dependent variable, should even out among the groups so that there would be no systematic bias favoring one group over another. In such a case, then, the two groups may be considered equivalent at the start of the experiment.

Christensen (1977) points out, however, that randomization may not always result in the selection of experimental and control groups that are equivalent in all respects, especially when a small number of subjects is used. Because random chance determines the assignment of subjects to experimental and control groups (and, therefore, the distribution of extraneous subject-selection variables to experimental and control groups), it is possible occasionally for the two groups to differ on some variables. Researchers often check this possibility by examining the groups after randomization to ascertain the equivalence of the groups on known extraneous variables. Christensen (1977) has indicated, however, that the probability of experimental and control groups being equivalent on extraneous variables is greater with randomization than with other methods of group selection and, therefore, randomization is a powerful technique for reducing systematic bias in subject assignment and thereby reducing the subject-selection threat to internal validity. In addition, randomization is an important prerequisite to unbiased data analysis, and many of the statistical techniques to be described in Chapter 5 are based on the assumption of random assignment to experimental and control groups.

A second technique for attempting to equate experimental and control groups in between-subjects experimental designs is matching. The experimenter could attempt to match the members of the two groups on all extraneous variables that were considered relevant to the experiment. Two groups could be assembled that would be equivalent at the start of the experiment on extraneous variables known to be correlated with the dependent variable. Because the rationale for matching groups is to reduce the possibility of subject-selection differences mimicking the effect of the independent variable on the dependent variable, it makes sense to match the groups on extraneous variables that could influence subjects' performance on the dependent variable. Thus, differences between the experimental and control groups on the dependent variable at the end of the experiment would not be attributable to differences between the groups on these extraneous variables.

A number of techniques are available for matching experimental and control groups on extraneous variables. Two common techniques employed are *matching the overall distribution* of the extraneous variables in the groups and *matching pairs of subjects* for assignment to experimental and control groups.

Overall matching is accomplished by assembling experimental and control groups that have similar distributions of the extraneous variables, that is both groups have about the same average and spread of each of the extraneous variables. For example, factors such as age, intelligence, level of education, and sex would be distributed about equally in the experimental and control groups. Each group could be assembled so that it would contain equal numbers of males and females; the age range and average age would be the same in each group; the average IQ and the range from the lowest to the highest IQ in each group would be about the same, and so on.

Although overall matching may appear on the surface to be an adequate technique for ensuring group equivalence, consumers of research should be aware that there are disadvantages to this technique. For example, one distinct disadvantage is that the combinations of extraneous variables in individual subjects may not be well matched for two groups. Although age and IQ may be the same on the average in the two groups, the older subjects may be more intelligent than the younger subjects in one group, whereas the younger subjects may be more intelligent than the older subjects in the other group. Although individual nuisance variables may appear to be equivalent in the two groups, the interaction of the nuisance variables in each subject in the two groups may not necessarily be the same.

Matching pairs of subjects for subsequent assignment to experimental and control groups is a more effective technique than overall matching. Matching pairs is accomplished by first selecting a subject for assignment to one group and then searching for another subject whose constellation of extraneous variables is essentially the same as for the first subject. Because no two people are exactly alike in all respects, matching is usually accomplished within certain limits on the extraneous variables. For example, the first subject may be a 21-year-old female college senior with an IQ of 115. To find her matched pair member for assignment to the other group, the experimenter would then look for a female college senior with an IQ between 112 and 118 in the age range from 20 to 22 years. The rest of the subjects would be paired in a similar fashion, with each pair having a unique pattern of the extraneous variables.

Once matched pairs have been assembled, the next step is to assign the pair members to the experimental and control groups. Although pair matching would equate experimental and control groups on the known extraneous variables selected for matching, it should not equate them with respect to any other extraneous variables overlooked by the experimenter. Therefore, assigning pair members to experimental and control groups only on the basis of some convenience may result in nonequivalent groups with respect to unknown extraneous variables. Suppose, for example, that the pairs were assembled by selecting subjects from two different clinical settings and matching one member from each setting to one member of the other setting. Then, for the sake of convenience, all pair members from one setting are assigned to the experimental treatment and all pair members from the other setting are assigned to the control group. The problem is that if there were any differences between the groups of subjects in the two settings on unknown extraneous variables, then these differences would result in a differential subject-selection threat to internal validity, despite the matching of the groups on the known extraneous variables.

Campbell and Stanley (1966) and Van Dalen (1966) have suggested, however, that matching pairs can be a powerful technique for ensuring group equivalence if that technique is *combined with randomization*. Members of matched pairs could be subsequently assigned *at random*, one pair member being assigned randomly to the experimental group and the other pair member to the control group. This combination of matching pairs and randomization would be used (1) to match pairs on extraneous variables that are known to be correlated with the dependent variable and (2) to reduce the probability of group differences on unknown extraneous variables through the random assignment of pair members to the two groups.

Consumers of research should be aware of some of the advantages and disadvantages both of randomization and of matching. Randomization is often preferred, for example, if a large number of subjects is available because it is difficult to match numerous pairs, especially if they must be matched on several extraneous variables. Therefore, it would be more efficient to randomize group assignment at the outset, as randomization alone decreases the probability of group differences with respect to both known and unknown extraneous variables.

Randomization is also generally preferred when more than one experimental group is to be compared with the control group. If, for example, three experimental groups were to be compared with one control group, then matched quadruplets rather than matched pairs would be needed. Matching quadruplets of subjects would present considerable difficulty to any experimenter, especially if the quadruplets were to be matched on several extraneous variables. It would be much more efficient to assign subjects randomly to each of the four groups at the outset than to try to match groups of four subjects for subsequent randomization.

The combination of matching pairs with subsequent randomization of pair members to experimental and control groups may be preferred by some investigators when only a small number of subjects is available for inclusion in the experiment. As indicated by Christensen (1977), the risk for failure to equate groups as a result of randomization is greater with a small number of subjects than it is with a larger number of subjects. Therefore, experimenters

may often feel more confident about group equivalence on known extraneous variables if pair matching is combined with subsequent randomization. Despite the disadvantages of overall matching and pair matching, many
experimenters apparently believe that matching alone is better than nothing
at all, as evidenced by the prevalence of articles in the research literature
that employ matching alone for assembling experimental and control
groups.

Thus far, we have discussed only reduction of the subject-selection factor
as a threat to internal validity in between-subjects experimental designs.
Readers should be aware that random assignment of subjects to experimental
and control groups also helps to reduce threats to internal validity arising
from history, maturation, pretesting, and regression. If any of these factors
would affect the performance of the experimental group on the dependent
variable, then they should also have a similar effect on the performance of
subjects in the control group when the two groups have been constructed on
the basis of random assignment. Any performance difference between randomly assembled experimental and control groups, then, would be attributable to the effect of the experimental treatment rather than to the effects of
these jeopardizing factors.

Mortality, however, is always a potential problem in any research design.
If mortality interacts with some extraneous variable (e.g., less motivated
subjects drop out; more motivated subjects remain in the experiment) then
randomization should, in the long run, ensure that mortality would be about
the same in both groups and that the same type of subjects would remain
after mortality. Because the extraneous variables (e.g., motivation) should be
about evenly distributed in the two groups, the likelihood of mortality being
different in the two groups is reduced with random assignment. Whenever
there is a high mortality rate in either group or a different rate of mortality in
the two groups, however, the consumer should be alerted to the researcher's
explanation of the mortality rate. Although differential mortality rates are
less likely to occur with randomization of subjects into experimental and
control groups, any time mortality does appear, it represents a significant
problem.

Randomization of subjects to experimental and control groups does not
ensure the reduction of the instrumentation threat to internal validity. Randomization would be a wasted effort on the part of an experimenter who
failed to pay careful attention to the calibration, reliability, and validity of
instrumentation employed for the measurement of the dependent variable.
Hardware instrumentation should be equivalent for all measurements made
before, during, and after any experimental treatments. The use of human
observers to measure a dependent variable is equally subject to scrutiny by
consumers of research. Authors should inform readers of the efforts made to
ensure that human observers were well trained and practiced in the use of
such devices as tests, rating scales, and behavioral observations. When
human observers evaluate the performance of subjects in both experimental
and control groups, it is desirable to have them do "blind" evaluations. That

is, the observers should test the subjects without knowledge of which group (experimental or control) the subjects were assigned to in order to reduce the possibility of observer bias in assessing the subjects' performances. The Rosenthal effect can best be reduced by withholding knowledge of group composition from persons who administer the tests or measurements. If more than one human observer is to be employed (especially if some observers test the experimental group and other observers test the control groups), it is advisable for the observers to be randomly assigned to test the experimental and control subjects in addition to being "blind" as to which group they are testing.

Between-subjects designs have been discussed so far only with regard to experimental research. Between-subjects designs are also common in descriptive research and many of the foregoing considerations, especially efforts to reduce mortality and instrumentation threats to validity, are applicable to descriptive research designs. In addition, there are other specific considerations unique to descriptive research that need to be addresssed.

Between-subjects designs are found in comparative research, in cross-sectional developmental research, and in surveys that compare the responses of different groups. Comparative research involves the description of criterion-variable differences between groups of subjects who differ with respect to some classification variable (e.g., stutterers vs. nonstutterers). Cross-sectional developmental research uses a between-subjects design because separate groups of subjects who differ with respect to age are compared (i.e., age is, in a sense, a classification variable). Some surveys are conducted for the purpose of comparing the interview or questionnaire responses of subjects who fall into different classifications (e.g., hearing aid users vs. nonusers).

Between-subjects descriptive research designs may be bivalent, in which case the classification variable is broken into two mutually exclusive categories (e.g., laryngectomees vs. speakers with normal larynges). Between-subjects descriptive designs may also be multivalent, in which case the classification variable is divided into categories that are ordered along some continuum (e.g., mild vs. moderate vs. severe hearing loss). Finally, between-subjects descriptive designs may include comparisons of subjects who are simultaneously categorized with respect to more than one classification variable (e.g., male vs. female; mild vs. moderate vs. severe mental retardation).

As is the case with between-subjects experimental designs, subject selection is a major consideration in between-subjects descriptive research designs. Consumers should recognize, however, that researchers cannot randomly assign subjects to different classifications in a descriptive study. Instead, the researcher has to select subjects who already fall within the various classifications (e.g., normal hearing vs. hearing-impaired subjects). The main strategy in between-subjects descriptive research design, then, is selection of subjects who fall into distinctly different categories of the classification variable but who are otherwise equivalent with regard to extraneous variables. This is, indeed, a formidable task. A comparison of some problems encountered and some strategies employed in designing between-subjects research studies with manipulable independent variables vs. classification variables may be found in Ferguson (1976, pp. 211–222).

The first step in this strategy is the definition of criteria for selecting subjects from each category of the classification variable. Consumers of research should pay careful attention to the manner in which subject-selection criteria are defined. Classifications must be constructed that are mutually exclusive, that is, subjects should fall into only one category with regard to each classification variable. For example, in a comparison of patients with cochlear hearing loss with patients with conductive hearing loss, all subjects must fit the definition of only one of the two groups. Patients who were found to have both a cochlear and a conductive component to their losses would have to form a third comparison group, that is, patients with mixed hearing losses. Consumers are likely to notice that researchers vary in the strictness with which they define subject-selection criteria. Compromises are often necessary in trying to establish well-defined groups and remain reasonably consistent with the actual characteristics of the subjects that are available for study.

Although some classification variables are relatively easy to categorize, others may require more elaborate criteria for defining mutually exclusive groups of subjects. Sometimes it may be necessary to employ several measures in a battery of selection tests in order to classify subjects. In many cases, a range of scores on a particular measure may be used to define arbitrary boundaries for classification. Consumers should examine the reliability and validity of tests used for subject classification in order to evaluate the effectiveness with which the researcher has assembled the groups of subjects.

The second step in the selection strategy of between-subjects descriptive research is the attempt to equate subjects on extraneous variables. Because subjects cannot be assigned randomly to the various classifications, consumers of research should realize that equivalence of groups on all extraneous variables is quite difficult to achieve. The inability to eliminate this subject selection threat to internal validity is one of the reasons that many researchers are reluctant to infer cause–effect relationships from descriptive studies.

Because random assignment to classifications is impossible, the best alternative is to try to minimize group differences on extraneous variables known to correlate with the criterion (dependent) variable. A common method for reducing extraneous variable differences is to match the various groups on the extraneous variables known to be most highly correlated with the criterion variable. Both overall matching and pair matching have been used for this purpose in between-subjects descriptive research. The advantages and disadvantages of these two techniques were discussed earlier. Neither technique fully eliminates subject-selection threats to validity, but many researchers consider using these techniques to be better than ignoring the problem of extraneous variables. The greatest problem, of course, is in overlooking relevant extraneous variables that could influence performance on the criterion variable.

Many between-subjects descriptive studies involve short-term measurement of the criterion variable that can be accomplished in a single setting. The effects of factors such as history, maturation, pretesting, regression, and mortality should not seriously threaten the internal validity of such comparisons. Observations that require longer testing times or more than one test session could be influenced by these factors. Good descriptive research designs will compensate for these factors by providing the subjects with rest periods, counterbalancing test orders, and carefully monitoring history and mortality problems. The earlier discussion of instrumentation in experimental between-subjects designs applies equally to between-subjects descriptive designs. Simply because a study is descriptive rather than experimental is no excuse for sloppy instrumentation. This is especially true of surveys in which the construction of the questionnaire or the behavior of the interviewer can easily bias the responses of subjects.

In summary, between-subjects designs compare the performance of different groups of subjects in experimental or descriptive research. In experimental work, the comparison is made between groups of subjects who are exposed to different treatments or levels of the independent variable. In descriptive research, the performances of subjects in different classifications are compared. Effective between-subjects designs include efforts to select groups that are equivalent regarding extraneous variables and attempt to control instrumentation artifacts and the influence of mortality.

Within-Subjects Designs

In within-subjects designs, the performance of the *same* subjects is compared in different conditions. In experimental research, the subjects are exposed to all treatments or levels of the independent variable. Longitudinal developmental studies are within-subjects descriptive designs because the same subjects are studied as they mature with the passage of time. Correlational studies also include within-subjects designs because each subject is measured on all of the variables that are correlated. Experimental within-subjects design will be considered first, and additional comments will be made about within-subjects descriptive research designs.

In the preceding discussion of between-subjects experimental design, emphasis was placed on evaluation of attempts to equate groups of subjects on extraneous variables. There is no problem with extraneous variables affecting the performance of one group of subjects and not the other in a within-subjects design because only one group of subjects participates. In other words, assignment of subjects to experimental and control groups is not a problem. The basic concern in evaluation of a within-subjects design is that all conditions should be equivalent except for the application of the various experimental treatments. Appropriate cautions should be taken to ensure that any changes in the dependent variable that are observed can be attributed to the effect of the experimental treatment rather than to the effect of factors such as history, maturation, and mortality.

Many of these threats to internal validity may be related to the temporal arrangements or sequence of the conditions of a within-subjects experiment. Therefore, a necessary strategy in within-subjects experimental design is the attempt to control what is sometimes termed "sequencing effect" or "order effect." Sequencing effect and order effect are not used consistently in the various textbooks on research design, but two distinct effects are usually identified regarding the temporal arrangement of experimental conditions. We will use the terminology employed by Christensen (1977) in describing these effects.

Christensen uses *sequencing effect* to describe the overall problem that occurs when subjects participate in a number of treatment conditions and their participation in an earlier condition may affect their performance in a subsequent condition. He differentiates between two types of sequencing effects. The first effect is called an *order effect*, that is, a general performance improvement or decrement that may occur between the beginning and end of an experiment. For example, subjects' performances might improve toward the end of an experiment because of the practice in the task that they receive simply by participating in earlier parts of the experiment. On the other hand, subjects may show a decrease in performance in the latter part of an experiment because of fatigue. In other words, short-term maturation may influence their performance on the dependent variable during the course of the experiment.

Christensen calls the second sequencing effect a *carry-over effect*. A carry-over effect is not a general performance change from the beginning to the end of an experiment but rather the result of the influence of a specific treatment condition on performance in the next condition. In other words, the results of one treatment condition may be carried over into the next condition. For example, in studies of temporary threshold shift (TTS) induced by presentation of intense noise, it is important that subjects be given sufficient time to recover from TTS before experiencing a subsequent noise exposure. Otherwise, performance in the subsequent condition would be affected by the carryover of TTS remaining from the first exposure. This carry-over effect may occur whenever exposure to one treatment condition either permanently or temporarily affects performance in subsequent conditions. Temporary carryover can often be minimized with a rest period between experimental condtions, but permanent carryover is a more serious problem that will be discussed later in this section.

There are two major techniques for reducing sequencing effects: *randomizing* and *counterbalancing* the sequence of experimental treatments. Randomization means the presentation of the experimental treatment conditions to the subjects in a random sequence. Random distribution of the treatments in the time course of the experiment would essentially wash out most sequencing effects in a within-subjects design. Sometimes, however, the experimenter may wish to examine the nature of a sequencing effect, and this cannot be done with randomization. Counterbalancing is a technique that enables the experimenter to control and measure sequencing effects by arranging all possible sequences of treatments and, then, randomly assigning subjects to each sequence. Any differences in performance attributable to the sequencing of treatment conditions could then be measured by examining the performances of subjects who participated in the different sequences. In a sense, the sequence of treatment conditions would become another independent variable that is manipulated by the experimenter.

In some cases, sequencing effects may involve such severe or permanent carryover that within-subjects designs are not appropriate. For example, Underwood and Shaughnessy (1975) list experiments on the effects of instructions as being generally inappropriate for within-subjects designs. Suppose an experimenter wished to study the differential effect of two types of instructions on subjects' performance of a certain task. One set of instructions contains information that may influence performance, but this information is withheld from the other set of instructions. If subjects always received the informative instructions last, a possible order effect might be introduced (i.e., subjects might warm up or become fatigued from the first to the second condition). If the sequence of instructions were randomized or counterbalanced, however, those subjects who received the informative instructions first would not be likely to forget those instructions when tested later with the noninformative instructions. In other words, there would be a permanent carry-over effect from the informative to the noninformative instructions.

Whenever carryover is likely to be permanent, a between-subjects design is more appropriate than a within-subjects design. In the example of the effects of instructions on performance, subjects could be randomly assigned to one of two groups: one group would receive the informative instructions, the other group would receive the noninformative instructions. Whenever a sequencing effect cannot be controlled by randomization or counterbalancing, between-subjects designs are usually considered more appropriate. Whenever sequencing can be well controlled, within-subjects designs are often considered to be more powerful than between-subjects designs because the subjects act as their own control group by participating in all experimental conditions.

In some cases it may be difficult for the consumer to decide whether a between-subjects design or a within-subjects design is more appropriate. Consumers should realize that the selection of the better alternative depends on a thorough understanding of the research problem and of the advantages and disadvantages of applying each design to that specific problem. The researcher and the consumer alike need to understand the substance of the problem through familiarity with the research and theoretical literature on the specific topic.

Longitudinal developmental research is an example of the application of a within-subjects design to descriptive research. The longitudinal design differs from the between-subjects cross-sectional design because the researcher follows the same subjects as they age or mature rather than measuring the performance of different groups of subjects selected from each age range. This within-subjects developmental design allows the researcher to study the rate of development directly for each subject as time passes and the subjects age or mature. Although the subject selection threat to internal validity may jeopardize a cross-sectional developmental design, this factor is not a threat to the internal validity of longitudinal studies because separate age groups are not studied.

Maturation plays a unique role in developmental research. Long-term maturation is actually the independent (or classification) variable that the investigator is studying. Therefore, it is not a threat to internal validity. Short-term maturation (i.e., fatigue or warm-up effects) could be a threat to internal validity, however, if care were not taken to make measurements in a systematic fashion at each measurement time. Short-term maturation effects are usually controlled by making all measurement sessions equivalent with respect to factors such as time of day and feeding schedules. History (and its interaction with other factors) could also threaten internal validity, and researchers generally take steps to monitor history carefully during a longitudinal study. For example, historical events such as recurrent middle ear infections or the separation of parents and children in a language development study should be carefully monitored and taken into account in reaching conclusions. Mortality must also be carefully scrutinized, as longitudinal studies are more prone to mortality because of their prolonged nature.

Correlational studies are also examples of within-subjects designs in descriptive research because they involve the application of a number of different measures to a group of subjects. Often these studies include rather short testing times so that factors such as history and long-term maturation do not threaten the internal validity of the studies. Sequencing effects can usually be controlled through randomization or counterbalancing the sequence of the tests administered.

In summary, within-subjects designs involve the comparison of the performance of the same group of subjects when tested under different experimental conditions, when followed over time in longitudinal research or when tested with different measures in correlational studies. Although differential subject selection is not a threat to internal validity in these designs, efforts must be made to minimize threats to internal validity such as history or maturation that may arise from the sequencing of measurements. The comments on instrumentation and mortality that were made in the section on between-subjects designs apply as well to within-subjects designs.

Mixed Designs

In many research studies more than one independent variable is considered. The effects of two or more independent variables on a dependent variable may be examined in an experimental study. More than one classification variable may be investigated in a descriptive study. In many of these cases, one independent variable is studied with a between-subjects comparison and the other independent variable is studied with a within-subjects comparison. Hence, a mixed design is employed that incorporates each of the two strategies.

In an experiment in which two independent variables are manipulated, it may sometimes be better to measure the effects of one independent variable with a between-subjects design and to measure the effects of the other independent variable with a within-subjects design. A descriptive study may incorporate a comparison of the correlation between two variables in one type of subject with the correlation between these two variables in another type of subject. A descriptive study may also incorporate a comparison of the longitudinal development of two different types of subjects. Combined descriptive–experimental studies often involve a within-subjects experimental study of the effect of an independent variable on a dependent variable with two different types of subjects. The experimental effect for one group would be compared to the experimental effect for the other group. All of these research studies would involve mixed designs because they incorporate both within-subjects and between-subjects comparisons.

Because mixed designs incorporate the strategies of both between-subjects and within-subjects designs, the foregoing discussion of both types of designs applies to the mixed designs. The cautions required to ensure group equivalence for between-subjects designs apply to groups compared in mixed designs. Similarly, the comments on randomizing or counterbalancing techniques apply to the within-subjects component of a mixed design. The instrumentation and mortality factors obviously merit attention in research using mixed designs.

It is important for consumers of research to be aware of the nature of mixed designs because of their high prevalence in the speech pathology and audiology literature. Consumers should be able to identify which part of a mixed design is a within-subjects comparison and which part is a between-subjects comparison in order to evaluate the attempts made by the researcher to minimize threats to internal validity. The examples shown in Chapters 2 and 7 may be helpful in illustrating the between-subjects and within-subjects components of mixed designs.

External Validity of Research Designs

The preceding discussion of research designs has focused on the problems of internal validity. Some comments are now in order with regard to external validity. External validity, or generalizability of results, is more difficult to deal with in a single research study than is internal validity. Also, as mentioned in Chapter 3, efforts aimed at increasing one type of validity may decrease the other type.

External validity concerns the ability to generalize research findings to other subjects, settings, measuring instruments, or experimental treatments. Efforts to increase internal validity often involve the narrowing or limiting of subject characteristics, research settings, measuring instruments, or experimental treatments. Therefore, the results of many research studies are limited in their generalizability. The results *may be generalizable*, in fact, to other subjects, settings, measurements, or treatments, but this cannot be assumed until it has been proven. In the meantime, researchers and consumers of research must *limit* the degree to which they try to generalize the results of an individual research article.

An important consideration in research design is to find solutions to the problem of extending findings beyond the limits of a single study. There are basically two tactics that are helpful in improving generalization to other subjects, settings, measurements, or treatments.

The first tactic is *random sampling* of subjects to be included in a study. Random sampling helps to improve generalization to the specific population of subjects represented by the group of subjects studied. Generalization of results is considered to be most feasible when the sample of subjects included in the study is a random sample of the population of interest. A random sample means that all subjects in the population have an equal probability of being selected for inclusion in the study. Although results of research studies using random samples have the best generalizability to the population of the same type of subjects, random sampling cannot help to extend generalization to other types of subjects or to other settings, measurements, or treatments.

Unfortunately, most investigators are unable to select random samples from the population of interest. Because the population is so large and widespread geographically, selecting a random sample is financially and practically unfeasible. The few studies in the speech pathology and audiology literature that have employed random samples have better generalizability (within the limits of type of subject, setting, instruments, and treatments) than those studies that are not based on random samples.

The second tactic is *replication*. Repeating a research study and finding the same results as in the first study is a powerful means of extending external valdity. A research result that can be replicated is stronger in external validity than a result that has not yet been replicated. Replication is a more practical technique than random sampling because it is more feasible for a researcher to repeat an experiment than to try to secure a random sample of a target population in the first experiment. Perhaps even more important, replication is more widely applicable than random sampling of subjects because it can help to extend generalization to other types of subjects as well as to other settings, measurements, or treatments.

Unfortunately, replication has not always been as common a practice in behavioral research as it has been in biological, medical, or physical sciences. But in recent years, more and more replication studies have appeared in the literature, perhaps indicating more sensitivity to the need for replications to extend the external validity of behavior research findings. Smith (1970) identified several reasons why researchers do not often replicate studies, including such factors as lack of time, funds, or available subjects; reluctance of some journals to publish replications of previous work; and development of new research interests by the investigator. In commenting on many of these reasons, Smith (p. 971) stated:

> . . . if the goal of scientific research is to render established truths, then the neglect of replication must be reviewed as scientific irresponsibility.

Smith further suggested that many of these barriers to replication can be overcome by obtaining replication data when the original study is conducted. A section on replication could then be added to the original article.

Sidman (1960) has discussed two major types of replication: *direct replication* and *systematic replication*. In direct replication, the investigator repeats the research with the same subjects or with a new group of comparable subjects in order to affirm the reliability of the original results or to test their generality within the limits of the subjects, settings, measurements, and treatments originally studied. Direct replication is an important technique for demonstrating generalization when it is impossible for an investigator to select a random sample from the population of interest. Consistency of results with direct replication helps to confirm generalization to comparable subjects performing under comparable conditions (i.e., settings, measurements, treatments).

In systematic replication, the research may be repeated under different conditions or with different types of subjects in order to extend generalization to other subjects, settings, measurements, or treatments. Some aspect of the subjects, setting, measurement, or treatment would be varied to include some new subject, setting, measurement, or treatment to which the investigator would like to generalize results. Systematic replication is, therefore, a powerful tool for extending external validity beyond the limits of a single research study. Consumers of research should consider the generalizability of research results as limited to the particular kinds of subjects, settings, measurements, and treatments used until such time as systematic replications demonstrate that the results are, in fact, more general. In some cases, of course, the limited generality of results may not pose a problem to consumers of research. The results of a study that used a particular measurement with a particular type of subject in a specific setting may be easily applied by professionals who normally use that particular measure with that kind of subject in that setting. Many research consumers, however, are interested in broadening the generality of research findings and will, therefore, be more interested in the implications of replication for the extension of external validity.

Many combined experimental–descriptive studies involve a form of systematic replication because they compare experimental effects for different kinds of subjects. The examples cited in Chapter 2 in the section, Combined Experimental–Descriptive Research, show how the experimental effect on one type of subject may be compared with the experimental effect on another type of subject.

There are several recent examples of replications that extend external validity in the speech pathology and audiology literature. Guitar (1976) included a direct replication in his correlational study of pretreatment factors associated with improvement in stuttering therapy and Monsen (1978) included a direct replication in his regression analysis of acoustic variables used to predict the intelligibility of deaf speakers. In both cases the direct replications showed results that were quite consistent with the results of the original studies, thus strengthening the generality of the original results within the limits of the same type of subjects, settings, and measures.

Systematic replications have also appeared as follow-up articles or have been included in an article reporting the replication along with the original results. Silverman (1976) provides an excellent example of a systematic replication in which an experiment on listener reactions to lisping was replicated with a different kind of subject used as listeners in order to extend generality regarding other subjects. Costello and Bosler (1976) evaluated generality to four other settings in their study of the efficacy of articulation therapy. Cottrell, Montague, Farb, and Throne (1980) examined generality to other measurements in their study of operant conditioning for improvement of vocabulary definition of developmentally delayed children by testing the degree to which their original results generalized to untrained vocabulary words within the same semantic classes. Courtright and Courtright (1979) examined external validity in regard to other treatments. They extended their earlier findings regarding imitative modeling as a language-intervention strategy by replicating an earlier study of modeling vs. mimicry and examining two other treatment variables associated with modeling—reinforcement and origin of the model—to determine their influence on the effectiveness of modeling.

In summary, external validity, or generality of results, is usually limited in any single research article. Random sampling and direct replication can help to improve generalization within the limits of type of subject, setting, measurement, and treatment. Systematic replication can help extend generalization to other kinds of subjects, settings, measurements, or treatments. As Hunter, Schmidt, and Jackson (1982, p. 10) have stated:

> *Scientists have known for centuries that a single study will not resolve a major issue. Indeed, a small sample study will not even resolve a minor issue. Thus, the foundation of science is the cumulation of knowledge from the results of many studies. There are two steps to the cumulation of knowledge: (1) the cumulation of results across studies to*

establish facts and (2) the formation of theories to place the facts into a coherent and useful form.

Hunter et al. (1982), then, have emphasized not only the empirical importance of external validity but also its theoretical importance, which is in consonance with Stevens' (1968) reminder of the schemapiric view of science. In other words, external validity is not only important in research design but also in the integration of rational and empirical evidence in the explanation of the laws of behavior.

Evaluation of Some Experimental Designs for Studying the Effectiveness of Therapy

In this section, much of the material discussed previously will be applied to the evaluation of experimental designs for studying the effectiveness of therapy. Many individuals express an interest in the analysis of therapy research because of the direct applicability of such research to clinical work. Also, much has been written about the validity of these designs (e.g., Campbell & Stanley, 1966). These designs incorporate within-subjects, between-subjects, or mixed comparisons and, therefore, serve to illustrate many of the concepts advanced in the earlier sections of this chapter.

In outlining the paradigms of the experimental designs to follow, we will adopt Campbell and Stanley's notation system (1966). The left-to-right orientation will indicate the progression of time from before to after therapy and the vertical orientation will indicate simultaneous occurrences. X will be the symbol for the administration of the experimental treatment and O will refer to the observation and measurement of the dependent variable. When subjects are randomly assigned to groups, R will precede the appropriate groups. When subjects are matched on known extraneous variables and subsequently assigned to groups at random, MR will precede the appropriate groups. When there is no formal means for certifying either of these attempts to equate groups in an experiment, dashed lines (− − − − − −) will separate the groups.

Weak Designs

Campbell and Stanley (1966) have identified several weak designs in educational research that may be applicable to the investigation of the effects of therapy in speech pathology or audiology. These experimental designs are weak in both internal and external validity. They are presented here to help the consumer of research to identify weak therapy research. They also may serve as a frame of reference for understanding the manner in which the stronger designs represent improvements on the weaker designs.

The One-Shot Case Study. The first weak design is what Campbell and Stanley called the one-shot case study and it can be diagrammed as follows:

X   O

In such a study, a single group is observed only once, after having been exposed to some treatment. For example, children with articulation disorders might be given an articulation test after therapy had been administered and their scores on this measure (dependent variable) used as an indication of the success of the therapy (independent variable). The major problem is that there is no reference point for comparison of the posttherapy scores on the articulation test; no pretest was administered and no control group was used. The *effects* of the articulation therapy cannot be evaluated because no comparison can be made to either pretherapy articulation performance or the performance of some group that did not receive therapy. Even if the articulation test scores were compared to existing norms, there is no basis for the conclusion that therapy affected the scores without pretherapy or control-group comparisons because no evidence is shown to indicate that articulation was better after therapy than it was before therapy. Campbell and Stanley have also pointed out that this design may suffer from the "error of misplaced precision" because careful data collection represents a wasted effort without the opportunity for comparison of the posttest scores with control group or pretest scores. The one-shot case study is fraught with threats to both internal and external validity when used as an experimental design for studying the effectiveness of therapy. It is extremely difficult, if not impossible, to draw valid conclusions from the results of a one-shot case study.

One-Group Pretest–Posttest Design. A second weak design discussed by Campbell and Stanley is the one-group pretest–posttest design, which may be diagrammed as follows:

$$O_1 \quad X \quad O_2$$

In such a design, one group is assembled, pretested, exposed to the experimental treatment, and posttested. This is a within-subjects design because all subjects are tested under two conditions: before and after therapy. For example, a group of children might be pretested on an articulation test, given articulation therapy, and then tested again after therapy on the articulation test. This design is more commonly found in the research literature and represents some improvement over the one-shot case study. But there are still numerous drawbacks to this design because of the threats to its internal and external validity.

The first problem concerns the effects of history because many events that could affect the posttest outcome may have occurred during the course of the experiment in addition to the experimental treatment. The stutterer in therapy may receive concomitant psychotherapy or may get a new job that increases his or her confidence in speaking situations. Maturation is also a threat because growth and development during the course of a study might affect the posttest, regardless of the application of the experimental treatment. Readers familiar with the process of spontaneous recovery in aphasia will understand this maturation threat. Testing represents still a third threat because the pretest may have increased the subjects' ability to perform well on the posttest.

Instrumentaion could be a threat if care is not taken to be sure that the pretest and posttest measures are equivalent. This is especially important when judgments of human observers are used in the pretest and posttest. For instance, the Rosenthal effect could operate if the human observers were biased in their observations by the belief that a change should have taken place as a result of the experimental treatment.

Statistical regression is a threat to internal validity when groups with extreme scores are retested. This would be important when subjects are selected because they had extremely poor pretest scores and were thereby considered good candidates for therapy. In such a case, regression toward the mean on a second test would be expected and could be a competing explanation for any performance gains after therapy. Threats to external validity would be primarily the interaction of selection or pretesting with the experimental variable, factors that are better controlled in the stronger designs to follow. Therefore, even though this design appears to be an improvement over the one-shot case study, it is still a weak design with many threats to both internal and external validity.

The Static-Group Comparison.   Another weak design is called the static-group comparison and can be diagrammed as follows:

$$X \quad O_1$$
$$\text{-----------}$$
$$O_2$$

In such a study, a group that has been exposed to the experimental treatment is compared to another group that has not, but no attempt is made to pretest the groups or to equate them by randomization or matching. This is a between-subjects design because two different groups are compared to each other. For example, children exposed to articulation therapy might be compared with children not exposed to such therapy to study the effects of therapy on their articulation performance.

There are two major problems with such a design. First, there is no pretest against which to compare posttest scores. Second, there is no formal means of certifying the equivalence of the groups on relevant extraneous variables, so any differences between the two groups may not be a result of the therapy program alone. Differential selection of subjects in the two groups would, therefore, be the greatest threat to internal validity because of lack of knowledge about extraneous variables in both groups. Also, any experimental mortality would seriously affect the internal validity of this design because there would be no way of certifying extraneous variables associated with mortality or what effect such variables would have had on the dependent variable in addition to the experimental treatment. Interaction of selection and mortality with the other factors would also threaten internal validity. The interaction of selection with the experimental variable would be the greatest threat to external validity, again because of the lack of knowledge about extraneous variables.

Nonequivalent Control-Group Design.   A fourth weak design is the nonequivalent control group design which can be diagrammed as follows:

$$O_1 \quad X \quad O_2$$
$$O_3 \qquad O_4$$

In such a study, one group is formed, pretested, exposed to the experimental treatment, and posttested, whereas another group is formed, pretested, not exposed to the experimental treatment, and posttested. This is a mixed design because it has both a within-subjects component (pretest vs. posttest) and a between-subjects component (experimental vs. control group). A difference between the two groups in the *improvement from pretest to posttest* would, then, be thought to be an index of the effect of the experimental treatment. This type of study might be done with naturally assembled groups because of the convenience of using one group intact as the experimental group and the other group intact as the control group. For instance, groups of subjects in two different clinics or schools might be compared. The subjects in one school would be exposed to the experimental treatment, whereas the subjects at the other school would be the control group receiving no treatment to compare the effect of therapy to no treatment. Sometimes this design is seen with the control group receiving a regularly scheduled therapy treatment to compare the effectiveness of a new treatment against the effect of an old treatment. Some studies have also used two control groups, one without treatment and another with the older treatment in order to make both comparisons.

This design may eliminate contamination of internal validity by the effects of history, maturation, and pretesting because of the introduction of a control group and may appear, therefore, to be a better design than the previous three, especially if the two groups perform similarly on the pretest. But there are problems involving the subject-selection factor and its interaction with the other factors that jeopardize internal validity. Because the groups have been selected on the basis of convenience rather than assembled on the basis of randomization or matching, it is possible that certain biases may arise from group composition that the experimenter cannot account for or measure. For example, if patients from a private clinic constituted one group and patients from a public clinic constituted the other, there might be important differences that related to their decision to attend a private vs. a public clinic. More affluent patients might attend the private clinic so that socioeconomic status would not be controlled as an extraneous variable. Private patients might be more motivated in therapy because they pay more for services rendered by the private clinic than do those patients in the public clinic. On the other hand, less affluent patients in a public clinic might be more motivated because they were striving to achieve better financial conditions and believed that better speech performance would help them to obtain better jobs. The main point is that the effects of these possible threats to internal validity due to differential selection of subjects in the two groups are unknown and, therefore, create a threat to internal validity. In addition, interaction of subject selection and other factors such as history, maturation, or mortality could also influence the results and thereby jeopardize internal validity.

Even though this design represents an obvious improvement over the previous three designs, it is not as strong in either internal or external validity as the designs in the next section. Unfortunately, the nonequivalent control-group design will probably find continued use in the literature because of its convenience, and readers should, therefore, be aware of the limitations inherent in this design.

Stronger Designs

Now that we have examined the pitfalls of some weak designs for studying the effectiveness of therapy, let us turn to the evaluation of stronger designs that illustrate some methods of reducing threats to internal and external validity.

Randomized Pretest–Posttest Control-Group Designs. Campbell and Stanley (1966) have outlined designs that include steps to ensure that (1) experimental and control groups are equivalent at the outset and (2) experimental and control groups are tested at equivalent time intervals to reduce threats to internal validity arising from factors such as maturation or regression.

The basic randomized pretest–posttest control-group design may be diagrammed as follows:

$$\begin{array}{cccc} R & O_1 & X & O_2 \\ R & O_3 & & O_4 \end{array}$$

In this mixed design, two groups are formed by randomly assigning half of the subjects to the experimental group and half to the control group. Both groups are pretested and posttested in the same manner at the same times. The factors that could jeopardize internal validity are well controlled in this design as the following discussion indicates.

History should be controlled because general historical events should theoretically have as much effect on the $O_1 - O_2$ difference as it does on the $O_3 - O_4$ difference because the groups are randomly assembled at the same time. There may be the possibility, however, of specific historical events differentially affecting one group and not the other (e.g., subjects in the experimental group meet for coffee between experimental sessions and influence each other's attitudes toward the experiment). Careful monitoring of such events can often preclude their threats to internal validity. Maturation and pretesting effects should be equivalent in both groups and affect the O_2 and O_4 scores by approximately the same amounts if randomization is used. Regression is not a threat, even if both groups have extreme scores on the pretest because both groups should evidence the same amount of regression as a result of random assignment. Differential subject selection is controlled because the groups have been randomly assembled and, therefore, extraneous variables should be randomly distributed among the subjects.

Attention must be paid to instrumentation and mortality, of course. Instrumentation problems would be minimized if careful calibration of equipment is achieved and if human observers are carefully employed by the researcher to preclude bias in their use of measurements. If mortality exists in any experiment, it poses a threat to internal validity. In this design, mortality should not generally affect one group more than the other because it should be present to the same extent in both groups if it is related to any extraneous variable (e.g., motivation). If, however, the researcher should note that the mortality rate is high or, perchance, that it is unevenly distributed between groups, he or she should undertake a replication of the experiment and also try to determine if any subject characteristics are related to mortality. Whenever mortality rates are high or unevenly distributed among groups in this or any research design, a serious threat may be posed to internal validity. But differential mortality is much less likely to occur with random assignment to experimental and control groups because the potential for attrition is randomly distributed.

In general, then, this design is strong in internal validity. There are also several variations on the randomized pretest–posttest control group design that may be considered. For example, matching may be used in conjunction with randomization to assemble the groups if there are certain extraneous variables that experimenters know should be controlled. The experimental and control groups would be formed by matching pairs of subjects on the known extraneous variables and, then, randomly assigning one member of each pair to the experimental group and the other member to the control group. Such a design could be diagrammed:

$$\text{MR} \quad O_1 \quad X \quad O_2$$
$$\text{MR} \quad O_3 \qquad\;\; O_4$$

The matching would equate pair members on extraneous variables known to be correlated with the dependent variable, and the random assignment of pair members to experimental and control groups should ensure that overlooked extraneous variables would be randomly distributed.

The randomized control-group design has been conceptualized by some researchers as a mixed design with a between-subjects independent variable (experimental vs. control groups) and a within-subjects independent variable (pretesting vs. posttesting). In this case, the *score* on whatever behavior is tested in the pretests and posttests would be the dependent variable. It has also been suggested (Campbell & Stanley, 1966) that the *gain in score* from pretest to posttest be considered the dependent variable. In that case, the *gain* of the control group would be compared to the *gain* of the experimental group and the experiment could be considered a simple bivalent experiment with just a between-subjects comparison of the control-group gain to the experimental group gain as an index of the effectiveness of therapy. The bivalent independent variable is therapy and assumes two values: presence vs. absence of therapy (analogous to the presence vs. absence of noise or earmold-venting samples shown in Chapter 2).

Using the pretest-to-posttest gain as the dependent variable, this design could be extended to a multivalent experiment by assembling groups that receive different values or different amounts of the experimental treatment (independent variable). For example, if the treatment involved practice drills with a certain behavior, several groups could each receive different amounts of practice or be drilled for different durations of therapy. Rather than simply comparing practice drills to no practice drills, the experimenter would be able to demonstrate changes in the dependent variable as a function of amount of practice drill. Such a design could be diagrammed as follows:

$$
\begin{array}{lllll}
\text{Group 1} & \text{R} & O_1 & X_1 & O_2 \\
\text{Group 2} & \text{R} & O_3 & X_2 & O_4 \\
\text{Group 3} & \text{R} & O_5 & X_3 & O_6 \\
\text{Group 4} & \text{R} & O_7 & & O_8 \\
\end{array}
$$

In this case, Group 1 might receive a certain amount of practice, Group 2 twice as much practice, Group 3 three times as much practice, and Group 4 would receive no practice and serve as the control group.

The design could be extended to a parametric design by studying the effects of two types of practice drills with varying amounts of each. For example, massed practice vs. distributed practice in three different amounts could be studied in the following paradigm:

$$
\begin{array}{llll}
\text{Group 1} & \text{R} & O_1 & X_{\text{Massed 1}} & O_2 \\
\text{Group 2} & \text{R} & O_3 & X_{\text{Massed 2}} & O_4 \\
\text{Group 3} & \text{R} & O_5 & X_{\text{Massed 3}} & O_6 \\
\text{Group 4} & \text{R} & O_7 & X_{\text{Distributed 1}} & O_8 \\
\text{Group 5} & \text{R} & O_9 & X_{\text{Distributed 2}} & O_{10} \\
\text{Group 6} & \text{R} & O_{11} & X_{\text{Distributed 3}} & O_{12} \\
\text{Group 7} & \text{R} & O_{13} & & O_{14} \\
\end{array}
$$

The first three groups would receive massed practice, with Group 1 receiving a certain amount, Group 2 twice as much, and Group 3 three times as much. Groups 4 though 6 would receive distributed practice, with Group 4 receiving the same amount of practice as Group 1 did, Group 5 receiving twice as much, and Group 6 receiving three times as much. Group 7 would receive no practice and would act as the control group. These designs may be expensive and difficult to administer, but they can be worth the effort because of the advantages of miltivalent and parametric experiments discussed in Chapter 2.

Although these equivalent pretest–posttest control-group designs are strong in internal validity, there are some restrictions on their external validity, mainly because of the interactions of some jeopardizing factors with the experimental treatment. The first problem with external validity involves the interaction of subject selection with the experimental variable. Although the simple main effect of subject selection as a threat to internal validity is minimized by random assignment of subjects to the experimental and control groups, it is possible that any demonstrated treatment effect may be valid only for the particular type of subjects studied in the investigation. For example, the results of a therapy study done with adult, male, college student stutterers attending a university speech clinic may be generalizable only to stutterers who are males, adults, college students, and attending a university clinic. Attempts to generalize to females, to children, to stutterers with less than a college education, or to stutterers attending other types of clinics may be unwarranted. Successful experiments in language therapy with mentally retarded children may not be generalizable to deaf or cerebral-palsied children. There is no guarantee, then, that generalization to subjects who are different from those studied in the original experiment will be valid. This does not mean that generalization never occurs; it simply means that it cannot be assumed until it has been proven. The possibility of the interaction of subject selection and the experimental treatment *limits* the generalizability to subjects who are equivalent to those in the original study until subsequent research demonstrates broader generalizability of the results.

One way to overcome this limitation and thereby extend generalization is to perform replications with other types of subjects as was mentioned earlier in this chapter. Replication of the experiment with different types of subjects would help to delineate the extent to which subject selection and the experimental treatment interacted by demonstrating the relative effectiveness of the treatment with various types of subjects.

Readers should recognize that such replication could be considered to be a combination of descriptive and experimental research because the experimental treatment would be manipulated by the researcher but the subject classification would not. The experiment would be replicated with subjects who differed in some classification variables such as age, sex, socioeconomic status, or type of pathology.

Such a replication of a randomized pretest–posttest control-group design could be diagrammed as follows:

$$\begin{array}{llllll} \textit{Initial experiment:} & R & O_1 & X & O_2 \\ \textit{Adults} & R & O_3 & & O_4 \end{array}$$

$$\begin{array}{llllll} \textit{Replication:} & R & O_5 & X & O_6 \\ \textit{Children} & R & O_7 & & O_8 \end{array}$$

In such a replication, the $O_1 - O_2$ difference would be compared with the $O_3 - O_4$ difference in the first experiment to examine the effect of the experimental treatment for the adult subjects. The replication with children would, then be run and the $O_5 - O_6$ difference would be compared to the $O_7 - O_8$ difference to examine the effect of the experimental treatment for the children. The replication would then be compared with the initial experiment to see if the same effect that was obtained with the adults could be generalized to children. Such systematic replication is the most promising method of reducing the threat to external validity posed by the interaction of subject selection and the experimental treatment. Otherwise, experimental results remain applicable only to subjects with essentially the same characteristics as those who participated in the original investigation.

A second threat to the external validity of the above designs is posed by the reactive effect of experimental arrangements. Experiments are usually novel events in the lives of subjects who participate in them, and experimental settings or situations are usually somewhat artificial. Subjects are often aware that they are participating in experiments, and they may differ in their attempts to discern the purpose of the experiment and in their conclusions regarding what the purpose is. The Hawthorne effect has always been thought to operate in experiments on human subjects as a threat to external validity. Government agencies now insist on protection of the rights of experimental subjects, and researchers must obtain informed consent from subjects before the experiment begins. Even if subjects agree to wait until after the experiment to be informed of its true purpose, they may have a preconceived notion of the purpose of the experiment and behave according to what they think the experimenter wants them to do (or does *not* want them to do!).

In many cases, it is not possible to control such reactive arrangements entirely, but they may be somewhat attenuated. For example, some studies may compare a placebo group to both the experimental and control groups to examine the effect of the suggestion to subjects that they are participating in an experiment. If the placebo group shows more improvement than the control group, a reactive arrangement may have accentuated improvement in the experimental group. Reactive arrangements are probably present in most experiments to the extent that subjects behave differently than they would if they did not know or believe they were in an experiment and the degree to which the experimental setting can be made more "natural' is important in reducing this threat to external validity. Systematic replication of the experiment in more "natural' settings may also help to extend the generalization of the results.

Still a third threat to external validity of the designs we have discussed so far is the interaction of pretesting with the experimental variable. It is possible that the pretest itself may sensitize the subjects to the possible effects that could be caused by the independent variable and make them more likely to show improvement. If the pretest does sensitize subjects to respond more to the experimental variable than would subjects who were not pretested, then the results cannot be generalized to subjects who have not had the same pretest. If the experimenter wishes to generalize only to subjects who will always have the same pretest, there is little problem with this factor. But suppose that someone in another clinic that does not use the same pretest wishes to use the treatment of an experiment. Can it be assumed that the same results will obtain without using the same pretest? Such generalization from any of the designs above cannot be made and only the next design is able to deal with the interaction of pretesting with the experimental treatment.

The Solomon Randomized Four-Group Design. Campbell and Stanley (1966, pp. 24–25) have discussed a design first used by Solomon in 1949 that is not only strong in internal validity but also makes a successful attempt to control one factor affecting external validity—the interaction between pretesting and the experimental treatment. The Solomon Randomized Four-Group Design may be diagrammed as follows:

$$
\begin{array}{llll}
\text{Group 1} & R & O_1 & X & O_2 \\
\text{Group 2} & R & O_3 & & O_4 \\
\text{Group 3} & R & & X & O_5 \\
\text{Group 4} & R & & & O_6 \\
\end{array}
$$

In the Solomon design, the subjects are randomly assigned to one of four groups. Group 1 receives the pretest, the experimental treatment, and the posttest. Group 2 is pretested, is *not* exposed to the experimental treatment, and is posttested (i.e., Group 2 acts as a traditional control group). Group 3 is *not* pretested, does receive the experimental treatment, and *is* posttested. Group 4 is *not* pretested, is *not* exposed to the experimental treatment, but *is* posttested. Because this design is an extension of the randomized pretest–posttest control-group design, comparison of Groups 1 and 2 is used to show the effect of the experimental treatment and has the same internal validity as the randomized pretest–posttest control-group design. In addition, by paralleling Groups 1 and 2 with Groups 3 and 4 (groups that are not pretested), the interaction of pretesting and the experimental treatment can be evaluated.

The statistical analysis of the results of the pretests and posttests of a Solomon design is complex and controversial because of the assymetry caused by removing the pretest for Groups 3 and 4. It is assumed that randomization should have resulted in essentially equivalent pretest scores (or *potential* pretest scores for the unpretested groups). Campbell and Stanley (1966, p. 25) suggest examining posttest scores only. Comparing the average scores on O_2 and O_5 to the average scores on O_4 and O_6 gives an index of the effectiveness of therapy. Comparing the average scores on O_2 and O_4 to the average scores on O_5 and O_6 gives an index of the influence of the pretest as a threat to internal validity. Comparing all four scores will indicate if there is an interaction between the pretest and the experimental treatment that threatens external validity. If the $O_2 - O_4$ difference is greater than the $O_5 - O_6$ difference, this would indicate that pretesting interacted with the experimental treatment, thereby precluding generalization to unpretested groups.

The Solomon design has been used in a number of investigations in educational psychology, but we have not yet seen its use in speech pathology and audiology. This is unfortunate because the Solomon design is one of the strongest therapy designs available, especially when combined with systematic replication. We hope that the Solomon design will find application in the speech pathology and audiology literature in the near future because it will pay off handsomely in improving therapy research.

Time-Series Designs.   A great deal of interest in the use of time-series designs has developed in recent years. Rather than using a single pretest and a single posttest with a large number of subjects, time-series designs employ repeated measurements of the dependent variable over an extended period of time with a single subject or a small number of subjects. The designs have found wide application in operant conditioning and behavior modification research. A number of examples of these designs can now be found in the speech pathology and audiology literature, especially in stuttering research.

Our interest here is in describing some of the basic principles in the design of time-series experiments for studying therapy effectiveness. Consideration of the role of time-series designs in behavioral analysis of communication disorders is beyond the scope of this book. Earlier general discussions of the application of behavioral principles in communication disorders are provided by Brookshire (1967), Sloane and MacAulay (1968), and Girardeau and Spradlin (1970). More recent accounts of behavior modification of communication disorders may be found in Lloyd (1976), Starkweather (1983), Ingham (1984), and McReynolds and Kearns (1983).

In describing the time-series design as a quasi-experiment, Campbell and Stanley (1966, p. 37) stated:

> The essence of the time-series design is the presence of a periodic measurement process on some group or individual and the introduction of an experimental change into this time series of measurements, the results of which are indicated by a discontinuity in the measurements recorded in the time series.

The simplest time-series design is the A-B design, which may be diagrammed as follows:

$$O_1 \quad O_2 \quad O_3 \quad O_4 \quad X \quad O_5 \quad O_6 \quad O_7 \quad O_8$$

$$\underbrace{}_{\text{A segment}} \quad \underbrace{}_{\text{B segment}}$$

In this design, repeated measurements of the dependent variable are made in the A segment (called a "baseline") before the experimental treatment is introduced. In the B segment (called the "experimental segment"), the experimental treatment is introduced and several more repeated measurements of the dependent variable are made. This is a within-subjects design because all subjects participate in two conditions—baseline and experimental segments. Comparison of a subject's performance in the baseline with his or her performance in the experimental segment indicates the effect of the experimental treatment on the dependent variable.

This design has many strengths. It also has a few weaknesses that may be overcome with some rather simple modifications. The strengths center on the fact that the repeated measurements of the dependent variable in the baseline provide relatively good control over the threats to internal validity posed by maturation, pretesting, regression, and instrumentation. In a sense, the subjects act as their own control group during the A (or baseline) segment of the design because the experimenter can examine their performances on the repeated measurements without an experimental intervention. If these baseline data are stable, maturation, pretesting, regression, and instrumentation should not threaten internal validity. Although this time-series design may appear, on the surface, to be similar to the one group pretest–posttest design, the repeated measurements in the baseline make it a substantially stronger design by reducing these threats to internal validity.

The A–B time-series design, however, does have a few weaknesses that merit attention. Even with a stable baseline, history may pose a threat because a historical event that does not occur during baseline but that does occur during the experimental segment may compete with the experimental treatment in affecting the dependent variable. Maturation could also pose a possible threat because maturation may not always start to affect performance at the outset of the A segment and progress in a linear fashion throughout the course of the experiment. Delayed maturation could, perhaps, begin toward the initiation of the B segment and mimic the effect of the experimental treatment on the independent variable.

Campbell and Stanley (1966) have suggested that the addition of a control group to a time-series design is one possible method for improving its internal validity. An A–B randomized control-group design may be diagrammed as follows:

$$
\begin{array}{c}
\text{R} \quad O_1 \quad O_2 \quad O_3 \quad O_4 \quad \text{X} \quad O_5 \quad O_6 \quad O_7 \quad O_8 \\
\text{R} \quad O_9 \quad O_{10} \quad O_{11} \quad O_{12} \qquad O_{13} \quad O_{14} \quad O_{15} \quad O_{16} \\
\underbrace{\hspace{4cm}}_{\text{A segments}} \qquad \underbrace{\hspace{4cm}}_{\text{B segments}}
\end{array}
$$

In this A–B randomized control-group design, subjects would be randomly assigned to two groups—experimental and control. This design would now be a mixed design because it has both within-subjects and between-subjects components. The experimental group would be observed several times in the baseline (A segment) and the experimental treatment would be applied in conjunction with more repeated measurements of the dependent variable in the B segment. The control group would be observed in baseline and also observed during a "pseudo-B segment" with no experimental treatment applied. In essence, it would be observed in two baseline segments. If the experimental group showed performance change in the B segment, but the control group did not, the possibility of history or delayed maturation affecting the behavior of one group and not the other would be greatly reduced.

The A–B design may also be strengthened by its extension to an A–B–A design that incorporates another baseline segment after the experimental treatment. The A–B–A design is often called a "reversal design" because of the reversal to baseline after completion of the experimental segment. An A–B–A design may be diagrammed as follows:

$$\underbrace{O_1 \quad O_2 \quad O_3 \quad O_4}_{\text{A segment}} \quad X \quad \underbrace{O_5 \quad O_6 \quad O_7 \quad O_8}_{\text{B segment}} \quad \text{(X Removed)} \quad \underbrace{O_9 \quad O_{10} \quad O_{11} \quad O_{12}}_{\text{A segment}}$$

In this design the A segment is followed by the B segment and then another baseline is introduced for observation of the subject's performance without the presence of the experimental treatment. This is a within-subjects design since no control group is used and all subjects participate in all conditions. A reversal design is often used to study a dependent variable that may be temporarily affected by the experimental treatment. If the treatment causes a temporary change in the dependent variable, removal of the treatment should cause performance to return to baseline level. Some dependent variables, on the other hand, are permanently affected by the experimental treatment and do not return to baseline levels in the second A segment. In therapy studies, it is desirable to produce a performance change that is maintained after the experimental treatment is removed so that improved behavior is continued beyond the therapy setting (Hersen & Barlow, 1976). Sometimes multiple-segment time-series designs are employed (e.g., A–B–A–B–A–B, . . . , A–B) to study long-term changes in behavior following experimental treatment. Performance on the dependent variable may return to baseline level in the first few reversals and then carry-over effects may be evident in improved performance during subsequent baseline segments. Such multiple-segment designs may be costly or time consuming, but are worthwhile efforts because short-term A–B–A studies may often obtain dramatic treatment effects with little or no carryover.

Baseline instability may threaten the internal validity of time-series designs. Instability could be the result of history, maturation, pretesting, regression, or instrumentation problems or of interactions among these factors. Also, the effects of these factors on the dependent variable may not be uniform with time and could, therefore, cause irregularities in the data that may be difficult to interpret. Of course, absolute stability of human behavior in a baseline segment can never be expected, so, the real difficulty centers on determining how much variability should be tolerated in the baseline segment. The question of deciding whether or not the baseline is sufficiently stable to allow the introduction of the experimental treatment may often be difficult to answer. As Christensen (1977, p. 228) has said:

> Of prime importance is the necessity of obtaining a stable baseline, because the baseline data serve as the standard against which change induced by the experimental treatment condition is assessed. The very essential question is, when has a stable baseline been achieved? This is a very difficult question to answer and is one that has no final answer.

Christensen (1977, p. 229) later suggested that one possible criterion for defining baseline stability would be to continue to monitor "baseline behavior until it is stable within a 5% range of the overall mean response." Many researchers may find this criterion too strict. Criteria used by different researchers for baseline stability are varied. Campbell and Stanley (1966) have described a number of possible baseline stability problems (see their Figure 3 and pp. 37–43) and their effects on the internal validity of time-series designs.

One particularly vexing problem in evaluating baselines occurs when the baseline performance systematically changes in the direction that would be expected during the experimental segment (e.g., stuttering decreases or fluency increases). In discussing baseline stability problems as one rationale for the use of statistical analysis of time-series data, Kazdin (1976, p. 270) has stated:

> . . . it is desirable in the A–B–A–B design to begin the intervention (B) phase only when a stable baseline rate of behavior has been achieved. If there is a trend in baseline, it should not be in the direction of the expected change, partially because this makes evaluation of subsequent phases difficult (and may indicate that the intervention is not needed). Yet it is not always feasible to achieve a stable baseline, as some investigators have lamented. . . . Further, sometimes a trend in baseline is in the direction of therapeutic change. Yet it may be desirable to accelerate the change.

Kazdin has outlined a variety of statistical procedures for analyzing the data of time-series designs, including statistical techniques that take into account changes or trends in baseline performance while evaluating the effect of treatment introduced in the experimental segment. Consumers who wish a more detailed discussion of baseline problems than can be presented here are urged to read Kazdin's chapter. It should be noted that he also summarizes many of the arguments against the use of statistical techniques for the analysis of time-series data. Despite the current popularity of time-series designs, the issue of baseline stability remains controversial as evidenced in the exchange of letters between Adams (1970) and Martin, Haroldson, and Starr (1971) concerning baseline stability in a stuttering experiment and in the arguments put forth by Starkweather (1971) against the use of baseline segments in stuttering research.

The external validity of time-series designs is sometimes cited as a problem by exponents of more traditional large sample designs because of the small number of subjects used and because of the complications that may arise if multiple treatments are applied to subjects. Because time-series designs involve an in-depth analysis of behavior that is quite time consuming, it is difficult to run them with large numbers of subjects. Critics of time-series designs believe that this may accentuate problems of the interaction of subject selection with the experimental treatment. Direct and systematic replications can often help to alleviate the external validity problem of subject selection. The problem of multiple-treatment interference is best alleviated by replications in which different treatments and treatment combinations are applied to individual subjects to assess their relative effectiveness.

The repeated testing done in time-series designs may be a reactive arrangement (Christensen, 1977) or may accentuate the interaction of pretesting with the experimental treatment, thereby limiting generalization to subjects who would normally undergo such repeated testing. This would not be a serious problem, however, if generalization were limited to subjects who were enrolled in relatively intensive or long-term treatment programs that would incorporate multiple testing as an integral part of therapy.

Time-series designs may be extended to include numerous combinations of experimental treatments and base line segments that may become quite complicated. Readers who are interested in a more detailed discussion of these designs than could be presented within the limitations of this book are referred to Hersen and Barlow (1976) and Cook and Campbell (1979) for reviews of various time-series designs and comparisons of the relative merits of time-series and traditional experimental designs.

Meta-Analysis of Therapy Research

In recent years, interest has developed in the possibilities for comparing therapy effectiveness across various studies that have been published. The technique of cumulating research findings across various studies is called "meta-analysis" (Hunter et al., 1982) and it has been applied to a number of different kinds of research, including studies of therapy effectiveness. In explaining the rationale for meta-analysis, Hunter et al. (1982, pp. 26–27) stated:

What is needed are methods that will integrate results from existing studies to reveal patterns of relatively invariant underlying relations and causalities, the establishment of which will constitute general principles and cumulative knowledge. . . . At one time in the history of psychology and the social sciences, the pressing need was for more empirical studies examining the problem in question. In many areas of research, the need today is not additional empirical data but some means of making sense of the vast amounts of data that have accumulated. Given the increasing number of areas within psychology and the other social sciences in which the number of available studies is quite large and the importance to theory development and practical problem solving of integrating conflicting findings to establish general knowledge, it is likely that methods for doing this will attain increasing importance in the future.

Hunter et al. (1982) have reviewed several different methods of meta-analysis, ranging from narrative review of studies to complex statistical comparison of the results of different studies that incorporate analyses of study characteristics, statistical corrections for factors such as test reliability, and weighting of the results of various studies according to their sample sizes. One important technique in meta-analysis of therapy studies is the evaluation of *effect size*, a method of standardizing across studies the measurement of the amount of pretherapy to posttherapy improvement. Effect size is often measured as the average pre–post difference in a dependent variable divided by the standard deviation of the pretherapy scores on the dependent variable. Calculating effect size in this way results in a reasonably comparable measure of improvement for all the studies that are compared. An effect size of zero indicates no improvement. An effect size of one indicates that the average of the posttest scores was one standard deviation higher than the average of the pretest scores. An effect size of two shows that the average posttest score increased two standard deviations above the average score on the dependent variable before therapy. In other words, the effect size allows the improvement results of all the studies to be expressed as a standard deviation relative to the pretherapy results.

Andrews, Guitar, and Howie (1980) recently published a meta-analysis of the studies concerned with the effects of stuttering therapy. They analyzed effect sizes for 116 dependent variables that had been examined in 42 studies of stuttering treatment that had included a total of 756 stutterers as subjects. The overall mean effect size for the 116 dependent variables was 1.3, indicating that stutterers had improved by 1.3 standard deviations relative to pretreatment measures on the average. Prolonged speech and gentle onset were the two therapy techniques that emerged with the best effect sizes from the meta-analysis.

There are a number of methodological problems in meta-analysis that must be dealt with. First, there is the manner in which the author selects the studies for inclusion in the meta-analysis. Consideration must be given to factors such as the author's attempts to judge the internal and external validity of the original studies, the sample sizes used in the studies, whether the studies were published in refered journals or in less selective media, and the types of dependent variables used to measure improvement. Second, there are complex statistical issues that must be dealt with in trying to weigh the equivalence of different studies. Consideration must also be given to different study characteristics such as sample size, method of measurement of dependent variables, kinds of statistics used to report results, type and length of treatments used in therapy, and selection criteria for including subjects in the studies. Hunter et al. (1982) have given extensive attention to a number of these and other problems in meta-analysis and provided an extensive bibliography of material relevant to meta-analysis. Andrews et al. (1980) have discussed some of these issues in relation to research on therapy effectiveness in speech pathology.

Ethics of Using Control Groups in Therapy Research

In concluding this discussion of research designs for studying the effectiveness of therapy, some comments are in order on the ethics of using control groups in therapy research. Some professionals have serious reservations about the ethics of withholding treatment from persons with speech or hearing problems, whereas other professionals believe that control groups should be used to confirm adequately the effectiveness of therapy.

A recent exchange of letters in the *Journal of Speech and Hearing Disorders* illustrates this controversy. Kushnirecky and Weber (1978, p. 106), in commenting on the validity of evidence in a study of therapeutic effectiveness, stated:

> . . . since *matched control subjects were not used, the data have limited interpretive value. It is possible that a control group may have shown that these children may have improved without intervention. Even if the children's rate of gain of language development equaled that of nonlanguage-delayed children, in the absence of controls, any conclusions concerning the effectiveness of the method are at best conjectures.*

Lee, Koenigsnecht, and Mulhern (1978, p. 107–108) replied that, in their opinion, the use of control groups

> . . . is impossible on ethical grounds. Kushnirecky and Weber should be strongly advised not to embark on research that withholds treatment from children who need it. . . . It would be unconscionable to withhold clinical training for any period of time from any child who needs it and would be likely to gain from it. This precludes designs in which one group of children receives treatment while treatment is withheld from a comparable group in order to show that the treatment produced results.

An editor's note appended to these two letters indicated that speech and hearing professionals do have an ethical obligation to provide treatment when possible but that they also have an ethical obligation to provide treatment that rests on "sound evidence" of its effectiveness. The editor's note also pointed out that control does not always mean withholding of treatment to a control group, as control can sometimes be accomplished with the use of multiple baselines (as in our discussion of time-series designs earlier in this chapter).

The major point illustrated by this exchange of letters is that a potential conflict of interest exists in our ethical obligations both to provide treatment and to demonstrate the effectiveness of treatment when the latter obligation may sometimes require the withholding of treatment to a control group. This is a difficult argument to settle, but there are compromises available for its possible resolution.

The use of time-series designs is one obvious approach and its potential for resolving this problem may be one of the reasons for the popularity of the time-series designs in recent years. Another possible solution lies in the use of waiting lists for construction of control groups. Many clinics have large case loads, therefore, staff clinicians often cannot accommodate all applicants immediately. Applicants for treatment could be randomly assigned to immediate treatment or to the waiting list and all applicants could be pre-tested at the time of application for therapy. At the end of the experiment, then, the control group on the waiting list could be used as the new experimental group in a direct or systematic replication of the study. This would be especially suitable when the experimental treatment can be accomplished in a relatively short time.

Despite these potential compromises, the issue of the ethics of withholding treatment from a control group remains controversial in a number of disciplines. Many professional and popular articles that have appeared in a number of journals and newspapers in recent years have presented a variety of opinions on these ethical issues. Cook and Campbell (1979) have discussed ethical concerns in withholding treatment from control groups and Hersen and Barlow (1976) have discussed ethical considerations in time-series designs. Readers who are interested in a more detailed discussion of these issues should consult the symposium on ethics and statistics in medical research that was published in the 18 November 1977 issue of *Science*. The whole topic of ethical responsibility in human research is controversial and widely written about; we expect that it will be some time before many of these issues are resolved to the satisfaction of the public and the professions alike.

Protection of Human Subjects in Research

A broader issue than the ethics of using control groups in therapy research also needs to be addressed: the protection of human subjects who participate in any research studies in speech pathology and audiology. In recent years, the scientific community and various governmental agencies have taken steps to safeguard the rights of human subjects participating in any kind of research. Past abuse of human research subjects is one reason for this concern, but even in the absence of actual abuse of human subjects, researchers and consumers of research need to be aware of the potential for physical or psychological harm to human subjects and of the need to protect the dignity and privacy of research participants.

The issue of protection of research subjects is complex, involving a balance of scientific concerns for the validity of results with humanitarian concerns for the rights of human subjects. Because of the importance of this issue, it is likely that considerable space will be devoted to protection of human subjects in future editions of textbooks on research design that are intended for producers of research. The consumer of research, for whom this book is intended, should also be aware of the problems involved in protecting human subjects' rights. We are fortunate to be able to take advantage of the work of two members of the American Sppech-Language-Hearing Association's Committee on Scientific Affairs, Dale Metz and John Folkins, who have prepared a paper on the protection of human subjects in speech and hearing research. They have kindly granted permission to reprint their original paper in its entirety in an appendix to this book. Therefore, rather than attempt to duplicate their efforts by trying to review these issues at length in this chapter section, we refer readers to Appendix A.

Summary

This chapter has provided an overview of research design considerations and suggested some possible techniques that may be used to reduce threats to internal and external validity of between-subjects, within-subjects, and mixed designs. Experiments designed to evaluate the effectiveness of therapy were reviewed and comments were made about their internal and external validity. Ethical considerations in therapy research were briefly discussed and the technique of meta-analysis of different therapy studies was briefly described.

Study Questions

1. Read the following article: Adams, M. R., & Hutchinson, J. (1974). The effects of three levels of auditory masking on selected vocal characteristics and the frequency of disfluency in adult stutterers. *Journal of Speech and Hearing Research, 17*, 682–688.
   (a) Did this study use a between-subjects or a within-subjects design?
   (b) What steps did the authors take to strengthen internal validity, given the type of design?
2. Read the following article: Lloyd, L. L., & Doherty, J. E. (1983). The influence of production mode on the recall of signs in normal adult subjects. *Journal of Speech and Hearing Research, 26*, 595–600.

(a) Did this study use a between-subjects or a within-subjects design?

(b) What steps did the authors take to strengthen internal validity, given the type of design?

3. Read the following article: Konkle, D. F., Beasley, D. S., & Bess, F. H. (1977). Intelligibility of time-altered speech in relation to chronological aging. *Journal of Speech and Hearing Research, 20,* 108–115.

   (a) Identify the manipulated and classification independent variables.

   (b) Which independent variables in this mixed design involved between-subjects and which involved within-subjects comparisons?

4. Read the following article: Kelly, J. F., & Whitehead, R. L. (1983). Integrated spoken and written English instruction for the hearing-impaired student. *Journal of Speech and Hearing Disorders, 48,* 415–422.

   (a) What factors could jeopardize the internal validity of this kind of therapy study?

   (b) What steps did the authors take to try to strengthen internal validity?

5. Read the following article: Peins, M., McGough, W. E., & Lee, B. S. (1972). Evaluation of a tape-recorded method of stuttering therapy: Improvement in a speaking task. *Journal of Speech and Hearing Research, 15,* 364–371.

   (a) Describe the design of this therapy experiment.

   (b) What features of this design would help to strengthen internal validity?

6. Read the following article: Reed, C. R. (1980). Voice therapy: A need for research. *Journal of Speech and Hearing Disorders, 45,* 157–169. What suggestions are made by Reed for studying the effectiveness of voice therapy?

7. Read the following article: Davey, B., LaSasso, C,, & Macready, G. (1983). Comparison of reading comprehension task performance for deaf and hearing readers. *Journal of Speech and Hearing Research, 26,* 622–628.
   Describe the between-subjects and within-subjects components of this mixed design and indicate which independent variables were manipulable and which were not.

8. Read the following article: Reich, A. & Till, J. (1983). Phonatory and manual reaction times of women with idiopathic spasmodic dysphonia. *Journal of Speech and Hearing Research, 26,* 10–18.

   (a) Describe the research design that was used.

   (b) What steps were taken to help improve internal validity?

9. Read the following article: Fein, D. J. (1984). Findings from the 1983 ASHA omnibus survey. *Asha, 26*(4), 45–48.

What technique did the author use to try to strengthen external validity?

10. Read the following article: Hanson, W. R., & Metter, E. J. (1980). DAF as instrumental treatment in progressive supranuclear palsy: A case report. *Journal of Speech and Hearing Disorders, 45,* 268–276. Describe how the baselines and experimental treatments were used to examine the three dependent variables in this time-series study.

11. Read the following letters to the editor: Adams, M. R. (1970). Some comments on "Time-out as punishment for stuttering." *Journal of Speech and Hearing Research, 13,* 218–220. Martin, R. R., Haroldson, S. K., & Starr, C. D. (1971). Time-out as punishment for stuttering: A reply to Martin Adams. *Journal of Speech and Hearing Research, 14,* 220–223.
    (a) Check the reference lists of these letters and find the original article discussed.
    (b) Examine the data in the original article and summarize the arguments for and against initiating the experimental segment after the completion of baseline measurements as outlined in the article and in both letters to the editor.

References

Adams, M. R. (1970). Some comments on "Time-out as punishment for stuttering." *Journal of Speech and Hearing Research, 13,* 218–220.

Andrews, G., Guitar, B., & Howie, P. (1980). Meta-analysis of the effects of stuttering treatment. *Journal of Speech and Hearing Disorders, 45,* 287–307.

Brookshire, R. H. (1967). Speech pathology and the experimental analysis of behavior. *Journal of Speech and Hearing Disorders, 32,* 215–227.

Campbell, D. T., & Stanley, J. C. (1966). *Experimental and quasi-experimental designs for research.* Chicago, IL: Rand McNally.

Christensen, L. B. (1977). *Experimental methodology.* Boston, MA: Allyn & Bacon.

Cook, T. D., & Campbell, D. T. (1979). *Quasi-experimentation.* Chicago, IL: Rand McNally.

Costello, J., & Bosler, S. (1976). Generalization and articulation instruction. *Journal of Speech and Hearing Disorders, 41,* 359–373.

Cottrell, A. W., Montague, J., Farb, J., & Throne, J. M. (1980). An operant procedure for improving vocabulary definition performances in developmentally delayed children. *Journal of Speech and Hearing Disorders, 45,* 90–102.

Courtright, J. A., & Courtright, I. C. (1979). Imitative modeling as a language intervention strategy: The effects of two mediating variables. *Journal of Speech and Hearing Research, 22,* 389–402.

Ferguson, G. A. (1976). *Statistical analysis in psychology and education* (4th ed.). New York: McGraw-Hill.

Girardeau, F. L., & Spradlin, J. E. (1970). *A functional analysis approach to speech and language.* (ASHA Monograph No. 14). Washington, DC: American Speech-Language-Hearing Association.

Guitar, B. (1976). Pretreatment factors associated with the outcome of stuttering therapy. *Journal of Speech and Hearing Research, 19,* 590–600.

Hersen, M., & Barlow, D. H. (1976). *Single case experimental designs: Strategies for studying behavior change.* New York: Pergamon.

Huck, S. W., Cormier, W. H., & Bounds, W. G. (1974). *Reading statistics and research.* New York: Harper & Row.

Hunter, J. E., Schmidt, F. L., & Jackson, G. B. (1982). *Meta-analysis: Cumulating research findings across studies.* Beverly Hills: CA: Sage Publications.

Ingham, R. J. (1984). *Stuttering and behavior therapy.* San Diego, CA: College Hill Press.

Kazdin, A. E. (1976). Statistical analyses for single-case experimental designs. In M. Hersen & D. H. Barlow (Eds.), *Single case experimental designs: Strategies for studying behavior change.* (pp. 265–316). New York: Pergamon.

Kerlinger, F. (1973). *Foundations of behavioral research* (2nd ed.). New York: Holt, Rinehart & Winston.

Kushnirecky, W., & Weber, J. L. (1978). Comment on Lee's reply to Simon. *Journal of Speech and Hearing Disorders, 43,* 106–107.

Lee, L. L., Koenigsnecht, R. A., & Mulhern, S. T. (1978). Reply to Kushnirecky and Weber. *Journal of Speech and Hearing Disorders, 43,* 107–108.

Lloyd, L. L. (Ed.). (1976). *Communication assessment and intervention strategies.* Baltimore, MD: University Park Press.

Martin, R. R., Haroldson, S. K., & Starr, C. D. (1971). Time-out as punishment for stuttering: A reply to Martin Adams. *Journal of Speech and Hearing Research, 14,* 220–222.

McReynolds, L. V., & Kearns, K. P. (1983), *Single-subject experimental designs in communicative disorders.* Baltimore, MD: University Park Press.

Monsen, R. B. (1978). Toward measuring how well hearing-impaired children speak. *Journal of Speech and Hearing Research, 21,* 197–219.

Sidman, M. (1960). *Tactics of scientific research.* New York: Basic Books.

Silverman, E. M. (1976). Listeners' impressions of speakers with lateral lisps. *Journal of Speech and Hearing Disorders, 41,* 547–552.

Sloane, H. N., & MacAuley, B. D. (Eds.). (1968). *Operant procedures in remedial speech and language training.* Boston, MA: Houghton Mifflin.

Smith, N. C. (1970). Replication studies: A neglected aspect of psychological research. *American Psychologist, 25,* 970–975.

Starkweather, C. W. (1983). *Speech and language: Principles and processes of behavior change.* Englewood Cliffs, NJ: Prentice-Hall.

Starkweather, C. W. (1983). *Speech and Language: Principles and processes of behavior change.* Englewood Cliffs, NJ: Prentice-Hall.

Stevens, S. S. (1968). Measurement, statistics, and the schemapiric view. *Science, 161,* 849–856.

Underwood, B. J., & Shaughnessy, J. J. (1975). *Experimentation in psychology.* New York: Wiley.

Van Dalen, D. B. (1966). *Understanding educational research.* New York: McGraw-Hill.

5
Organization
and Analysis
of Data

TERI A. DENSON

Introduction

The purpose of this chapter is to describe some basic terms, concepts, and procedures used in organizing and analyzing data derived from research in speech pathology and audiology. Our intention is to delve into the "whats" and "whys" of data manipulation so that the reader will have background for understanding what research results mean. This chapter will not be concerned with extensive details about formulae, calculations, or other "hows" of data manipulation. For a more detailed treatment of the methods of data analysis, the reader is referred to standard texts in statistical methods, two of which are included in the reference list at the end of this chapter. Also, the reader is reminded that Chapter 8 provides many examples of the way researchers in speech pathology and audiology organize and analyze their data for publication purposes.

Rationale for the Use of Data-Manipulation Techniques

Data organization and analysis techniques are statistical tools that assist the researcher in drawing conclusions and making inferences from a study. Experimental and descriptive studies both employ data organization or analysis procedures to aid in answering research questions by indicating how plausible certain conclusions are in light of the obtained data. Because many of the same statistical techniques may be used to analyze either experimental or descriptive data, the type of data organization or analysis employed does not indicate whether a study is experimental or descriptive.

The organization and analysis techniques for empirical research are commonly referred to as "statistics" because they are derived from a branch of mathematics by that name. However, the term "statistics" also refers to the numeric descriptors of a *sample*, as opposed to the companion term "parameter," which refers to the numeric descriptors of the *population* from which a sample is drawn. In this usage, then, the term "statistics" may be defined as computed estimates of parameters because it is only rarely that an entire population can be studied directly.

To illustrate, suppose that we wished to know the average number of articulation errors made by children at age five years. The average number of errors made by all five-year-old children (i.e., the population of interest) would be a parameter. We could never test all of the five-year-olds who speak English to get a direct measure of this population characteristic. So, we would select a sample of five-year-old speakers of English, say 200, and determine their average number of articulation errors. The average number of articulation errors made by this sample of five-year-olds would be a statistic and could be used in estimating the parameter. In other words, a statistic is a number describing a sample characteristic and a parameter is a number describing a population characteristic.

Levels of Measurement

The measurements made in a research study are conventionally presented in some numerical form in a research article. In order to discuss procedures for the organization and analysis of numerical research data, we must first define measurement and identify some important properties of the measurements that researchers make. Stevens (1946, p. 677) stated:

> . . . *measurement, in the broadest sense, is defined as the assignment of numerals to objects or events according to rules. The fact that numerals can be assigned under different rules leads to different kinds of scales and different kinds of measurement. The problem then becomes that of making explicit (a) the various rules for the assignment of numerals, (b) the mathematical properties (or group structure) of the resulting scales, and (c) the statistical operations applicable to measurements made with each type of scale.*

Stevens (1946) first described four scales (or levels) of measurement and later expanded on their applicability in psychophysical research (Stevens, 1951). Although there is some debate among statisticians (Haber, Runyon, & Badia, 1970) regarding the number, characteristics, and appropriateness of Stevens' scales, his original measurement scheme has remained influential in modern statistical treatment of data and will be used in this discussion.

Stevens' four levels of measurement are: *nominal, ordinal, interval,* and *ratio*. Table 5.1 shows defining characteristics and examples for each of the four levels of measurement. Knowing what level of measurement has been

TABLE 5.1 LEVELS OF MEASUREMENT

Scale	Defining Characteristics	Examples
Nominal	Mutually exclusive categories or named groupings	Pass/fail criterion on screening test Type of nonfluency (prolongation vs. repetition) Type of hearing loss (conductive, sensorineural, or mixed) Stimulus categories (meaningful vs. meaningless syllables) Subject characteristics (stutterer vs. nonstutterer) Phoneme production (correct vs. incorrect)
Ordinal	1. Mutually exclusive categories or named groupings 2. Ranks or ordered levels	Rated severity (mild, moderate, severe) Stimulus complexity (easy, moderate, difficult) Socioeconomic status (low-, middle-, upper class) Rank in class (e.g., first, second, third, etc.) Ranking of members of a group by rated degree of any subject attribute (e.g., perceived degree of vocal hoarseness)
Interval	1. Mutually exclusive categories or named groupings 2. Ranks or ordered levels 3. Equivalence of units throughout scale or constant distance between adjacent intervals	Personality-, achievement-, or intelligence scores Ratings obtained with many equal-appearing interval scales (e.g., semantic differential scales) Fahrenheit and Celsius temperatures
Ratio	1. Mutually exclusive categories or named groupings 2. Ranks or ordered levels 3. Equivalence of units throughout scale or constant distance between adjacent intervals 4. Equivalence of ratios among scale values can be determined 5. A true zero point exists on the scale	Vowel duration Voice onset time Sound frequency Sound intensity Acoustic impedance Subglottal air pressure

used to assign numerals to objects or events is an important step in ascertaining the appropriateness of the procedures used to organize and analyze the data.

If data are best organized by grouping them into equivalent but mutually exclusive *categories* or *named groupings* such as diagnostic descriptions, then those data are termed "*nominal*." If, in addition to being grouped by category, the categories (and the data that fall within them) can be arranged in *ranks* or *levels* such as "greatest" to "least" or "most severe" to "least severe," then those data are termed "*ordinal*." The next level contains those data that can, in addition to being categorized and ranked, be given a value on a *numerical scale* with equivalent interval size between units throughout the range of scale. These data are termed "*interval*." Finally, the fourth level of data is termed "*ratio*" because, in addition to the characteristics enumerated previously, these data are arranged on a scale with a true *zero point* and ratios can be computed between units. Physical measures commonly fall into this last category.

Thus, if the data from a study are categorized, they are probably at the *nominal* level; if they are presented as ranks or in some order, they are probably at the *ordinal* level. If the data are in numerical form such as test scores, they are probably either *interval* or *ratio* data.

Organization of Data

Characteristics of Data

Whenever measures on one or more variables are obtained in a research study, the obtained values form a *distribution*. The distribution may be one of categories (for nominal data), ranks (for ordinal data), or score values (for interval or ratio data). All distributions have two basic characteristics— central tendency and variability. Before proceeding with any analysis of research results, the researcher usually ascertains the characteristics of the distribution of data from the study and provides this information to readers so that they may examine the organized data to see the overall pattern of the results. There are two ways to provide such information: (1) through graphic or tabular presentation and (2) through calculation of summary statistics.

Tabular and Graphic Presentation

Many researchers represent the distribution of data in some graphic form for inspection before performing further analysis. Such a presentation has the advantage of showing the contours of a set of data by using frequencies or magnitude indicators without laboriously describing each value. Among the ways used to present information graphically are frequency tables, histograms, frequency polygons, and cumulative frequency distributions.

To illustrate some of these basic data-organization techniques, a set of

TABLE 5.2 HYPOTHETICAL EXAMPLE OF CONVERSION OF RAW SCORES INTO A FREQUENCY AND CUMULATIVE FREQUENCY TABLE USING GROUPED DATA

Raw Scores								Grouped Scores Score	Frequency f	Cumulative Frequency cum f
4 4 3	6	8	8	2	5			10	5	80
7 9 2	7	4	5	6	6			9	6	75
3 8 3	6	3	4	5	9			8	9	69
6 5 4	1	4	7	8	4			7	11	60
2 4 2	10	1	2	5	3			6	16	49
5 8 6	7	5	6	5	7			5	13	33
7 9 5	7	6	9	5	6			4	8	20
5 6 8	9	8	7	5	5			3	5	12
6 7 6	9	10	6	7	8			2	5	7
6 8 6	7	10	10	10	6			1	2	2
									$N = 80$	

hypothetical data is shown in Table 5.2. The data for 80 subjects are first presented in raw form, just as they might appear in the researcher's notes. The data are then *grouped* in a frequency table so that, for each score value, the number of cases obtaining that score is shown in the frequency (*f*) column. The cumulative frequency (cum *f*) column shows, for each score value, the number of cases that obtained scores *at* or *below* that value. Thus looking at the score of 6, we note that 16 subjects received scores of 6 and 49 subjects received scores at or below 6.

In some instances, when the researcher is working with a fairly small number of values and wishes to keep individual subject data on a number of variables together, the use of *ungrouped* data is feasible. This type of organization would simply show the score values listed in order rather than showing the *f* and cum *f* columns. In addition, the mechanics of calculating some of the indices to be shown later would be altered somewhat from the examples given in this chapter.

Figures 5.1(*a*) through 5.1(*d*) show how this hypothetical set of scores can be presented graphically. Figure 5.1(*a*) shows a histogram, or bar graph, of the scores. Note that the midpoint of each bar is directly above the score value on the horizontal axis of the graph. If we were to take these midpoints, record them on a graph, and connect these points with straight lines, the results would be the frequency polygon shown in Figure 5.1(*b*). Figure 5.1(*c*) shows a frequency curve of the same data. The major difference between the polygon and the curve is that the curve smooths out the distribution somewhat, as shown by the manner in which the curve passes between or close to

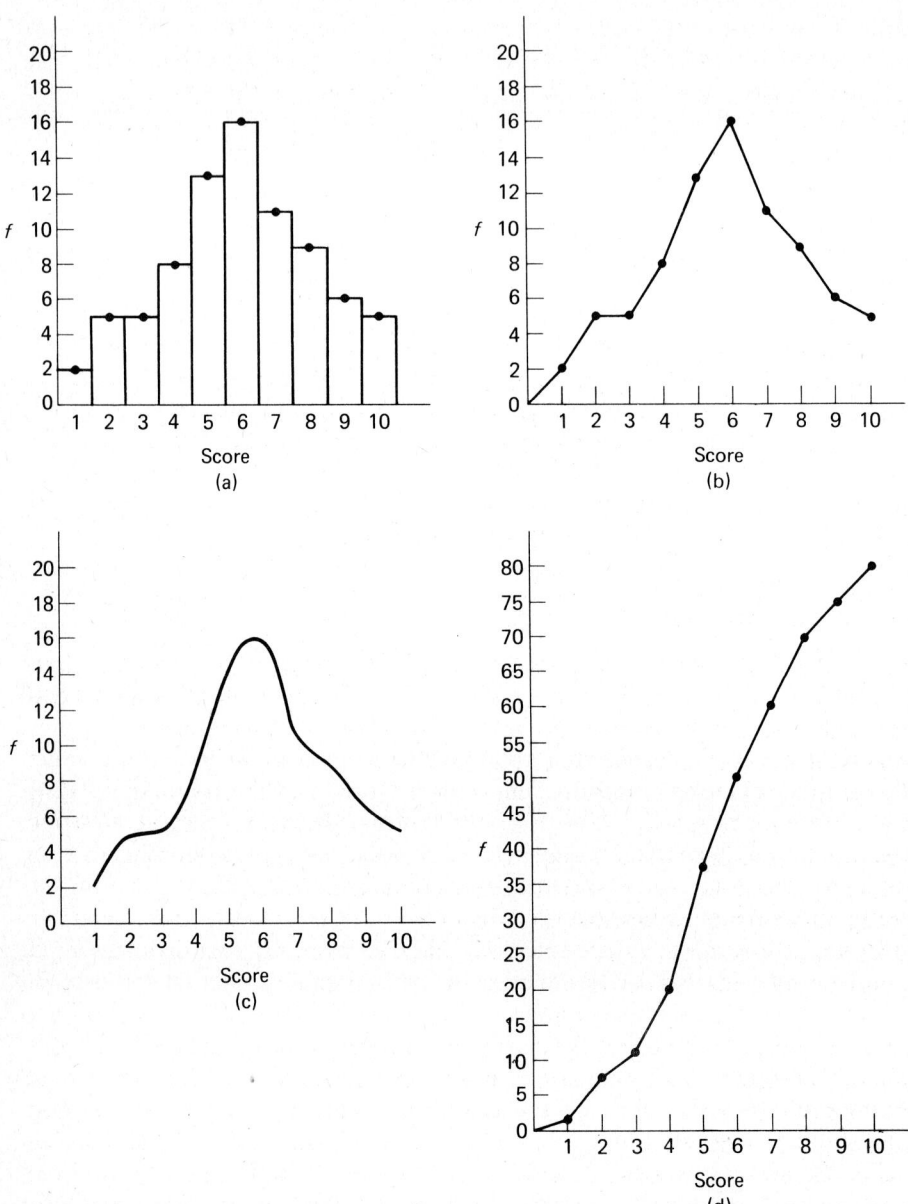

Figure 5.1   Graphic presentation of test scores: (*a*) Histogram of scores. (*b*) Frequency polygon of scores. (*c*) Frequency curve of scores. (*d*) Cumulative frequency polygon.

rather than right through the points corresponding to the observed frequencies. Finally, Figure 5.1(d) shows a cumulative frequency polygon. This is a graphic representation of the cumulative frequency (cum f) column rather than the frequency (f) column in Table 5.2. The reader will note that one distinctive characteristic of cumulative polygons (or curves) is that the curve or polygon is always either ascending or stable; it *never* descends. In contrast, the frequency curves or polygons in Figures 5.1(b) and 5.1(c) go up and down to show the frequency with which cases occur at each possible score point.

The selection of a tabular or graphic format depends partly on the researcher's style and partly on the requirements of the data. No matter which format is chosen, the material should: (1) accurately represent the data, (2) be clearly labeled to permit interpretation, and (3) relate to the textual narrative of the report. Although tabular or graphic presentation of research results is not appropriate or feasible in some cases, it can be used with great effectiveness and is a popular way of summarizing information and showing trends in data, especially when supplemented by other analyses.

Basic Summary Statistics

The second way to organize research data is to summarize them in numerical form. Because summary statistics are the foundation on which most data-analysis techniques rest, the selection of appropriate summary statistics is critical to the clear reporting of research findings. These statistics describe the characteristics of the data by answering the following questions: What is the average or typical value in the distribution? and How much variety or dispersion is there in the values represented by the distribution? Although graphs and tables can provide a pictorial presentation of answers to these questions, the summary statistics present more precise quantitative information that is amenable to further data analysis. Summary statistics include measures of central tendency and measures of variability.

Measures of Central Tendency.   There are three common measures of central tendency—the mode, the median, and the mean. The *mode* is the most frequently occurring score in a distribution. The *median*, or middlemost score, can be determined as long as the data can be ranked. The median describes the point in the distribution that separates the upper half of the data from the lower half. It is determined by counting how many scores there are and finding out which score is in the middle of the distribution. If the median is 40, then you know that one-half the scores in the distribution are below 40 and one-half are above 40. The last index of central tendency is the *mean*, or arithmetic average, of the values in a set of data. It is found by adding up all the values and dividing by the number of values there are in a set of data. Table 5.3 illustrates the calculation of these three measures of

TABLE 5.3 DETERMINING MEASURES OF CENTRAL TENDENCY

Scores X	f	cum f	fX	
10	5	80	50	
9	6	75	54	
8	9	69	72	
7	11	60	77	
6	16	49	96	
5	13	33	65	
4	8	20	32	
3	5	12	15	
2	5	7	10	
1	2	2	2	
			$\Sigma fX = 473$	

$$Mean = \bar{X} = \frac{\Sigma f(X)}{N} = \frac{473}{80} = 5.91$$

$Mode$ = the most frequently occurring score = 6.0.

$Median$ = the score separating the upper half of the cases ($\frac{1}{2}$ N) from the lower half of the cases.

In this instance, it is the point separating the upper 40 cases from the lower 40 cases.

Inspection of the cum f column shows that this point is somewhere between a score of 5 and a score of 6.

The exact value, by interpolation, is 5.43.

central tendency for the hypothetical set of grouped data presented in Table 5.2.

Readers will note that Table 5.3 and other tables in this chapter contain statistical formulae and notation. These are presented for illustrative purposes for those readers who wish to examine the calculation of these statistics, and they were derived from two basic statistics texts (Guilford, 1965; Siegel, 1956). There are numerous alternative formulae and notation conventions for most statistical calculations; readers should not feel that one type of notation or one formula is inherently superior to other techniques for obtaining the same information.

Measures of Variability. The other major category of summary statistics includes those that indicate the amount of dispersion, spread, or variability in a set of data. Known as indices of variability, the major statistics in this category include: the *range*, the *variance* (σ^2), the *standard deviation* (SD or σ), and the *semi-interquartile range* (Q).

The *range* is simply the spread from the lowest value to the highest value in a distribution of data. It can be expressed in several ways, including: "scores ranged from _____ to _____" "the range was _____ points." The smaller the range, the less variability there is in a distribution; conversely, the larger the range, the more variability there is in a distribution.

The *variance* is determined by finding the mean of the values in a distribution and determining how far each value in the distribution deviates from the mean. Then these deviation scores are each squared to deal with the fact that half of the deviation is negative (i.e., below the mean) and half is positive (i.e., above the mean). If these deviation scores were not squared, their sum would always be zero and, therefore, useless. Then the squared deviation scores are summed and averaged to compute the variance. The variance cannot be presented in the original units of measurement because of the squaring, so it is not usually used as an absolute index of how the data spread out from the mean. But the variance does have two particularly important uses in data organization and analysis.

First, the variance is a most important number that represents variability and is used in the calculation of some statistics that will be described later in this chapter. These statistics include the correlation coefficient for analyzing relationships among variables and the analysis of variance for analyzing differences between groups of subjects. Second, the square root of the variance is a useful measure of the average amount by which all of the scores deviate from the mean of a distribution, and it is presented in the original units of measurement. This average amount of dispersion of the scores in a distribution is called the *standard deviation* (SD) and it is a most important statistic for organizing the data of a study. A small SD indicates that the scores in the distribution did not spread out from the mean very much, that is the group was relatively homogeneous. A large SD, on the other hand, indicates a wide dispersion of scores from the mean of the distribution, that is the group was more heterogeneous.

The interpretation of the SD depends on what statisticians call the normal curve model and assumes that the values in the distribution are symmetrically arranged on either side of the mean. The normal curve model and its uses will be discussed later. The last measure of variability, the *semi-interquartile range,* is used if the values in a distribution are *not* symmetrically arranged around the central tendency and it indicates one-half the range of the middle 50% of the scores in the distribution. Table 5.4 illustrates calculation of some measures of variability for the set of grouped data presented in Tables 5.2 and 5.3.

Use of Measures of Central Tendency and Variability.   By comparing the indices that an author presents for central tendency, the reader can ascertain the overall pattern of a given distribution of data. For instance, if the data are balanced or symmetrical in the way that they are distributed around the measures of central tendency, the values for the central tendency indices should be quite similar. However, if the mean and median are very different in value, then the distribution is *skewed.* A skewed distribution is one in which scores cluster around either a very high value (negative skew) or a very low value (positive skew). Examples of various distribution shapes and their measures of central tendency are shown in Figure 5.2. (*a–c*).

If data are severely skewed, then the reader should immediately know that this affects the applicability of various subsequent procedures for data analy-

TABLE 5.4 DETERMINING MEASURES OF VARIABILITY

X	f	cum f	fX	$X - \bar{X}$	$(X - \bar{X})^2$	$f(X - \bar{X})^2$
10	5	80	50	+4	16	80
9	6	75	54	+3	9	54
8	9	69	72	+2	4	36
7	11	60	77	+1	1	11
6	16	49	96	0	0	0
5	13	33	65	−1	1	13
4	8	20	32	−2	4	32
3	5	12	15	−3	9	45
2	5	7	10	−4	16	80
1	2	2	2	−5	25	50
			$\Sigma fX = 473$			$\Sigma f(X - \bar{X})^2 = 401$

$\bar{X}$ (from Table 5.3) = 5.91   median = 5.43   mode = 6.0

Statement of range = "the scores ranged from 1 to 10."

Standard deviation = SD = $\sigma = \sqrt{\dfrac{\Sigma f(X - \bar{X})^2}{N}} = \sqrt{\dfrac{401}{80}}$

$$= \sqrt{5.01} = 2.23$$

Semi-interquartile range = Q = $\dfrac{\text{P75} - \text{P25}}{2}$.

P75 = (calculation not shown) is the point separating the upper 25% of the cases from the lower 75% of the cases. For these data, P75 is 7.0.

P25 = (calculation not shown) is the point separating the upper 75% of the cases from the lower 25% of the cases. For these data, P25 is 4.0.

Q = one-half the range of the middle 50% of scores

$$\frac{7.0 - 4.0}{2} = \frac{3.0}{2} = 1.5.$$

[a]For convenience sake, the mean has been rounded to 6.0 for calculation of the deviation scores $(X - \bar{X})$.

sis. Moreover, depending on the scale from which the data are derived, the skewness may be due to a ceiling or basement effect caused by an unwise or incorrect choice of methods to produce the information derived from a research study. In addition to detecting skewness in a distribution, examination of central tendency can indicate the comparability of data generated by different studies.

Distributions having large standard deviations and Q values are said to be platykurtic because the pictorial representation of the distribution would be a flattened curve. On the other hand, distributions with small standard deviations and Q values are called leptokurtic because the graphic presentation

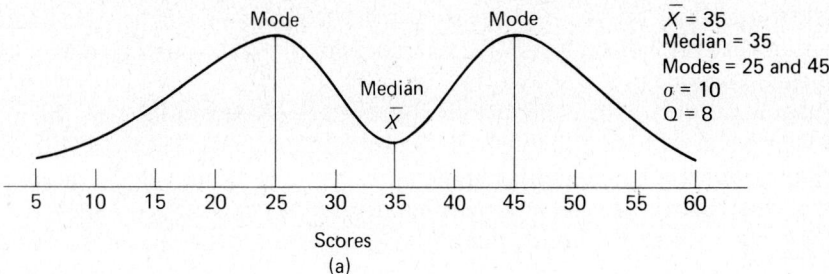

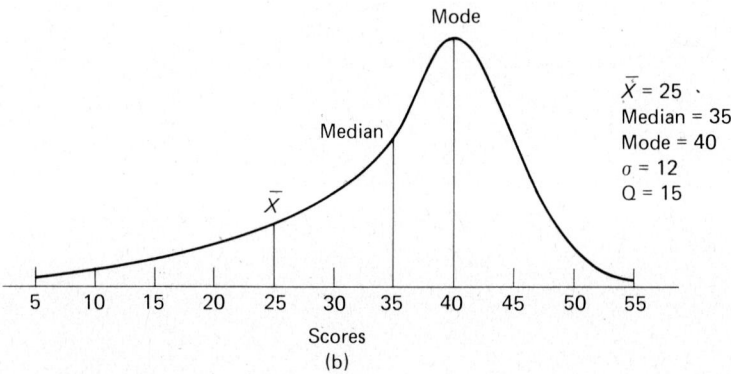

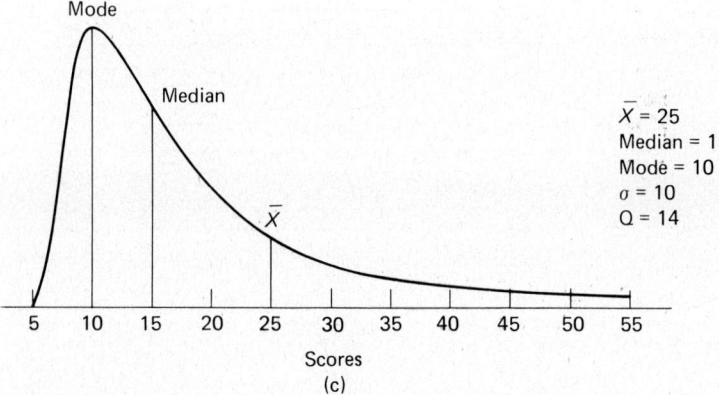

Figure 5.2   Various shapes of distributions: (*a*) A bimodal distribution. (*b*) A negatively skewed distribution (mean significantly lower than median). (*c*) A postively skewed distribution (mean significantly higher than median).

yields a peaked curve. A normal distribution is mesokurtic because it is neither very flat nor very peaked. Examples of distributions showing various types of variability are shown in Figure 5.3 ($a-c$).

In general, if the SD is about one-fourth to one-sixth as large as the range, the sample is typical of that usually found in most statistical work. Likewise, if the SD is about one-and-one-half times as large as the semi-interquartile range, the distribution is not significantly skewed (Guilford, 1965).

In a good research report, the author provides all the summary statistics

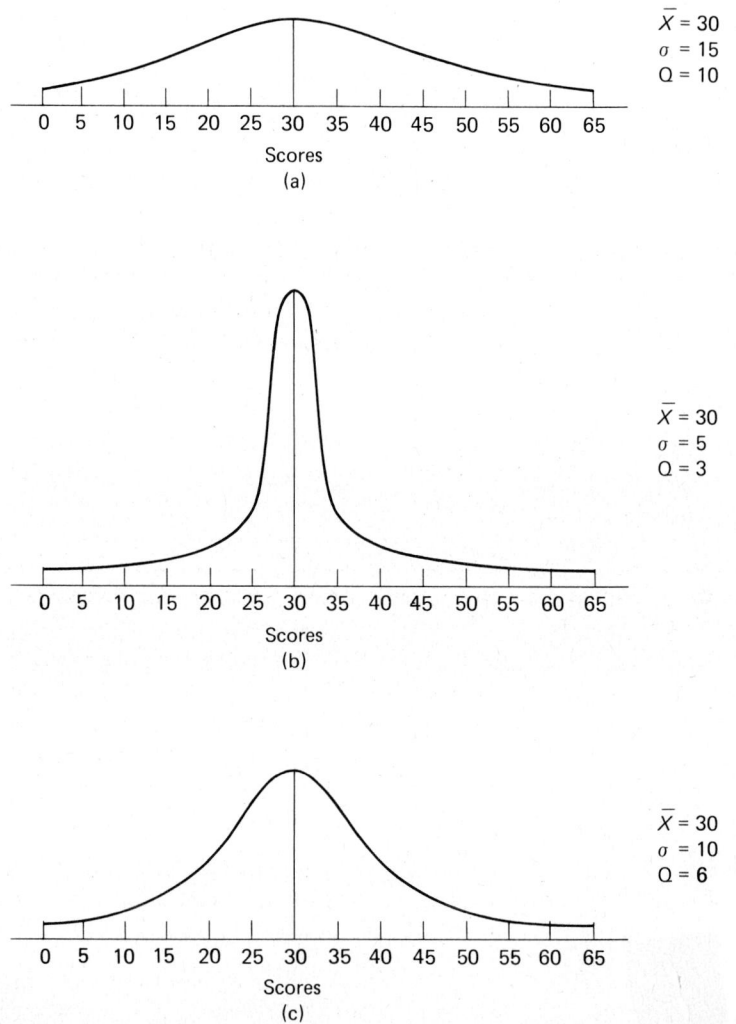

Figure 5.3 Distributions showing various types of variability: (*a*) A platykurtic distribution. (*b*) A leptokurtic distribution. (*c*) A mesokurtic distribution.

appropriate for the data from the study. Often, the mean and SD will be used to describe the central tendency and the variability for a set of data. If the distribution is skewed, then the median and the semi-interquartile range are often reported. Ideally, both the mean and median should be reported as indices of central tendency so that the reader can see the extent to which a set of data is skewed or symmetrical. Likewise, both the SD and the semi-interquartile range should appear. These four indices tell a great deal about the data. Careful examination of these summary statistics can indicate which statistical procedures should be used to analyze the data.

In many research designs, organization of data and presentation of summary statistics are sufficient for answering the questions posed by the study. It is important to realize that the absence of statistical analysis in the form of significance tests or other procedures does not indicate an unsophisticated or unimportant contribution. The converse is also true. The researcher should select and present only those procedures and indices that are sufficient for his or her purposes and that are the most justifiable and parsimonious for the data. Moreover, in some studies, application of certain planned procedures is abandoned after an initial examination of the data in graphic and summary statistic form. This should not be interpreted as an indication of laziness on the part of the researcher but rather as a possible indication that the author realized that further analysis could not change what the data themselves indicated and could, in fact, mislead the reader.

In many cases, however, the presentation of graphs or score distributions and summary statistics is a prelude to further data analysis. Such analysis may have been planned in advance (*a priori*) or may have been selected after examining the data (*a posteriori*). Most studies use *a priori* methods because these procedures enable the researcher to have some specified level of confidence in the conclusions regarding research questions or hypotheses that were posed in the first place. *A posteriori* methods are applied cautiously by most researchers because they may draw attention away from the major research questions and because of certain technical difficulties encountered in their use. For our purposes, we will assume that most analyses have been planned in advance to answer the questions or test the hypotheses posed in a study.

Analysis of Data

Basic Concepts of Data Analysis

Appropriate Methods.   As indicated previously, selection and application of data-analysis techniques beyond summary statistics is determined partly by the research questions of a study and partly by the level of the data yielded by the research. Basically, analysis techniques may be either *correlational* or *inferential*, depending on whether they are used to describe existing relationships or differences among data. In addition, the choice of the exact analysis procedure also depends on the number of variables being examined, the size and characteristics of the samples used, and the type of research plan in effect. Techniques of data analysis seem to be amenable to classification and description by "families" based on their derivation and their methodological assumptions. Because this is not a statistics text, each member of the procedural "families" will not be discussed at length. Instead, a summary of which procedures fit into the various situations described appears in Table 5.19 (at the end of the chapter).

For our purposes, it is sufficient to indicate that the various families of data-analysis techniques are more or less powerful (able to detect trends or differences in data), more or less well known, and more or less respected. However, each has unique characteristics that set it apart from the others and make it particularly useful in the right circumstances. Later sections of this chapter will describe each of these techniques and give some examples of how they may be used in speech pathology and audiology research.

The Normal Curve Model.   We have previously referred to statistical procedures based on assumptions of the normal curve model, and it is appropriate to summarize the basic concepts of the model before proceeding.

The normal curve model is a construct based on the observation that measures of physical or psychological variables derived from large numbers of people (or animals) tend to form a characteristic type of distribution when graphed. This distribution is the familiar symmetrical, bell-shaped curve that shows a concentration of values in the middle of the distribution with fewer and fewer values as the extremes are approached (Figure 5.4). The generalizability of this curve and its mathematical properties were first described by Gauss and it is sometimes known as a Gaussian curve. Because it is the kind of distribution that data typically resemble, it also became known as a "normal" curve.

Inspection of Figure 5.4 reveals the symmetry of a normal distribution. It can be seen that most cases fall in the middle of the distribution, with fewer cases seen at the lower and higher score values at the extreme right- and left-hand sides of the distribution. About two thirds of the cases fall within plus-or-minus 1 SD of the mean; 95% of the cases fall within plus-or-minus 2 SDs of the mean; and 99% of the cases fall within plus-or-minus 3 SDs of the mean. Although a perfect Gaussian or normal distribution is never attained in practice, there is enough resemblance between it and the actual obtained-data distributions to warrant its adoption as a mathematical model for statistical procedures that are used to analyze relationships and differences. The extent to which actual data resemble the model determines the usefulness of the model and statistical procedures derived from it. If data do not approximate a normal distribution in the way they occur in a sample or population, then the normal curve model and the statistical procedures based on it are simply not applicable. Therein lies the necessity to ascertain whether the assumptions of the model and methods based on it fit the particular set of

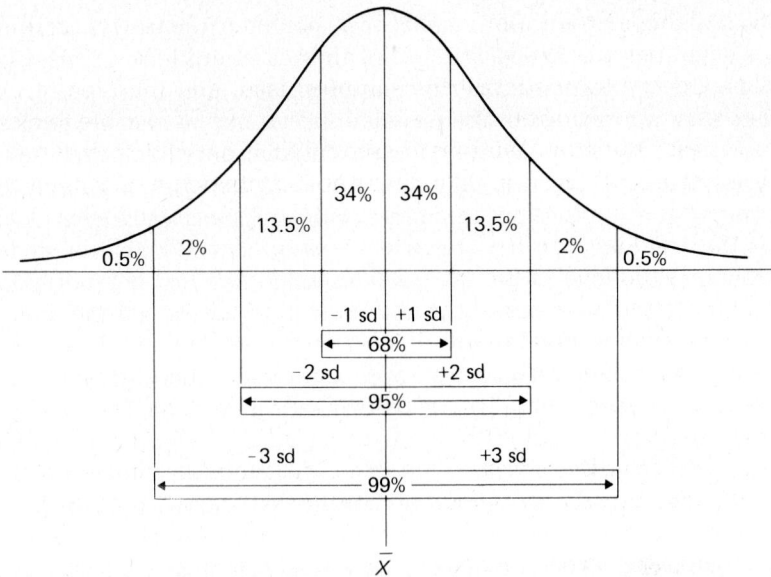

Figure 5.4 Normal distribution with percentages of cases falling within SD bands.

data to be analyzed. These considerations lead us to a discussion of statistics based on a normal curve model (*parametric statistics*) vs. statistics that are not based on a normal curve model (*nonparametric statistics*).

Parametric and Nonparametric Statistical Procedures. Parametric statistics are based on certain assumptions about the population from which the sample data were obtained. Because population quantities are often called parameters and sample quantities are often called statistics in statistical work, the term "parametric statistics" has been applied to data-analysis procedures that rest on certain assumptions about the population.

There are several assumptions about the population, and the sample drawn from it, that underlie the use of parametric statistics:

1. The population parameter should be normally distributed.
2. The level of measurement of the parameter in question should be interval or ratio.
3. When there are two or more distributions of data to be analyzed (e.g., two groups of subjects are tested or one group of subjects is tested under two different conditions) the *variances* of the data in the two different distributions should be about the same.
4. The sample should be fairly large. There is no agreed-on, absolute definition of "large," but most statisticians consider 20 or 30 subjects to be large enough.

When all of these assumptions can be met, parametric statistics are appropriate for data analysis. If one or more of these assumptions is seriously violated, parametric statistics may be inappropriate.

When assumptions about the populations cannot be met, researchers use nonparametric statistics. Nonparametric statistics are often called "distribution-free" statititics because they do not rest on assumptions about the distribution of the population parameter. Nonparametric statistics deal with data at the nominal or ordinal level of measurement. When a researcher has interval- or ratio-level data, but realizes that they are not normally distributed (or fail to meet one of the other assumptions listed), the data can be *transformed* from interval or ratio level to nominal or ordinal level in order to be used in a nonparametric test. For example, internal-level scores could be classified as "pass" or "fail" by using a cutoff score on the interval scale. Another alternative would be to rank-order all the subjects on the basis of their interval-scale scores and then use their ranks as the data for a nonparametric statistical analysis. Of course, if the original data were already nominal or ordinal, then a nonparametric statistical procedure would have to be used instead of a parametric procedure.

Although it may appear that the use of nonparametric alternatives to parametric statistical analysis is always the "safest' way to analyze data, this is not really true. Parametic statistics are more powerful (i.e., more sensitive to differences and relationships) than nonparametric tests; therefore, they are preferred when the assumptions listed can be met. Throughout the rest of this chapter, we generally will describe a parametric procedure for each particular kind of analysis and then consider nonparametric alternatives to each parametric statistic.

Testing a Null Hypothesis.   Statistical analysis is concerned with making decisions about the existence vs. the nonexistence of differences between groups or relationships among variables. This is usually done by examining the plausibility of a *null hypothesis* in light of obtained data. A null hypothesis is a hypothesis that states that there is no difference between groups or no relationship among variables. A simple null hypothesis may state, for example, that there is no difference between the means of two groups of subjects (e.g., stutterers vs. nonstutterers) on some dependent variable. The mean of the sample of strutterers would be compared to the mean of the sample of nonstutterers to decide how plausible that null hypothesis is. If the means of the two groups are about the same, then, it is plausible that the null hypothesis is true and the researcher could accept it. If, however, the means of the two groups are quite different, it does not seem plausible that the null hypothesis is true, and the researcher could reject it. The concept of testing a null hypothesis is the basis for *statistical inference* and underlies all of the methods for testing differences to be discussed subsequently in this chapter. Inferential hypothesis testing can also be applied in analyzing relationships, as will be seen later.

Status of Null Hypothesis

Researcher's Decision	Null Hypothesis Is True	Null Hypothesis Is False
Accept Null Hypothesis	Correct Decision	Type II Error
Reject Null Hypothesis	Type I Error	Correct Decision

Figure 5.5 Contingencies involved in making a decision about a null hypothesis.

Type I and Type II Errors. When a researcher makes a decision about a null hypothesis, one of four things can happen: the hypothesis can be true or false and the researcher can accept or reject it. Figure 5.5 illustrates the contingencies of this situation.

Inspection of Figure 5.5 reveals that there are two possible correct decisions that a researcher can make: accepting a true null hypothesis and rejecting a false null hypothesis. There are two possible incorrect decisions: rejecting a true null hypothesis (called a *Type I* error) and accepting a false null hypothesis (called a *Type II* error).

If a researcher concludes on the basis of the sample data that two groups are different, the decision will either be correct (if the groups are different) or a Type I error (if the groups are not different). If a researcher concludes on the basis of the sample data that the two groups are not different, the decision will either be correct (if the two groups are not different) or a Type II error (if the two groups are different). Statistical analysis helps the researcher to make the decision about a null hypothesis by indicating the probability that a decision to reject a null hypothesis is a Type I error. Statistical analysis can also help a researcher to make a decision to accept a null hypothesis by indicating the probability of making a Type II error. Unfortunately, the probability of making a Type II error is not as easily determined as the probability of making a Type I error. Consumers of research are more likely to find analyses of the probability of making a Type I error in articles that report group differences and are less likely to find analyses of the probability of committing a Type II error in articles reporting no differences between groups or conditions.

The Level of Significance. The probability of making a Type I error is called the *level of significance*. When a researcher decides to reject a null hypothesis and conclude that there is a difference between two sets of data, he or she does so because the statistical test comparing the two sets of data indicates that the probability of making a Type I error in rejecting the null hypothesis is quite small. This probability is expressed by stating the level of significance (sometimes called "alpha") associated with the comparison.

Stating the level of significance indicates the degree of confidence that the researcher has that the difference seen in the sample data would not have occurred by chance alone. In fact, the level of significance is sometimes called the "level of confidence" for the comparison. The comparison of two data sets may be a between-subjects comparison, for example, the comparison of the means on some dependent variable for stutterers vs. nonstutterers. The comparison of the two data sets may be a within-subjects comparison, for example, the comparison of the means on some dependent variable of stutterers tested under two different experimental conditions.

If the statistical analysis shows that it is highly improbable that an obtained sample difference would have occurred if the null hypothesis were true, then the researcher will reject the null hypothesis because the probability of committing a Type I error is small. If, however, the statistical analysis shows that it is not improbable that an obtained sample difference would have occurred if the null hypothesis were true, the researcher will not reject the null hypothesis because the probability of committing a Type I error is not small enough. How small must the probability of committing a type error be for a researcher to reject the null hypothesis? In other words, what must the level of significance be for a comparison of sample groups of data for a researcher to conclude that the groups of data are different?

Although there is no absolute answer to the question of what level of significance should be adopted, there are conventional preferences that have evolved. The most frequently used levels of significance are 0.05 and 0.01. These figures mean that the probability of committing a Type I error is 0.05 (5 chances in 100) or 0.01 (1 chance in 100). In other words, if the level of significance yielded by a statistical analysis indicates that the difference between the data sets could have resulted by chance (if null hypothesis were true) only 5 times out of 100, then, the null hypothesis will be rejected and the difference will be called "significant at the 0.05 level." Sometimes the level of significance is indicated by using the letter p (for probability) and then stating the value of the probability of committing the Type I error. For example, a researcher might state: "The difference between the two groups was significant ($p = .05$)." Selection of the 0.05 vs. the 0.01 level of significance by an investigator is arbitrary. Because the 0.01 level of significance indicates less chance of a Type I error than the 0.05 level, it is stricter or more conservative than the 0.05 level of significance. In other words, other things being equal, a larger difference between two sets of sample data must be found to reach the 0.01 level of significance than to reach the 0.05 level of significance.

The selection of a level of significance is a complicated process, a discussion of which is beyond the scope of this chapter. In general, however, if the study is in a previously unexplored domain or is one in which the researcher is trying to identify possibilities for further study at a later time, then, a more lenient level of significance may be reasonable. If, on the other hand, the researcher is examining well-developed hypotheses or replicating a study, a stricter level of significance may be desired.

Two final remarks about significance levels are in order. First, many consumers of research interpret the term "significant" to mean a result that has clinical relevance or theoretical meaning. This is not necessarily true. A very small difference between groups that has little or no clinical relevance or theoretical meaning may be statistically significant, in the sense that it is highly improbable to occur if the null hypothesis were true. Perhaps in that sense the term "significant" is inappropriate and the term "level of confidence" is a better one because it simply indicates the confidence that the researcher has that the result did not simply occur by chance. Whether or not a statistically significant difference between two groups of data also has theoretical or clinical significance is a rational matter that is more often treated by an author in a discussion section of an article than in the results section. Second, it should be pointed out that there are many researchers who prefer not to analyze results with statistical significance testing procedures. Proponents of this point of view prefer to rely on replication studies and stronger rational examination of the meaning of their research results. Carver (1978) recently presented this point of view in a lengthly criticism of statistical-significance testing. Consumers of research should realize, then, that not all research articles will include statistical-significance tests and that the absence of such tests does not necessarily mean that the results are not clinically or theoretically significant or that the researcher has been faulty in the data analysis. It may simply mean that the particular researcher is in Carver's camp in opposition to statistical-significance testing.

One- and Two-tailed Tests.   Another important consideration in evaluating the results of data analysis is whether the researcher has chosen a one-tailed (directional) test or a two-tailed (nondirectional) test. This decision is made in relation to the questions or hypotheses posed in the study. If the researcher has made a directional hypothesis, he or she applies one-tailed tests. Examples of statements calling for one-tailed tests include: "Scores of group X will be higher than scores of group Y," "Scores will be significantly below average," and "There will be more persons in the X category than in the Y category." If the researcher is considering questions or hypotheses that are nondirectional, she or he applies two-tailed tests. Examples of statements calling for two-tailed tests include: "There will be a difference in scores betweeen group X and group Y," "Scores will be significantly different from the average," and "There will be different number of persons in the X category than there is in the Y category."

Consumers of research should be aware that two-tailed tests are more strict or conservative than one-tailed tests. That is to say, a greater difference between groups must be found to call the difference significant when using a two-tailed test. A somewhat smaller difference may not be significant with a two-tailed test, but may be significant when analyzed with a one-tailed test. Typically, one-tailed tests are used when the researcher has some reason to suspect in advance that the difference between groups or conditions should be in one direction. There is some controversy about when it is appropriate to select the more liberal one-tailed test, and more conservative statisticians and researchers generally recommend the more stringent two-tailed tests. For example, Cohen (1969) strongly advises researchers to avoid one-tailed tests. Consumers should expect to find both one-tailed and two-tailed tests in the literature, however, and they should realize that significant differences found with two-tailed tests are, in a sense, more significant than those found with one-tailed tests.

Degrees of Freedom.   The importance of sample size in the selection and application of a particular analysis procedure is highlighted by the concept of degrees of freedom. To interpret the results of a given statistical procedure, the researcher must know the degrees of freedom (*df*) in the data before tables of statistical significance can be used. In a most basic sense, *df* indicate the number of values in a set of data that are free to vary once certain characteristics of the data are known. Generally, if the mean or the sum of a set of scores is known, then the *df* are equal to the number of scores in each distribution minus 1 ($df = n - 1$).

The formula for determining the number of the *df* varies according to the procedure employed for analysis and the number of the *df* should always be reported when analyses are described and interpreted. In a table or in the text of the results section of an article, the *df* are usually listed as an accompaniment to the outcome of the particular data-analysis procedure that was used. A discussion of the techniques for calculating *df* for all the various analysis procedures is beyond the scope of this text. Consumers of research, however, should be aware of the fact that each analysis procedure must take into account the correct number of *df* in determining statistical significance. Authors usually show *df* in the results section to demonstrate to the editors and to readers more familiar with statistical analysis that the *df* were correctly accounted for in the analysis.

The following sections will examine how some of the commonly used parametric and nonparametric analysis procedures are utilized in speech pathology and audiology studies. Procedures are grouped under two major headings: (1) methods for analyzing relationships and (2) methods for describing differences. The reader will find it useful to refer frequently to Table 5.19 while reading these sections because this table summarizes these analysis procedures regarding: (1) the level of measurement for which each is appropriate, (2) whether the procedure analyzes differences or relationships, and (3) whether the procedure is parametric or nonparametric. Although this table is not a complete list of all statistical methods employed in speech pathology and audiology research, it does give an organized overview of those common procedures considered in this chapter.

Methods for Analyzing Relationships

Often the researcher wishes to determine the strength and direction of relationships that exist in a set of data or simply whether some overall

TABLE 5.5 SCORE PAIRS FOR THREE SETS OF 10 SUBJECTS

	Illustration A			Illustration B			Illustration C	
Subjects' Initials	Score on First Variable	Score on Second Variable	Subjects' Initials	Score on First Variable	Score on Second Variable	Subjects' Initials	Score on First Variable	Score on Second Variable
RB	4	16	CJ	21	8	DS	21	2
CS	6	14	DD	53	5	BC	83	1
JD	8	17	NS	14	9	WD	45	7
WM	3	13	IV	67	6	MC	17	4
SV	2	11	TY	82	4	HC	62	8
BP	7	18	BH	98	1	DR	91	3
BD	1	12	GS	34	10	AT	37	9
TM	5	15	JF	47	7	JN	99	6
FD	10	19	RF	94	2	RP	72	5
MC	9	20	TD	76	3	JF	56	10

association does occur among variables in a given sample or population. To do this, two or more sets of scores or ranks or classifications are derived from a particular sample and subjected to analysis.

The relationship between two variables can be described graphically using a scattergram or scatterplot. Each subject has a pair of scores or ranks on the variables, and these are plotted on a bivariate graph with the axes representing the variables under study. Table 5.5 shows three sets of score pairs for 10 subjects. The corresponding scatterplots for these data sets appear in Figure 5.6.

Examination of the scatterplot will reveal the *direction* of the relationship. If the scores on one variable tend to *increase* as the other variable increases, the relationship is *positive* (Figure 5.6a). If one variable *decreases* as the other variable *increases*, the relationship is *negative* (Figure 5.6b). These relationships are shown by the direction in which the plot moves across the graph as in Figure 5.6(a–c). Moreover, the density with which the data points on the plot are clustered together reveals the *strength* of the relationship. Figures 5.6(a) and 5.6(b) show points tightly clustered, indicating a strong relationship whereas Figure 5.6(c) shows a wide dispersal of points, indicating a weak relationship.

Although scatterplots are useful, they do not give a precise index of association between variables. For this reason, most relationships are reported as *correlation coefficients*. Many types of coefficients exist, depending on the methods used to obtain them, but the two most common ones are the *Pearson Product-Moment Correlation Coefficient* (a parametric index) and the *Spearman Rank-Order Correlation Coefficient* (a nonparametric index). Occasionally, a partial, multiple, biserial, point biserial, tetrachoric, or phi correlation may be cited, but these indices are interpreted in essentially the same way as the Pearson and Spearman indices.

Correlation coefficients have two components: a sign and a numeric value. The sign indicates the *direction* of the relationship ($-$ = a negative or inverse relationship; $+$ = a positive relationship). The numeric value indicates the *strength* of the relationship and may take on an absolute value ranging from .00 (no relationship) to 1.00 (a perfect relationship). Thus correlation coefficients can range from -1.00 (a perfect negative relationship) to $+1.00$ (a perfect positive relationship), as shown in the interpretive guide in Figure 5.7.

One point of confusion in interpreting these indices lies in the fact that the strength and direction of the coefficient are independent. Commonly, we think of negative numbers as being less desirable or significant than positive numbers; this is *not true* of correlation. For instance, if we were given the two correlation coefficients:

$$r_{ab} = -.79$$
$$r_{ac} = +.63$$

and asked which describes a *stronger* relationship, the answer is $r_{ab} = -.79$, even though it is a negative coefficient. Incidentally, the subscripts *ab* and *ac* are a statistical convention for telling the reader which variables are being

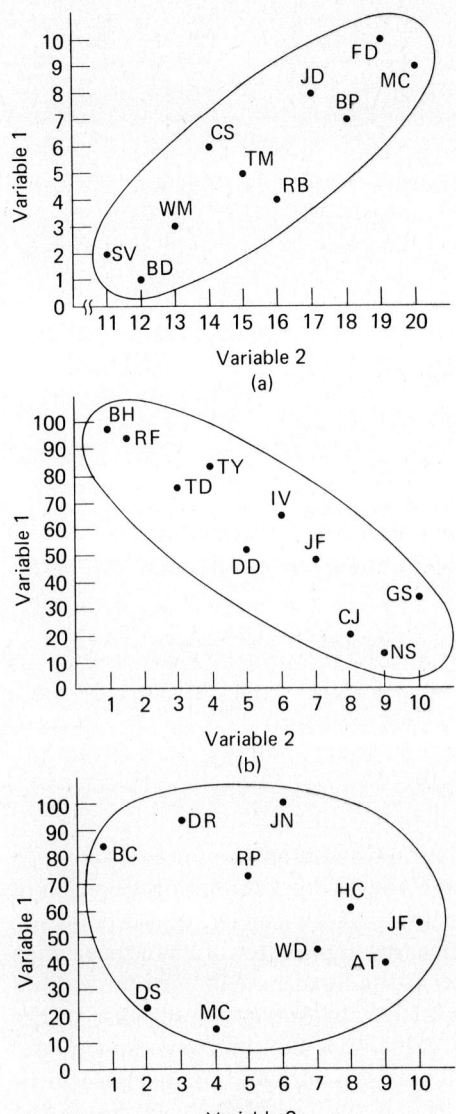

Figure 5.6 Graphic presentation of relationships: (*a*) Scatterplot for data in Illustration A (Table 5.5). (*b*) Scatterplot for data in Illustration B (Table 5.5). (*c*) Scatterplot for data in Illustration C (Table 5.5).

correlated; in this case r_{ab} is the correlation between two variables, a and b, whereas r_{ac} is the correlation between two variables a and c.

Moreover, the coefficients

$$r_{ad} = -.43$$
$$r_{bc} = +.43$$

indicate relationships of the *same strength*, even though the relationship between variable a and variable d is inverse and the relationship between variables b and c is positive.

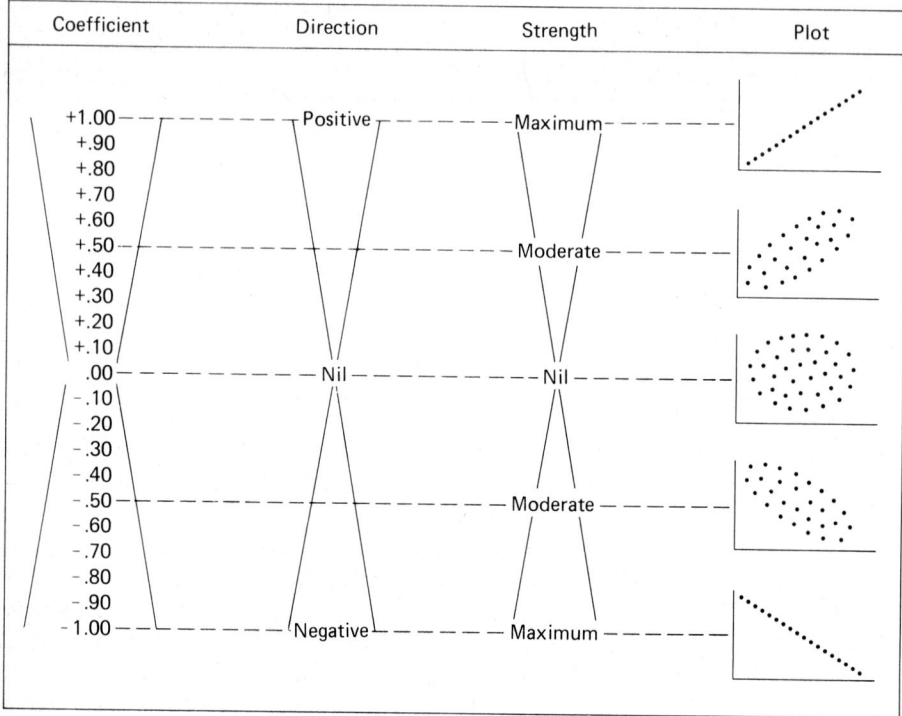

Figure 5.7 Interpretive guide for correlation coefficients.

The Pearson Product-Moment Correlation Coefficient uses actual scores in the calculation, whereas the Spearman Rank-Order Correlation Coefficient requires that ranks or scores converted to ranks be used in the calculation. Generally, the Pearson coefficient applies to sample sizes of 25 or more with data at the interval or ratio levels, whereas the Spearman is used for ordinal data or when the sample size is below 25. No matter which of these or the other methods listed earlier is used, the researcher should clearly specify the procedure selected for analyzing particular sets of data. For purpose of illustration, both the Pearson and Spearman indices have been computed (Table 5.6) for the illustrative data sets in Table 5.5.

Rather then reporting entire lists of correlation coefficients showing relationships between variable pairs in a multivariate study, many researchers present these data in a *table of intercorrelations* or in a *correlation matrix*. This way, the reader can, by locating the desired variable pairs in the row and column headings, find the correlation between those two variables. Table 5.7 shows a correlation matrix for five variables. By consulting the table, the reader can see that the correlation of variable *b* with variable *d* is −.60, and so forth. Note that the entries in the table are duplicated below the underlined diagonal values. For that reason, the shaded portion often does

TABLE 5.6 CORRELATION COEFFICIENTS FOR DATA OF ILLUSTRATIONS A, B, AND C LISTED IN TABLE 5.5 AND GRAPHED IN FIGURE 5.6

Data Set	Pearson r	Spearman Rho
A	+.91	+.92
		(Very strong positive correlation)
B	−.93	−.93
		(Very strong negative correlation)
C	−.10	−.13
		(Very weak correlation)

not appear in research reports. In addition, the underlined diagonal values represent the correlation of each variable with itself and, therefore, equal +1.00, a perfect positive correlation.

When correlation coefficients are reported, the researcher may accompany this by some statement of the *statistical* significance of the index, that is, whether or not the correlation coefficient is *significantly different from zero*. Because statistical significance may be obtained for very small correlations if the sample is large enough, small correlation coefficients should be interpreted cautiously. For example, for a sample size of 200, a correlation of plus or minus .14 is considered statistically significant (Guilford, 1965, p. 581). However, the *practical* usefulness of this index is limited because it is, at best, a modest correlation.

To evaluate the practical meaning of a correlation coefficient of a given magnitude, a statistic known as the Index of Determination is often used. This index, commonly known as r^2, is the square of the correlation coefficient and it gives an indication of the actual amount of overlap between two variables in terms of shared variance. For example, a correlation, $r_{de} = +.50$ indicates that there is actually only a 25% ($.50^2$) overlap between the variables d and e in terms of variance accounted for. This is illustrated by Figure

TABLE 5.7 A HYPOTHETICAL CORRELATION MATRIX

Variable	a	b	c	d	e
a	1.00	.64	.14	−.39	.04
b	.64	1.00	.79	−.60	.43
c	.14	.79	1.00	.98	.16
d	−.39	−.60	.98	1.00	−.37
e	.04	.43	.16	−.37	1.00

5.8 which shows two variable domains—domain G and domain H. If the correlation between the two variables (G and H) is $r_{gh} = +.60$, then this indicates that 36% ($.60^2$) of the two domains actually overlap, leaving a full 64% of the domain variability unaccounted for. Figure 5.8 also illustrates the Indices of Determination for correlations of $-.30$ and $+.20$. The shaded areas represent the amount of variance that overlaps or that is shared by the two variables; the white areas with question marks indicate the variance that is not accounted for by the correlation. The reader can readily see that the

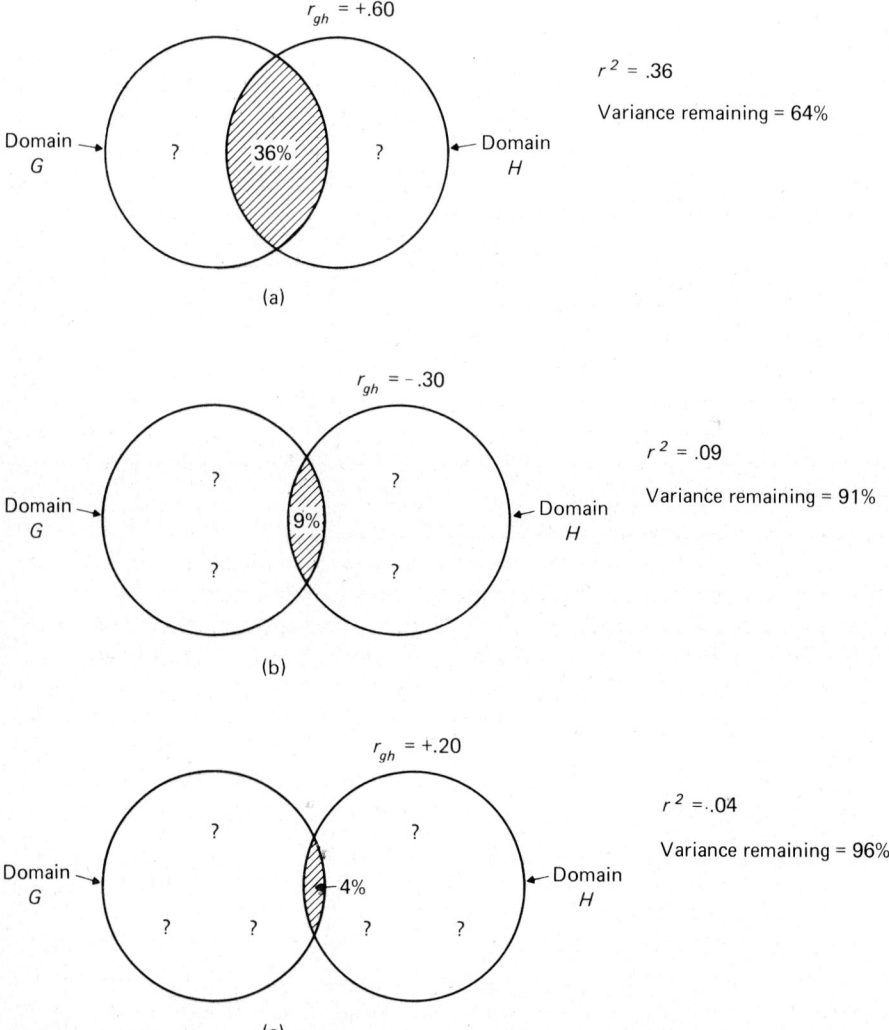

Figure 5.8   The index of determination as an indication of the variance shared by two variables.

statistical significance of a correlation is only one indication of its quality and that the r^2 value can be a more pragmatically useful index for judging the meaning of the correlation.

Another consideration necessary for proper interpretation of correlation coefficients is that correlation does *not* imply that a cause–effect relationship exists between the variables being correlated. Thus, if variable *a* and variable *b* are correlated, this should be interpreted to mean that they *co*-relate, or vary together in some describable way so that as one variable moves in one direction, the other *tends* to move in the same direction (for a positive relationship) or the opposite direction (for a negative relationship). One does not necessarily *cause* the other to vary.

In addition to ascribing causality to correlations, there exists another common *mis*interpretation of correlation coefficients. This is the direct translation of a coefficient into a percentage or proportion. Often, students tend to think that if we knew the correlation between two variables was +.58 and had data for one of these variables, we would correctly predict what the data for the other would 58% of the time. This is *not* correct, and researchers who make these kinds of statements are being inaccurate. Instead, a +.58 correlation indicates that there is a moderately positive relationship between two variables so that, in general, the individuals who had high scores or rankings on one variable would probably tend to have high scores or rankings on the other. Note the qualifiers: "in general," "probably," and "tend to" in the preceding statement. These indicate the tentative nature of interpretation of correlation coefficients as well as the possibility that, unless the relationship is *perfect*, there will be some cases in any sample or population that do not behave in the same way as the majority.

In addition to allowing researchers to understand the relationships among variables, correlational analysis allows researchers to make predictions of the value of one variable from knowledge of the values of other variables. For example, a research study may be concerned with prediction of some criterion performance such as degree of success in a treatment program (designated a dependent variable) from knowledge of factors such as subject characteristics, pretherapy test scores, prognostic indicators, or severity of disorder (designated as independent variables). To accomplish this, the researcher assembles data for a sample of subjects and correlates all of the independent variables with the dependent variables. Often, the independent variables are termed *predictor* variables and the dependent variables are termed *predicted* variables because of the direction of the prediction. The relationships, expressed as correlation coefficients, can be presented in tables of intercorrelations showing how each variable relates to each other variable and to the criterion. In rare instances, a single factor emerges as having such a strong relationship with the criterion that it can be used as the sole predictor in a regression equation. Most of the time, however, the array of correlations indicates that several variables should be used in combination to predict the criterion more closely than any single variable could.

The researcher then sets out to find the best linear combination of predictors, that is, one that acknowledges the unique relationship of each predictor with the criterion, minimizes the overlap (correlation) among predictors, and maximizes the combined strength of the predictors. Rather than attempt this task of finding the optimum combination of predictors through trial and error, the researcher uses a statistical technique known as multiple-regression analysis. In brief, this technique mathematically enables the researcher to determine the *order* in which predictor variables should be entered in a prediction equation to maximize prediction; assigns a *weight* to each predictor variable entered into the equation; and (in a stepwise multiple regression) indicates the *contribution* of each new added variable to the predictive validity of the equation. By the use of these methods, the researcher may initially examine the relationships among each of 20 variables themselves. The researcher may then conclude the analysis by specifying three or four variables that can be combined in a given order and with given weights in a regression equation to best predict the criterion.

The success and meaning of multiple regression analysis depends on a number of factors the researcher must consider. These factors include: (1) care in selection of the initial variables for the analysis, (2) the reliability and validity with which the variables are measured, (3) the size and representativeness of the sample used for study, (4) the reliability and validity of the criterion measure, and (5) the practicality of gathering all of the predictor data appearing in the equation. Multiple-regression analysis is a popular and appealing data-manipulation procedure. Unfortunately, the attractiveness of this procedure often results in its misuse.

The correlation and regression methods discussed above give quantitative descriptions of the strength and direction of association among variables that can be assigned ranks or score values. Occasionally, however, the researcher is faced with the task of ascertaining if there is an association between two or more variables when at least one of them is a nominal variable. This is especially pertinent to studies using questionnaire or demographic data that can be reported as frequencies in categories but cannot satisfactorily be expressed in ordinal or interval scales.

To organize such nominal-level data, the researcher may present them in *contingency tables.* The categories used for one variable are listed across one axis of the table, whereas those for a second variable are listed along the other axis. Contingency tables can also be generated for more than two variables, but they are somewhat awkward and are not found as often in the research literature. The entries in the table are the frequencies with which subjects had that particular combination of values. Table 5.8 shows a contingency table having 2 rows and 2 columns, which is, thus, known as a 2 × 2 contingency table. Hypothetical data on pass–fail performance of speakers with normal palate and cleft palate are entered in the cells of Table 5.8.

Although contingency tables are useful on their own, they are usually accompanied by further data analysis that enables the researcher to deter-

TABLE 5.8   A 2 × 2 CONTINGENCY TABLE
ILLUSTRATING DATA FROM HYPOTHETICAL
PERFORMANCE OF SPEAKERS WITH AND WITHOUT
CLEFT PALATE ON SOME CATEGORICAL PERFORMANCE
MEASURE

	Cleft Palate	Normal Palate
Passed	3	17
Failed	13	6

$$\chi^2 = 9.39$$
$$C = .44$$

mine if significant relationships exist among the variables. Two common analysis techniques that may be applied to such data are the chi square (χ^2) and the contingency coefficient (C)

Application of chi square to the data in the contingency table discussed above yields a value of 9.39. Consulting a table of chi square values required for the .01 level of statistical significance shows that the required value for this set of data having 1 df is 6.64 (Siegel, 1956, p. 249). Thus, this chi square would be statistically significant beyond the .01 level, indicating that there is a relationship between the two categorical variables that could only have occurred by chance less than 1 time in 100.

Briefly, a chi square analysis requires that the actual observed (O) frequencies listed in the contingency table be compared to expected (E) frequencies generated during the analysis or postulated by the researcher earlier on the basis of some theory or prior experience with similar data. If the discrepancy between what was actually observed in the study and the estimates given by the expected values is large enough, the resulting chi square value will reach statistical significance. The reader will note that the outcome of the analysis must be evaluated by consulting statistical tables of significance using the df determined from the data. These significance tables give the minimum values of the chi square statistic needed with various df to permit the conclusion that there is a statistically significant relationship between or among the variables in question. The chi square analysis does *not* indicate the strength of any relationship that exists nor the direction of that relationship. Chi square indicates only the extent to which the relationship is outside the realm of chance or normal probability. The contingency coefficient is used to measure the extent or strength of the relationship and can be computed by a formula that employs the chi square value. The contingency coefficient for the data in Table 5.8 is $C = 0.44$, and this coefficient would be interpreted in much the same way as the other correlation coefficients discussed earlier except that the upper limit for C for a 2 × 2 table is .707, not 1.0.

Although chi square is often used for ascertaining the presence of significant bivariate relationships, it can be extended to multivariate situations as long as a subject's data can be classified within one value or category in each variable. Thus, chi square can be used for a 2 × 3 × 5 contingency table or a 3 × 6 × 2 × 7 contingency table. The only difficulties lie in finding a way to present these data and interpret the meaning of three-way and four-way relationships.

Although chi square is used to determine the presence of relationships in nominal-level data, it is an extremely flexible procedure that can also be used as a method for analyzing *differences* in groups. In this sense, the method provides a link between procedures that show relationships and those that describe differences. The major difference among the applications of this procedure lies in the nature of the questons or hypotheses examined, as we will see in the next section.

Methods for Analyzing Differences

Many research problems in speech pathology and audiology concern differences between (or among) groups of subjects. For example, a researcher might ask if there is a difference between normal-hearing and hearing-impaired children on a particular language measure. Other problems concern differences between (or among) conditions for the same group of subjects. For example, a researcher might ask if there is a difference between hearing impaired subjects' speech-discrimination scores before and after auditory training. In other words, researchers are concerned about the analysis of between-subjects differences and within-subjects differences. In analyzing the between-subjects and within-subjects differences, researchers want to determine if the differences are large enough in the sample data to rule out the probability that they could be attributed to chance or sampling error. The procedures of statistical inference are used to make such an analysis for determining the statistical significance of differences between-subjects and within-subjects. In other words, the researcher will examine the probability of making a Type I error in concluding that there is a between-subjects or a within-subjects difference.

Table 5.19 (at the end of this chapter) summarizes many of the common analysis procedures and the situations in which they are applicable. The table indicates the level of measurement for which each procedure is applicable and shows which procedures are parametric and which are nonparametric. Also indicated is whether the procedure is applicable to between-subjects comparisons (i.e., independent samples tests) or within-subjects comparisons (i.e., related samples tests). Some of the statistical tests are also identified as appropriate for comparing only two samples or for comparing more than two samples of data.

We will first consider statistical methods that are used to ascertain the significance of the difference between *two groups of data* on a *single dependent variable*. These procedures could be used to compare two different groups of subjects, like stutterers vs. nonstutterers, or to compare one group of subjects under two different conditions, like stutterers speaking in quiet vs. noise. In other words, these procedures can be used to make between-subjects comparisons (i.e., to compare independent or uncorrelated samples) or to make within-subjects comparisons (i.e., to compare related or correlated samples).

In the two-group one-variable analysis situation described above, the basic parametric procedures for determining the significance of differences are the z-ratio and the *t*-test. The z-ratio is used when the samples are large (30 or more) and the *t*-test is applicable for smaller samples. Basically, both of these methods (and their various subroutines) examine a theoretical distribution of *differences* in means to determine how the observed differences derived from a particular study compare to the average differences in a theoretical distribution. If the observed difference departs markedly from the average difference in the theoretical distribution, it is judged significant at a given level of significance (usually the .05 or .01 level, as described earlier). This is accomplished through the use of established formulae and tables available in statistical texts.

In the case of the z-ratio, the values required for statistical significance are 1.96 (.05 level) and 2.58 (.01 level) for two-tailed tests and 1.65 (.05) and 2.33 (.01) for one-tailed tests. With the *t*-test, the values required for statistical significance vary according to the number of degrees of freedom available for the data and require the consultation of a table showing significant *t*-values for different degrees of freedom. The researcher who uses these procedures should cite both the z-ratio or *t*-value obtained for the data in the study and the z-ratio or *t*-value required for statistical significance at the level chosen for the study.

Table 5.9 shows examples of the application of the z-ratio to compare means from two different groups and to compare the pretreatment and posttreatment means from a single group. Similar examples for the *t*-test appear in Tables 5.10 and 5.11. In the examples in Tables 5.9 and 5.10, it is the *mean* of the group or groups that is examined rather than individual subject values. The *t*-test for correlated groups shown in Table 5.11 uses mean pair differences and deviations of pair differences in the calculations.

Also listed in these tables are the null hypotheses (H_0) and their alternates (H_1, H_2, etc.) that are tested with each statistical procedure. Each statistical procedure considers the probability of the hypothesis (H_0) that there are no differences between the groups of scores. If the obtained statistic indicates that this null hypothesis is highly improbable (i.e., the statistic reaches the significance level), then the H_0 is rejected in favor of one of the alternative hypotheses listed.

When the assumptions required for the use of parametric methods cannot

TABLE 5.9 SUMMARY TABLE FOR z-RATIO

	Illustration Different Groups				Illustration Same (Correlated) Groups		

$$H_0 : M_1 = M_2$$
$$H_1 : M_1 \neq M_2$$

$$H_0 : M_1 = M_2$$
$$H_1 : M_1 \neq M_2$$

	Group 1		Group 2			Testing 1		Testing 2
N	35		41		N	40		40
M^*	29.5		31.2		M	53.1		55.4
σ	5.3		4.8		σ	7.9		8.1
σ_M	.91		1.76		$r_{M_1 M_2}\dagger$	—	.80	—
σ_{D_M}	—	1.18	—		σ_M	1.3		1.3
					σ_{D_M}	—	.83	—

Formula for z-ratio: $z = \dfrac{D_M}{\sigma_{D_M}}$

(where $D_M = M_2 - M_1$) $= \dfrac{31.2 - 29.5}{1.18}$

$$= 1.44.$$

Formula for z-ratio: $z = \dfrac{D_M}{\sigma_{D_M}}$

(where $D_M = M_2 - M_1$) $= \dfrac{55.4 - 53.1}{.83}$

$$= 2.77.$$

The z-ratio of 1.44 is less than that required for statistical signficance at the .05 level (1.96) for a two-tailed test. Therefore the difference in the two means is not significant and could have occurred by chance more than 5 times in 100.

The z-ratio of 2.77 exceeds that required for statistical significance at the .01 level for the two-tailed test (2.58). Therefore, the difference in means between the two testings is statistically significant and could have occurred by chance less than 1 time in 100.

Decision: accept H_0.

Decision: reject H_0; accept H_1.

*Either M or $\bar{X}$ can be used to represent the mean score.
†Correlation between testing 1 and testing 2 derived during prior analysis and used in calculating σ_{D_M}.

be met (e.g., the data are not in interval or ratio scales, or sample sizes are extremely small), the researcher would apply analogous nonparametric procedures to the data. Among them are the Wilcoxon Matched-Pairs Signed-Ranks Test for changes within a group over time and the Mann–Whitney U Test that examines differences between groups. The values reached by use of these procedures must be compared with values in appropriate tables. As with the z-ratio and t-test, both the observed and the required values should be reported. Examples of the Wilcoxon and the Mann–Whitney procedures

TABLE 5.10 SUMMARY TABLE FOR t-TEST
(UNCORRELATED GROUPS)

$$H_0 = \bar{X}_1 = \bar{X}_2$$
$$H_1 = \bar{X}_1 > X$$

Directional hypotheses; call for one-tailed test.

	Group 1	Group 2
N	21	23
$\bar{X}$	15.7	13.5
σ	3.7	3.9
*Σx^2	287	349
$X_1 - \bar{X}_2$	2.2	

Formula for t
(difference between
uncorrelated means):

$$\frac{\bar{X}_1 - \bar{X}_2}{\sqrt{\left(\frac{\Sigma x^2_1 + \Sigma x^2_2}{N_1 + N_2 - 2}\right)\left(\frac{N_1 + N_2}{N_1 N_2}\right)}}$$

t for these data = 1.88 df for these data = 42

t required for 42 df one-tailed test = 1.68 (.05 level)

The t-value of 1.88 exceeds that required for statistical significance at the .05 level for a one-tailed test with 42 df. Therefore, the difference in means between the two groups is statistically significant and would have occurred by chance less than 5 times in 100. The mean of Group 1 is significantly larger than the mean of Group 2.

Decision: reject H_0; accept H_1.

*Information derived during analysis; calculations not shown.

are found in Tables 5.12 and 5.13. A more detailed description of nonparametric methods for describing differences is found in Siegel (1956).

We will now consider situations in which there are more than two groups for comparison and more than two conditions under which each group is tested. The parametric statistical procedure used for these situations in most studies is the *analysis of variance* (usually abbreviated ANOVA). The statistic calculated in ANOVA is called the *F-ratio* and the outcome of the analysis is usually reported in the form of a summary table. Interpretation of an F-ratio requires consultation of special significance tables. However, the summary table should present the value of F required for significance (or the p

TABLE 5.11 SUMMARY TABLE FOR t-TEST (CORRELATED GROUPS)

$$H_0 = \bar{X}_1 = \bar{X}_2$$
$$H_1 = \bar{X}_1 \neq \bar{X}_2$$

Note: This procedure tests for differences in score pairs rather than means.

Raw Data for 18 Subjects

	Subject	Pretest	Posttest	Subject	Pretest	Posttest
$N = 18 \; \bar{X}_1 = 21.8 \; \bar{X}_2 = 22.7$	a	23	28	j	28	27
	b	24	22	k	27	27
	c	16	18	l	18	15
	d	15	16	m	21	23
	e	18	23	n	26	27
	f	16	18	o	19	25
	g	21	20	p	21	19
	h	25	23	q	26	26
	i	26	28	r	23	24

Information derived from these data during analysis includes:

$$M_d = 1.0 \qquad \Sigma x^2_d = 110$$

t-test formula: $\quad t = \dfrac{M_d}{\sqrt{\Sigma x^2_d / N(N-1)}}$

t for these data = 1.69.

t required for statistical significance (two-tailed test; $df = 17$)
    2.1 (at the .05 level);
    2.9 (at the .01 level).

The t-value of 1.69 is less than that required for statistical significance with 17 df at the .05 level for a two-tailed test. Therefore, the difference in the scores received on pretest and posttest is not statistically significant and could have occurred by chance variation more than 5 times in 100.

Decision: accept H_0.

---

value of each reported F) and the appropriate number of df for each comparison.

We cannot provide a detailed explanation of the assumptions underlying ANOVA and the procedures for calculating F-ratios. However, we will try to present the overall logic of ANOVA as a test for differences among several means. If there is a difference among a set of group means, the variance

TABLE 5.12 SUMMARY OF WILCOXON MATCHED-PAIRS SIGNED-RANKS TEST (T)

$$H_0 = \Sigma \text{Ranks}_1 = \Sigma \text{Ranks}_2$$
$$H_1 = \Sigma \text{Ranks}_1 \neq \Sigma \text{Ranks}_2$$

Subject	Score Before Treatment X_1	Score After Treatment X_2
a	14	16
b	17	17
c	18	23
d	15	20
e	16	14
f	12	11
g	16	18

This procedure determines an index known as T for the data and compares this value to those required for statistical significance at various levels.

The value of T for these data = 6.

T required = 2 (.05 level); 0 (.02 level).

Note: In this procedure the observed T must be *smaller* than the required value to be significant.

The observed T is larger than that required for statistical significance at the .05 level. Therefore, the shift in scores between pretesting and posttesting is not significant and could have occurred by chance more than 5 times in 100.

Decision: accept H_0.

between the groups will be significantly larger than the variance *within each of the groups.* The variance between the groups can be thought of as the variance of the group means around the *grand mean* of all the scores.

For instance, a researcher might ask if children of different ages would differ in their performance on some language task. Using a cross-sectional developmental approach, the researcher assembles four age groups (5-, 6-, 7-, and 8-year-olds), with 100 children in each group, and assesses the performance of these 400 children using a one-way ANOVA design (see Table 5.14). This ANOVA is called a one-way ANOVA because there is only one independent (classification) variable. In other words, the structure of an ANOVA, or the number of "ways" it tests for mean differences, is determined by the structure of the independent variables in the research study.

Within each age group, there will be some variation among the 100 children

TABLE 5.13   SUMMARY OF MANN–WHITNEY U TEST (U)

$$H_0 = \text{Ranks}_1 = \text{Ranks}_2$$
$$H_1 = \text{Ranks}_1 \neq \text{Ranks}_2$$

Hypothetical raw data for two samples of 10 subjects on a vocabulary test.

Group 1	Group 2
10	25
25	23
20	14
16	12
14	20
12	20
15	15
23	17
16	18
12	22

The U value for these data = 34.5.

The required value of U at the .05 level = 23;
.01 level = 19.

Note: The observed value of U must be *smaller* than the required value to be statistically significant at that level.

The observed U is larger than that required for statistical significance at the .05 level. Therefore, the difference between Groups 1 and 2 is not statistically significant and may have occurred by chance more than 5 times in 100.

Decision: accept H_0.

tested so that there will be an age-group mean and an age-group variance for each of the four age groups. If the variance *between the age-group means* (relative to the grand mean) is much larger than the variance *within each age group*, then there will be a significant difference among the age groups as shown by the F-ratio. The F-ratio that results from such an ANOVA is the ratio of the between-groups variance (called Mean Square between groups or MS between) to the within group variance (called MS within). When the between-groups variance is much larger than the within-groups variance, the F-ratio is large and reaches statistical significance when it is large enough for the appropriate number of *df* and alpha level. When the between-groups variance is not larger than the within-groups variance, the F-ratio is small and does not reach statistical significance. A table summarizing a possible ANOVA for the hypothetical cross-sectional study discussed above is shown in Table 5.15.

TABLE 5.14 REPRESENTATION OF A ONE-WAY ANOVA DESIGN FOR COMPARING THE MEANS OF FOUR AGE GROUPS

	Independent (Classification) Variable = Age			
	Group A (5-year-olds)	Group B (6-year-olds)	Group C (7-year-olds)	Group D (8-year-olds)
Dependent (criterion) variable	$\bar{X}_a$ σ_a $N_a = 100$	$\bar{X}_b$ σ_b $N_b = 100$	$\bar{X}_c$ σ_c $N_c = 100$	$\bar{X}_d$ σ_d $N_d = 100$

H_0 = there are no differences in the means of the four groups.
H_1 = there is a difference among the means of the four groups.

If there is only one independent or classification variable in a study (i.e., age or clinical diagnosis), then the data form a one-way-classification problem, and a one-way ANOVA is performed with the resulting F-ratio reported, as in the example in Table 5.15. The F-ratio is the ratio of a between-groups value called the mean square (MS between) to the within group mean-square (MS within) value, which are calculated during the analysis.

Let us now proceed to a more complex situation that takes the basic problem outlined above one step further. Suppose our researcher felt that the

TABLE 5.15 SUMMARY TABLE FOR ONE-WAY ANOVA (USING EXAMPLE FROM TEXT)

Components	Sum of Squares	Degrees of Freedom (df)	Mean Squares	F-Ratio
Between groups (ages)	53.19	3	17.73	3.1
Within groups	2265.12	396	5.72	
Total	2318.31	399		

$$F = \frac{\text{MS between}}{\text{MS within}} = \frac{17.73}{5.72} = 3.1$$

F_{required} (3/396 df) = 2.62 (p = .05)
     3.83 (p = .01)

The observed F-ratio of 3.1 falls between that required at the .05 level and that required at the .01 level. Therefore, there is a statistically significant difference among the four groups. This difference could occur by chance less than 5 times in 100 but more than 1 time in 100.

Decision: reject H_0; accept H_1.

children's sex was also a factor involved in language performance. The research design would then be constructed so that in addition to the four age categories, each age group would be divided into a group of males and a group of females. The researcher now has a 4 by 2 design (often abbreviated 4 × 2), and the resulting data would be analyzed using a two-way ANOVA in which one variable of interest is age and the other is sex. Hypothetical data for a 4 × 2 design are shown in Table 5.16 with a list of the statistical hypotheses that would be evaluated. The researcher is, then, asking more than one question in the analysis, namely:

1. Is there a difference in language performance among children of different ages?

2. Is there a difference in language performance among children of different sexes?

Both of these questions concern so-called *main effects* in the ANOVA. In addition, another question has been implicitly introduced: Is there an *interaction* of age and sex with respect to language performance? Thus, might

TABLE 5.16 REPRESENTATION OF A 2 × 4 DESIGN SUITABLE FOR A TWO-WAY ANOVA

	Independent (Classification) Variable Age of Subjects			
	Group A (5-year-olds)	Group B (6-year-olds)	Group C (7-year-olds)	Group D (8-year-olds)
Males	$\bar{X}_{ma}$ σ_{ma} $N_{ma} = 50$	$\bar{X}_{mb}$ σ_{mb} $N_{mb} = 50$	$\bar{X}_{mc}$ σ_{mc} $N_{mc} = 50$	$\bar{X}_{md}$ σ_{md} $N_{md} = 50$
Females	$\bar{X}_{fa}$ σ_{fa} $N_{fa} = 50$	$\bar{X}_{fb}$ σ_{fb} $N_{fb} = 50$	$\bar{X}_{fc}$ σ_{fc} $N_{fc} = 50$	$\bar{X}_{fd}$ σ_{fd} $N_{fd} = 50$

H_0 (for main effect of sex): there are no differences between the means of the male and female groups.

H_1 (for main effect of sex): there are differences between the means of the male and female groups.

H_0 and H_1 for main effect of age take the same form as above.

H_0 (for age by sex interaction): there are no differences between the means of various ages by sex groups.

H_1 (for age by sex interaction): there are differences between the means of various ages by sex groups.

males and females show a different pattern of language performance across ages? Therefore, ANOVA has to examine three sources of variance in this problem—variance across age (MS age), variance across sexes (MS sex), and variance owing to the interaction of age and sex (MS age × sex)—and compare each of these three sources of variance with the variance within the eight groups (MS within groups). There will then be three F-ratios calculated: the F-ratio for age; the F-ratio sex; and the F-ratio for the interaction. Any, all, or none of these might be statistically significant. The summary table for the example we have discussed is shown in Table 5.17. The information in the table that is most pertinent to the consumer of research is in

TABLE 5.17 SUMMARY TABLE FOR TWO-WAY ANOVA (USING EXAMPLE FROM TEXT)

Components	Sum of Squares	Degrees of Freedom (df)	Mean Squares	F-Ratios
Between groups (ages)	54.00	3	18	5.8**
Between groups (sexes)	12.10	1	12.1	3.9*
Interaction of age × sex	38.10	3	12.7	4.1**
Within groups	1215.20	392	3.1	
Total	1319.40	399		

*p < .05
**p < .01

Calculation of F-Ratios		Required F-Ratios for Significance		
F for age	$= \dfrac{18}{3.1} = 5.8$	2.62	3.83	(df = 3 , 392)
F for sex	$= \dfrac{12.1}{3.1} = 3.9$	3.86	6.70	(df = 1 , 392)
F for age × sex interaction $= \dfrac{12.7}{3.1} = 4.1$		2.62	3.83	(df = 3 , 392)
		.05	.01	
		Level of significance		

The obtained F-ratios can be evaluated as follows:
  F for main effect of age indicates significant differences among ages
  F for main effect of sex indicates significant differences between sexes
  F for interaction of age and sex indicates significant interaction effect

TABLE 5.18 HYPOTHETICAL ROW AND COLUMN MEANS ILLUSTRATING MAIN EFFECTS OF AGE AND SEX ON LANGUAGE PERFORMANCE AND INTERACTION OF AGE AND SEX

Sex of Subjects	Age of Subjects				
	Group A (5-year-olds)	Group B (6-year-olds)	Group C (7-year-olds)	Group D (8-year-olds)	Ages Combined
Males	12.0	16.0	21.0	24.0	18.25
Females	17.0	20.0	23.0	23.0	20.75
Sexes combined	14.50	18.00	22.00	23.50	

the far right column where the F-ratios appear. These can be compared with the required values given below the body of the table to determine their statistical significance. In addition, a frequent notation for indicating level of significance appears in the table: the use of the single asterisk (*) to denote statistical significance at the .05 level, and the use of the double asterisk (**) to denote statistical significance at the .01 level.

We should now return to the notion of interaction and deal with it in a bit more detail. We have seen that once the researcher moves away from designs having a single independent or classification variable to designs having several independent or classification variables, concern for the main effects of each of these variables is supplemented by consideration of the interaction between or among the variables. These interactions are aptly named because

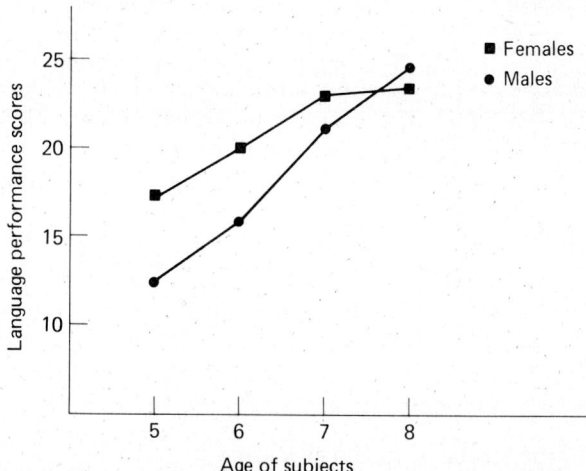

Figure 5.9 Graphic plot for visualizing interaction of two independent (classification) variables in a hypothetical two-way (4 × 2) ANOVA problem.

interaction variations are not attributable to any of the main effects acting *alone* but rather to the *joint action* of two or more variables. Sometimes, interactions are called crossover effects because of the way they show up in graphic representations of data. In the hypothetical example used earlier, sex and age showed a significant interaction. This is illustrated in Table 5.18 and Figure 5.9 that show the performances for the various ages and sexes. Note that the plots for sex and age are *not* parallel; although females *generally* have a higher performance than males, the female performance advantage is not the same at each age, and by age 8, male and female scores are essentially equivalent. That is to say, the performance difference between males and females decreases as the subjects' ages increase to 8 years when males catch up to females.

Every field of research has identified and studied variables that tend to interact. In our hypothetical example we have considered a so-called two-way interaction. In a design using three variables, both two-way and three-way interactions must be examined. For instance, a speech pathology or audiology study might look at the effects of sex, clinical classification, and length of time in treatment on some outcome variable. The ANOVA for this situation would consider the following main effects and interactions:

1. Sex (S)
2. Clinical classification (C)
3. Length of time in treatment (T)
4. S × C interaction
5. S × T interaction
6. C × T interaction
7. S × C × T interaction

From a practical standpoint, most studies do not involve interactions of more than three variables. Not only are more complex interactions difficult to interpret but also the sample size and other design considerations required for such studies present difficulties for the researcher. Moreover, interaction effects should be carefully evaluated when reporting research results. In fact, in some research studies, interaction effects may be more important than main effects. Often ANOVA will show both significant main effects and significant interaction effects.

Once a researcher has, though application of ANOVA procedures, shown that a significant difference occurs among the groups in the study, further analyses may be conducted to ascertain the location of the significant differences among the groups. Historically, *t*-tests were used to compare pairs of means following determination of a significant F-ratio. However, newer procedures are often used instead of *t*-tests for various mathematical and logical reasons. Among these are the Tukey, Duncan, Newman-Keuls, and Sheffé procedures. The reader may often find that research reports contain references to these analyses following ANOVA in order to identify specific significant differences.

The application of nonparametric methods to designs that lend themselves to ANOVA procedures is found in speech pathology and audiology research when data are in the form of nominal or ordinal scales, making use of such methods imperative. As noted in Table 5.19, the nonparametric procedures that more or less parallel the parametric ANOVA are the Kruskal-Wallis One-Way ANOVA by Ranks (H), the Friedman Two-Way ANOVA by Ranks (x_r^2), the Cochran Q test, and a chi square test for independent samples. Discussion of each of these methods can be found in Siegel (1956). H and x_r^2 both test the hypothesis that a number of samples (groups) have been drawn from the same population and, hence, have similar average values in rank. Cochran's Q tests whether frequencies or proportions from correlated groups (or repeated measures on a single set of subjects) differ across occasions. The chi square test for independent samples tests the hypothesis that different samples come from the same population; it is useful for data that can be presented as frequencies.

This overview of methods for describing differences will close with a very brief description of still another variety of analysis included here because it may be mistakenly confused with ANOVA. It is Analysis of Covariance (or

TABLE 5.19 SUMMARY OF SELECTED ANALYSIS PROCEDURES

Level of Measurement		Methods of Analyzing Relationships	Methods for Analyzing Differences		
			Related Samples		Independent Samples
Nominal	Nonparametric methods	Contingency Coefficient (C) Chi Square (χ^2)	Cochran Q Test		Chi Square Test for Independent Samples (χ^2)
Ordinal		Spearman Rank-Order Correlation Coefficient (Rho)	Two Samples	Wilcoxon Matched-Pairs Signed-Ranks Test (T)	Mann-Whitney U Test
			More Than Two Samples	Friedman Two-way ANOVA	Kruskal-Wallis One-way ANOVA
Interval or ratio	Parametric methods	Pearson Product-Moment Correlation Coefficient (r)	Two Samples	t-Test for Correlated Groups z-Ratio	t-Test for Independent Groups z-Ratio
		Multiple-Regression Analysis	More Than Two Samples	ANOVA (F) ANCOVA (F)	ANOVA (F) ANCOVA (F)

ANCOVA for short), and it is used in studies in which one of the independent or classification variables is related inextricably to the dependent variable. The analysis itself controls for the co-relation of the two variables by virtue of the method used to compute the F-ratios and the outcome is interpreted in the same manner as ANOVA results. An example of a situation requiring the use of ANCOVA would be one in which subjects' verbal aptitude is an independent classification variable and vocabulary scores are a dependent variable in a study of the comparative effects of training programs for language-disordered children. Because verbal aptitude is significantly related to vocabulary scores, the ANCOVA would control for this relationship in determining whether significant differences in vocabulary scores existed as a function of the program independent of verbal aptitude.

Summary

This chapter has considered the organization and analysis of data derived from empirical research. Methods for organizing data, including basic summary statistics, were discussed after a brief description of levels of measurement and a statement of a basic rationale for using data-manipulation techniques in speech pathology and audiology research.

Data analysis techniques were described in two sections. The first summarized methods for analyzing relationships, including correlation indices, chi square techniques, and multiple regression analysis. The second section summarized methods for analyzing differences, including z-ratios, t-tests, ANOVA, and ANCOVA and their nonparametric counterparts.

Discussion of the techniques stressed the basic logic and meaning of each procedure for a consumer of research and gave less attention to the actual calculations that would interest readers who plan to do research. The reader interested in more detailed treatment of the methods mentioned in this chapter is directed to the basic statistical textbooks cited in the references. Chapter 8 shows illustrative examples from the speech pathology and audiology literature of many of the data organization and analysis techniques discussed in this chapter. A checklist for evaluating the results section of an article is also shown in Chapter 8.

Study Questions

1. Read pages 21–30 in Chapter 3 of: Siegel, S. (1956) *Nonparametric statistics for the behavioral sciences.* New York: McGraw-Hill.
   (a) Write a brief summary of Siegel's discussion of each level of measurement.
   (b) Siegel's examples of each level of measurement come from psychology and sociology. Find analogous examples of each level of measurement in speech pathology and audiology.

2. (a) Which measures of central tendency and variability are usually reported when the distribution of data is normal?
   (b) Which measures are usually reported when the distribution is skewed?

3. Examine the data in each of the following tables:

   Table 1 in: Adam, M. R., & Hayden, P. (1976). The ability of stutterers and nonstutterers to initiate and terminate phonation during production of an isolated vowel. *Journal of Speech and Hearing Research, 19,* 290–296.

   Table 2 in: Samar, V. J., & Sims, D. G. (1984). Visual evoked-response components related to speechreading and spatial skills in hearing and hearing-impaired adults. *Journal of Speech and Hearing Research, 27,* 162–172.

   Which measures of central tendency and variability were used in each table to summarize the distribution of the data?

4. Examine the data in each of the following figures:

   Figure 2 in: Siegel, G. M., & Kennard, K. L. (1984). Lombard and sidetone amplification effects in normal and misarticulating children. *Journal of Speech and Hearing Research, 27,* 56–62.

   Figure 1 in: Wingfield, A., Lombardi, L., & Sokol, S. (1984). Prosodic features and the intelligibility of accelerated speech: Syntactic vs. periodic segmentation. *Journal of Speech and Hearing Research, 27,* 128–134.

   (a) How are the means displayed in each of these figures?
   (b) Summarize, in your own words, what differences among the means are displayed in these figures.

5. (a) Describe what is meant by the strength and direction of a relationship between two variables.
   (b) How are these two aspects of a relationship demonstrated in a scattergram?
   (c) How are they demonstrated in a correlation coefficient?

6. Examine the data in the following table:

   Table 2 in: Stitt, C. L., & Huntington, D. A. (1969). Some relationships among articulation, auditory abilities, and certain other variables. *Journal of Speech and Hearing Research, 12,* 576–593.

   (a) Which correlation coefficient was used to analyze the relationships among the variables listed in this table?
   (b) Which correlations were significantly different from zero at the .05 level? At the .01 level? At the .001 level?

(c) Which pair of variables showed the strongest relationship? Which pair showed the weakest relationship?

7. Examine the data in the following table and the analysis in the accompanying paragraph:

   Table 2 in: Conrad, R. (1973). Some correlates of speech coding in the short-term memory of the deaf. *Journal of Speech and Hearing Research, 16,* 375–384.

   (a) What technique was used to analyze the relationships among the variables?
   (b) Which pairs of variables showed significant relationships?
   (c) Which pairs of variables did not show significant relationships?

8. (a) What are Type I and Type II errors?
   (b) Is it possible to make *both* types of error at the same time in reaching a decision about the plausibility of a null hypothesis? Why or why not?

9. Under what circumstances would it be more appropriate to use nonparametric statistics instead of parametric statistics?

10. Examine the data in the following tables:

    Tables 1 and 2 in: Santo Pietro, M. J., & Rigrodsky, S. (1982). The effects of temporal and semantic conditions on the occurrence of the error response of perseveration in adult aphasics. *Journal of Speech and Hearing Research, 25,* 184–192.

    (a) What summary statistics were used to describe the central tendency and variability in each task and condition?
    (b) What statistical test was used for each comparison?
    (c) Which tests showed significant differences and which did not?

11. Examine the data in the following table:

    Table 2 in: Hubbard, D. J., & Kushner, D. (1980). A comparison of speech intelligibility between esophageal and normal speakers via three modes of presentation. *Journal of Speech and Hearing Research, 23,* 909–916.

    (a) What technique was used to analyze the differences between-subjects and within-subjects?
    (b) Were there any significant main or interaction effects?

References

Carver, R. P. (1978). The case against statistical significance testing. *Harvard Educational Review, 48,* 378–399.

Cohen, J. (1969). *Statistical power analysis for the behavioral sciences.* New York. Academic Press.

Guilford, J. P. (1965). *Fundamental statistics in psychology and education* (4th ed.). New York: McGraw-Hill.

Haber, A., Runyon, R. P., & Badia, P. (Eds.). (1970). *Readings in statistics.* Reading, MA: Addison-Wesley.

Siegel, S. (1956). *Nonparametric statistics for the behavioral sciences.* New York: McGraw-Hill.

Stevens, S. S. (1946). On the theory of scales of measurement. *Science, 103:* 677–680.

Stevens, S. S. (1951). Mathematics, measurement, and psychophysics. In S. S. Stevens (Ed.), *Handbook of experimental psychology* (pp. 1–49). New York: Wiley.

Part II
Evaluation of the Components of a Research Article

Overview

The main purpose of Part II is to show how the principles discussed in Part I can be applied to the evaluation of research. It is in Part II, then, that the reader is provided the guidelines for analyzing and critically evaluating the four basic parts of the research article.

The four chapters of Part II cover the Introduction, Method, Results, and Discussion sections of a research article. The journals published by the American Speech-Language-Hearing Association (ASHA)—as well as many other journals of interest to speech pathologists and audiologists—follow the style specified in the current edition of the *Publication Manual of the American Psychological Association*. The manual states (American Psychological Association [APA], 1983, p. 21):

> *Journal articles are usually reports of empirical studies, review articles, or theoretical articles. Reports of empirical studies are reports of original research. They typically consist of distinct sections that reflect stages in the research process and that appear in the sequence of these stages:*
> • introduction: *development of the problem under investigation and statement of the purpose of investigation;*
> • method: *description of the method used to conduct the investigation;*
> • results: *report of the results that were found; and*
> • discussion: *interpretation and discussion of the implications of the results.*

Thus, we will follow the APA style suggestions in outlining the various parts of a research article in this part of the book.

Although much has been written about methods and statistical analyses in a number of texts, relatively little attention has been devoted to the evaluation of the research problem itself. Chapter 6 presents the guidelines for evaluating the introductory part of the research article. Emphasis here is placed on assessing the adequacy of the rationale for the study, on deciding if the literature citations support the need for the study, and on evaluating the research questions or hypotheses. Numerous examples, drawn from the speech pathology and audiology literature, are used throughout this chapter and the chapters that follow. The chapter concludes, as do the other chapters in this part, with an Evaluation Checklist.

A brief word is necessary here about the Evaluation Checklists. Our intention in presenting the Checklists is to help the reader *focus* on those *key* elements of an article that deserve special and careful attention. We recognize that it is unlikely that most consumers of research will conduct the type of intensive analysis suggested by the Checklists, at least not in ordinary circumstances. We also recognize that because of the variety of research designs found in the literature, not all items on the Checklists will be applicable to all research reports. This is especially true for the Method Checklist. Nevertheless, the Checklists represent a didactic device that should be useful to the consumer, the would-be researcher, the researcher preparing a report of his or her study, and editorial consultants.

Chapter 7 deals with the Method section of the research article. It is in this section of the article that threats to internal and external validity are identified; thus, the Method section is of vital importance to the critical evaluator. Chapter 7 is divided into the three typical components of a Method section: subjects, materials, and procedures. The reader is urged to pay careful heed to how subjects are selected, how they are assigned to treatment groups, the reliability and validity of any tests used in the research, the research design employed, and whether the design reduces confounding threats to internal and external validity. The Checklist at the end of the chapter again serves to focus on those critical features of the Method section that require the careful attention of the reader.

The next chapter is concerned with the results section of an article. Nothing is introduced in Chapter 8 that has not already been treated in Chapter 5. The whole point of this chapter is simply to illustrate the concepts and principles detailed earlier. We were concerned about possible overlap and redundancy in Chapters 5 and 8, but we decided that when it comes to the evaluation of a Results section, one probably cannot be too redundant. The major topics covered in this chapter deal with the adequacy of figures and tables, with the appropriateness of the statistical treatment, and with the evaluation of an author's interpretation of the data analysis.

The final chapter of Part II outlines the criteria to be used in evaluating the Discussion and Conclusions section of the research article. Here as in the

Introduction section of an article, remarkably few guidelines are available to the critical evaluator. Yet, the Discussion and Conclusions section represents the culmination of a particular research effort and frequently is of considerable interest to the practitioner because of the possible implications for clinical practice. Some of the questions that are addressed in this chapter: Are the conclusions fairly and accurately drawn from the results? Are the limitations of the study identified? Are there implications for research, theory, or for application and do these implications stem from the data? Are comparisons with previous research fair and objective? The checklist concludes Chapter 9.

Reference

American Psychological Association. (1983). *Publication manual of the American Psychologcal Association* (3rd ed.). Washington, DC: Author.

6

The Introduction Section of the Research Article

Introduction

We have emphasized previously the importance of the problem in initiating and designing a research study. The Introduction section of the research article is of the utmost importance to the critical reader of the research literature. It is in this section that the researcher presents the rationale for doing the research. If the author fails in this task, the remainder of the article may founder as well. It cannot be emphasized too strongly that the research problem, as described in the introduction to the article, is the thread that ties together the Method, the Results, and the Discussion sections. In essence, the good introduction is very much like a legal brief. Just as a legal brief is designed to convince the judge or jury, so, too, is the introduction designed to convince the reader of the need and the value of the study being proposed.

The various components of the introduction to a research article are:

1. Title
2. Abstract
3. General statement of the problem
4. Rationale for the study
5. Review of the literature
6. Specific purposes, research questions, or hypotheses

These six components do not always appear as separate entities in this order in every research article. Different authors have different writing styles and preferences for the organization of the introduction. Each of these components is identified in one form or another in the *APA Publication Manual* (APA, 1983, pp. 22–25) as a key part in writing the introduction to a research article. Therefore, we will identify, describe, and exemplify each of these six components of the introduction in this chapter.

Title of the Article

The introduction to a research article actually begins with the title of the article. The title is important because it is the first thing the reader sees. It alerts the reader to an article that may be of professional interest. The title should identify the general problem area, including the specification of independent and dependent variables and the target population.

The *APA Publication Manual* (APA, 1983, p. 22) states that the "title should summarize the main idea of the paper" and that it should be "fully explanatory when standing alone" because a title has two main functions. The title informs readers about the article and is used as the basis for indexing the article in the journal's index and in the various abstracting services and journals (e.g., *dsh Abstracts*).

Three examples of research article titles are shown in Excerpts 6.1, 6.2, and 6.3.

EXCERPT 6.1

Effects of Stimulus Repetition Rate and Frequency on the Auditory Brainstem Response in Normal, Cochlear-impaired, and VIII Nerve/Brainstem-impaired Subjects.

SOURCE: Fowler, C. G., & Noffsinger, D. (1983). *Journal of Speech and Hearing Research*, **26**, 560–567.

The title shown in Excerpt 6.1 is long, but complete. It identifies the independent variables (stimulus repetition rate and frequency), the dependent variable (auditory brainstem response), and the target populations (normal, cochlear-impaired, and VIII nerve/brainstem-impaired subjects). The reader should have no difficulty in knowing what the article is about, and the article can be indexed quite well from the title alone.

EXCERPT 6.2

The Perception of Nonverbal Vocal Cues of Emotional Meaning by Language-disordered and Normal Children.

SOURCE: Courtright, J. A., & Courtright, I. C. (1983). *Journal of Speech and Hearing Research*, **26**, 412–417.

The title shown in Excerpt 6.2 is shorter, but it still conveys the essence of the study. The article is a comparison of abilities of normal and language-disordered children to interpret emotional meaning from nonverbal vocal cues.

EXCERPT 6.3

Acoustic Patterns of Apraxia of Speech.

SOURCE: Kent, R. D., & Rosenbek, J. C. (1983). *Journal of Speech and Hearing Research,* 26, 231–249.

Even a very short title can fully inform the reader about the nature of a study. In the six words of Excerpt 6.3, Kent and Rosenbeck have told us what their study is about. A reader would know immediately if the article is of interest and an abstracting service could do a reasonable job of indexing the article from the title.

In summary, the title of an article should capture the essence of the topic that was investigated. It should be concise, well written, and should identify the variables studied and the target population.

The Abstract

Many journals require a short abstract that briefly summarizes the major points of the article. The *APA Publication Manual* (APA, 1983, pp. 23–24) suggests that an empirical research article should contain an abstract of 100–150 words that describes the problem, the subjects, the method, the findings, and the conclusions. The manual further states that the abstract should be accurate, self-contained, concise, specific, comprehensive, and readable. It should be aimed at increasing the audience and the future retrievability of the article. Abstracts are not easy to write. Important, precise information must be packed into a small space. But the importance of the abstract is highlighted by the following statement (APA, 1983, p. 23):

> A well-prepared abstract can be the single most important paragraph in the article. An abstract (a) is read first, (b) may be the only part of an article that is actually read (readers frequently decide, on the basis of the abstract, whether to read the entire article), and (c) is an important means of access in locating and retrieving the article.

The abstract shown in Excerpt 6.4 is an example of an abstract that covers considerable ground in a small space. The first sentence states the purpose and identifies the subjects. The next few sentences describe the method and results; the last sentence deals with implications of the findings.

EXCERPT 6.4

The purpose of this study was to compare deaf speakers' ($n = 4$) laryngeal behavior during voiced and voiceless consonant productions to that of normal hearing subjects ($n = 4$). Laryngeal behavior during these two speaker groups' productions of six word-initial stop plosives (/b d g p t k/) and fricatives (/v z ð f s θ/) was visually observed by means of a flexible fiberoptic nasolaryngoscope (fiberscope). The visualizations and their acoustic correlates were audiovisually recorded. The audiovisual recordings were analyzed by means of both frame-by-frame categorical judgments of laryngeal behavior and broad phonetic transcriptions of the accuracy/inaccuracy of consonantal voicing. Results indicated that deaf speakers' laryngeal behavior during production of those consonants perceived as *accurately* voiced was comparable to that of normal speakers, whereas deaf speakers' laryngeal behavior during production of consonants perceived as *inaccurately* voiced generally differed in various ways from normal. Findings seem to suggest that some aspects of deaf speakers' atypical laryngeal behavior associated with inaccurately voiced consonants may be due to an aberrant linguistic system while other aspects may be due to inadequate laryngeal motor control.

SOURCE: Mahshie, J. J., & Conture, E. G. (1983). Deaf speakers' laryngeal behavior. *Journal of Speech and Hearing Research, 26,* 550–559.

The abstract shown in Excerpt 6.5 also deals concisely and clearly with the study reported thereafter. The purpose of the study is described, subjects

---

EXCERPT 6.5

The purpose of this study was to examine stutterers' and nonstutterers' fluent voice onset time (VOT) and fundamental frequency (F_0) contour measures from target syllables located at the beginning of a carrier phrase. Ten adult male stutterers were matched within one year of age with 10 adult male nonstutterers. Oscillographic and spectrographic analyses of subjects' VOT and F_0 at vowel onset, average vowel F_0, and speed and range of F_0 change were obtained from fluent productions of 18 stop consonant-vowel syllables. Results showed that VOTs for voiced stops and the range of F_0 change for voiceless stops were associated with significant between-group differences. All other dependent measures were not significantly different between the two groups. When compared with past research, these findings indicate that greater differences emerge between stutterers and nonstutterers when measures of fluency are taken at the beginning than in the middle of a carrier phrase. Implications for future research are discussed.

SOURCE: Healey, E. C., & Gutkin, B. (1984). Analysis of stutterers' voice onset times and fundamental frequency contours during fluency. *Journal of Speech and Hearing Research, 27,* 219–225.

and method are briefly treated, results are summarized, and a conclusion is briefly presented.

A word of caution: the adequacy of a research article cannot be evaluated simply by reading the abstract. The purpose of the abstract is to provide an overview of the article so that the reader can determine quickly if the article should be read. What may seem on the basis of the abstract to be an exciting and original contribution to the literature may on closer inspection of the article itself turn out to be a poor study, both conceptually and methodologically. The only way to determine the quality of a research study is to read the whole article.

General Statement of the Problem

We have identified four major components in the text of the introduction to a research article. Although these components are frequently woven together in the introduction and may not receive separate subheadings to help the reader identify them, the evaluation process is facilitated if the reader can identify these components for the purpose of analysis.

The first component is the general statement of the problem. Here the author sets forth the topic of the article, including the major variables and the target population. The problem can be described in a variety of ways and different authors have different preferences and styles.

The general statement of the problem lends perspective to the specific empirical operations of a research article. It provides a context for the specific purpose, method, and results to make the conclusions meaningful. The general problem statement may be a short first paragraph or it may run through a few initial paragraphs, including references to previous research, to help establish the context of the research.

A simple, straightforward general problem statement is shown in Excerpt 6.6. In a short paragraph, the author clearly states what general issues will be addressed. The concept of speech intelligibility will be analyzed, the variables that influence it will be identified, and their relative importance will be considered. Later in the article, the author describes a study of the influence of specific syntactic and phonologic variables in the oral speech intelligibility of deaf children.

EXCERPT 6.6

The oral speech intelligibility of hearing-impaired individuals has long been the fulcrum of the discussion on how they should be educated, and yet it is a concept that is difficult to define and about which there are many questions, both unanswered and unposed. Because the oral speech intelligibility of hearing-impaired children is likely to remain an important issue, it is worthwhile to try to analyze the concept in great detail, to pinpoint the many factors which influence it, and to understand the extent to which they do so.

SOURCE: Monsen, R. B. (1983). The oral speech intelligibility of hearing-impaired talkers. *Journal of Speech and Hearing Disorders, 48,* 286–296.

The example in Excerpt 6.7 shows the opening two paragraphs of a study of aging and the acoustic reflex. This general problem statement includes citations of previous research literature and a brief summary of some previous findings that help to provide a context for the research reported later in the article. The summary of previous research findings sets the stage for the current investigation.

EXCERPT 6.7

Recent reports have indicated that the aging process alters selected aural acoustic-immittance[1] characteristics of the middle-ear transmission system (Alberti & Kristensen, 1972; Handler & Margolis, 1977; Jerger, Hayes, Anthony, & Mauldin, 1978; Jerger, Jerger, & Mauldin, 1972; Silman, 1979b; Silman & Gelfand, 1979; Thompson, Sills, Recke, & Bui, 1979, 1980). The results from these studies revealed the following general characteristics as a function of increasing age.

1. Static-immittance changes are minimal to ~ 60 years.
2. Acoustic-reflex thresholds for tonal stimuli increase, decrease, or remain unchanged, depending upon the study.
3. Acoustic-reflex thresholds for broadband noise increase or remain unchanged, again depending upon the study.
4. The magnitude of the acoustic-reflex growth tends to be reduced.

As an extension of the acoustic-reflex studies on young adults from this laboratory (Wilson, 1979; Wilson & McBride, 1978; Wilson, Steckler, Jones, & Margolis, 1978), the present investigation was undertaken to clarify some of the controversies regarding the influence of the aging process on acoustic-reflex characteristics. In addition, it was of interest to document the variability of the various middle-ear immittance measurements and to study the relationship between conductance and susceptance during the reflexive state.

[1]Throughout this paper, the use of *immittance, admittance,* or *impedance* implies aural acoustic-immittance, aural acoustic-admittance (acoustic mmho = $m^3/10^8Pa\cdot s$), or aural acoustic-impedance (acoustic ohm = $10^5Pa\cdot s/m^3$).

SOURCE: Wilson, R. H. (1981). The effects of aging on the magnitude of the acoustic reflex. *Journal of Speech and Hearing Research, 24,* 406–414.

Excerpt 6.8 shows the first three paragraphs of a study of developmental disfluency and emerging grammar. The first paragraph identifies the relationship under investigation, the second paragraph shows the lack of knowledge of this relationship, and the third paragraph sets forth the general plan for studying the problem.

EXCERPT 6.8

Young children in the process of learning to talk display varying degrees of disfluent speech (Adams, 1932; Branscom, Hughes, & Oxtoby, 1955; Davis, 1939, 1940a, 1940b; Egland, 1955; Johnson, 1955; Métraux, 1950; Silverman, 1971, 1972a, 1972b, 1973). As language learning and the development of fluent speech co-occur during the preschool years, a question exists as to what extent observed disfluent behavior in nonstuttering children is related to their emerging language.

Parental reports of the existence of disfluency from the moment children begin to use two-word phrases during the second year of life are common, but few systematic explorations of this period of developmental disfluency have been made. Several investigators have reported on group data with preschool children, using the 2-year-old child as the lower limit of their population (Davis, 1939; Johnson, 1955; Métraux, 1950; Hughes, Note 1). There are no published studies that describe either the frequency of disfluency types used by 2-year-old children or subsequent changes in the distribution of disfluency types with development. No studies have used longitudinal data to investigate variation in individual patterns of disfluency observed during early language acquisition.

The purpose of this longitudinal study was to describe the characteristics of developmental disfluency in the spontaneous speech of four nonstuttering children as language developed from single words through early multiword utterances. In a related study, the same data were examined to determine if developmental disfluency covaried over time with the emergence of specific semantic-syntactic structures in each child's speech during the early acquisition of grammar.

SOURCE: Colburn, N., & Mysak, E. D. (1982). Developmental disfluency and emerging grammar: I. Disfluency characteristics in early syntactic utterances. *Journal of Speech and Hearing Research, 25,* 414–420.

In all of these introductory statements, the essence of the general problem area is defined along with an implicit or explicit statement of the importance of the problem. Literature citations are used, if necessary, to buttress the authors' position. As we will see later, the reader's substantive background in the area investigated plays a critical role in the evaluation of the introductory section. Familiarity with the theory and data concerning a particular topic is necessary for the reader to evaluate the arguments developed in an introduction. Even the novice reader, however, should be able to follow the *logic* of the arguments presented and should understand the importance of the general problem.

The Rationale for the Study

The rationale for the study constitutes the second component of the text of the introduction and should stem from the general statement of the problem. The rationale presents the reasons for doing the particular study. It is here that the author justifies the selection of the particular independent and dependent variables studied with the specific population. Because it is impossible to investigate all aspects of the general problem in one research study, the rationale presents the case for studying selected aspects of the problem and may identify limitations imposed on the study.

The major question that the critical reader needs to ask about the rationale is whether the reasons for doing the study are clearly and explicitly stated and documented with literature citations. A variety of reasons are offered by investigators to support the importance and need for the study. The author may cite and attempt to document the inadequacy of previous research in the area under investigation. Another reason for doing the research is to follow-up on previous research or to resolve conflicting or inconclusive results reported by other investigators. Still another reason offered by researchers is to provide empirical data related to theoretical aspects of the phenomenon under question. Finally, the rationale may be based on the paucity or absence of previous research in a given area. Any one or combination of these reasons might be used to develop a need for the study.

Excerpt 6.9 is from a study concerning the use of contralateral masking in auditory brainstem response (ABR) measurement. Humes and Ochs developed their rationale on two bases. First, they cited the results of previous research that were conflicting with regard to the necessity for contralateral masking during the measurement of ABR. Second, the authors pointed out the importance of masking effects in the clinical interpretation of ABR measurements. Their first two paragraphs present the problem and review some recent studies that showed different results. The third paragraph points to the clinical importance of the problem and identifies subjects with profound unilateral hearing loss as an important population for consideration of crossover brainstem responses and interaural attentuation for the click stimuli used in ABR testing.

EXCERPT 6.9

Over the past 10 years, numerous investigators have examined the effects of a variety of parameters on the auditory brainstem response (ABR), that is, the series of neuroelectric potentials measured from the scalp within 10–12 msec following the presentation of transient acoustic stimuli (e.g., Davis, 1976; Fria, 1980). Much of this research activity has led, either directly or indirectly, to the establishment of clinical procedures for measurement of the ABR. One stimulus-related variable that has been studied recently is the introduction of masking noise to the contralateral or nontest ear. Existing literature is unclear as to whether masking of the nontest ear is necessary for clinical measurement of the ABR. Finitzo-Hieber, Hecox, and Cone (1979), for example, obtained ABRs from two adults with unilateral deafness. No identifiable responses were observed when stimulating the poorer ear at levels of 110–117 dB peak equivalent sound pressure level (p.e. SPL re: 20 μPa). The authors concluded, therefore, that contralateral masking may not be necessary with ABR. Chiappa, Gladstone, and Young (1979), on the other hand, recorded recognizable waveforms of increased latency upon stimulation of the poorer ear in two cases of complete unilateral hearing loss when the nontest ear was not masked. The addition of masking to the nontest (better) ear abolished the recorded response. Based on these findings, the latter authors recommended the use of contralateral masking in clinical situations.

Chiappa et al. (1979) also studied the effects of contralateral masking on the ABR of normal-hearing young adults. Click-evoked ABRs were obtained from 12 normal hearers in both unmasked and masked conditions for a stimulus presentation level of 60 dB SL. The masking stimulus was a broadband noise presented at a "sensation level" (SL) of 60 dB. The reference used to establish SL, however, was not specified. That is, it was unclear if 60 dB SL referred to a threshold for the noise, or if it was referenced to a level sufficient to mask a 60 dB SL click. Nonetheless, Chiappa et al. (1979) were unable to observe any effect of the contralateral masking noise on the latencies and amplitudes of the ABR in normal hearers. They noted, however, that there was some change in the shape of the waveform in several subjects brought about by the addition of masking to the nontest ear.

The effects of presenting a masking noise to the nontest ear on the response obtained from the test ear are critical to the successful interpretation of the ABR in clinical settings. One must be aware of the limitations on the use of the unmasked and masked ABRs in order to localize a lesion effectively or to establish the degree of impairment accurately. In view of the foregoing, the present study evaluated in more detail the effects of contralateral masking on the ABR. The effects of contralateral masking on the ABR of normal hearers were studied in a systematic fashion using a variety of stimulus and masker intensity levels. In addition, four subjects with profound unilateral sensorineural hearing loss were studied. From the latter subjects we obtained information regarding the existence of a crossover brainstem response and the estimation of interaural attenuation for click stimuli.

SOURCE: Humes, L. E., & Ochs, M. G. (1982). Use of contralateral masking in the measurement of the auditory brainstem response. *Journal of Speech and Hearing Research 25*, 528–535.

The introductory paragraphs shown in Excerpt 6.10 present the general and specific rationales from a study of airflow characteristics of normal and hearing-impaired speakers' fricative productions. The first paragraph presents a general rationale for studying speech physiology in order to understand better the speech production problems of hearing impaired speakers. The subsequent paragraphs review some of the important literature on speech physiology with the hearing impaired. The fourth and fifth paragraphs present a more specific rationale for studying the aerodynamics of fricative production. Both basic considerations about the nature of aberrant speech production and applied considerations about remediation of the speech of hearing-impaired persons are entertained in this rationale.

EXCERPT 6.10

Identification of the factors which contribute to the reduced speech intelligibility of some hearing-impaired persons has been addressed primarily from an acoustic and/or descriptive frame of reference. Findings have included errors or disorders in prosody (phrasing and intonation), articulation, vowel duration, breath control, timing, tension/harshness, nasality, breathiness/weakness, pitch control, pitch register, and rate of syllable articulation (Boone, 1966; Hudgins, 1934; Hudgins & Numbers, 1942; Markides, 1970; Miller, 1946; Monsen, 1974; Silverman, 1960; Stevens, Nickerson, & Rollins, 1983; Subtelny, 1976). The descriptions of the speech errors of the hearing impaired are generally consistent, but fail to identify the underlying nature of the reduced speech intelligibility. The study of speech physiology, however, can provide insights relative to the fundamental properties of speech production. Zimmermann and Rettaliata (1981) have suggested that analyses of the physiological parameters of speech produced by hearing-impaired persons are important because they may lead to a better understanding of the speech errors which reduce intelligibility and may assist in the development of remediation procedures designed to modify aberrant physiological patterns.

Early investigations into the physiology of speech produced by the hearing impaired appear to have focused primarily on the respiratory mechanism. Authors such as Hudgins (1934, 1937) and Rawlings (1936) reported that many of the speech and voice deficits exhibited by the hearing impaired were directly correlated with aberrant respiratory characteristics. Hudgins and Numbers (1942), however, concluded that the intelligibility of hearing-impaired speakers depended not only on respiratory behaviors but also on proper coordination between respiratory and articulatory mechanisms.

Recent physiological investigations regarding the speech of the hearing-impaired have included measures of respiratory kinematics (Forner & Hixon, 1977; Whitehead, 1983), laryngeal dynamics (Mahshie, 1980; Metz & Whitehead, Note 1), and interarticulatory timing (Huntington, Harris, & Sholer, 1968; McGarr & Harris, 1983; McGarr & Löfqvist, 1982; Rothman, 1977). These investigations have focused primarily on one physiological component of the speech mechanism and have utilized relatively small numbers of subjects, usually because of the invasive and/or highly sophisticated nature of the data collection procedures. Despite the limitations, there is mounting evidence from these investigations that some hearing-impaired speakers significantly mismanage and fail to coordinate the biomechanical aspects of speech properly. The data from many of these investigations also suggest that a relationship exists between aberrant biomechanical functioning and the degree of speech intelligibility exhibited by the hearing-impaired individual.

Data regarding the aerodynamic components of speech produced by the hearing impaired also have been reported (Gilbert, 1974; Hutchinson, Kornhauser, Beasley, & Beasley, 1978; Hutchinson & Smith, 1976; Whitehead & Barefoot, 1980). The study of speech aerodynamics in the hearing impaired is critical because measures of airflow and/or air pressure are a direct reflection of the management of the entire physiological process for speech. Furthermore, the specific measure of airflow during speech production is accomplished with a noninvasive procedure which allows for data collection on a large number of subjects with relative ease. Gilbert (1974) and Hutchinson and Smith (1976) have reported both differences and similarities between hearing-impaired and normally hearing speakers for measures of airflow and/or air pressure during production of plosive consonants. Because of the large variability in speech production skills within the hearing-impaired population, Whitehead and Barefoot (1980) categorized hearing-impaired adults on the basis of overall speech intelligibility and degree of hearing loss. These authors reported consistent similarities in measures of airflow for plosive consonants between normally hearing and intelligible hearing-impaired speakers and consistent differences between semi-intelligible hearing-impaired speakers and both the normally hearing and intelligible hearing-impaired groups.

Presently, there appear to be very few data regarding the aerodynamics of fricative consonants produced by hearing-impaired adults (Hutchinson & Smith, 1976). Such information is necessary in order to gain a better understanding of the dynamics regarding the physiological management of speech by hearing-impaired persons. The purpose of the present study, therefore, was to investigate the patterns of airflow for fricative consonants produced by hearing-impaired young adults categorized according to speech intelligibility and degree of hearing loss.

SOURCE: Whitehead, R. L., & Barefoot, S. M. (1983). Airflow characteristics of fricative consonants produced by normally hearing and hearing-impaired speakers. *Journal of Speech and Hearing Research, 26,* 185–194.

In the example shown in Excerpt 6.11, Young developed a rationale for studying articulation effort. His rationale was based on a careful review of previous research studies and a critical analysis of their results and limitations. His first two paragraphs review the previous studies and point to their discrepancies and the third paragraph describes some procedural problems with such studies. Finally, in the fourth paragraph, he states his goals as a consequence of his review and analysis.

EXCERPT 6.11

Recent studies by Locke (1972) and Parnell and Amerman (1977) have shown that judgments of articulation effort are associated with phonological acquisition, frequency of occurrence of sounds in English, and pattern of children's substitutions. An earlier study by Malecot (1955) was concerned with force of articulation as a factor in the lenis-fortis distinction.

Although all three studies employed similar paried-comparisons procedures to rank selected consonants on an articulation effort dimension, the results were greatly discrepant. Parnell and Amerman (1977) and Malecot (1955) used a VCV context and had observers voice each stimulus. A correlation (tau) between the 12 consonants common to both studies generated a nonsignificant index of .15. (Malecot's study is described in a brief paragraph and the procedures must be inferred.) Locke (1972) employed a CV stimulus and had observers whisper. In comparison with the 13 consonants in common ranked by Parnell and Amerman's whispered task, Locke's ranks generated a correlation (tau) of −.18, also nonsignificant. Daniloff (1973) and Parnell and Amerman (1977) have suggested how important procedural differences among the three studies may have accounted for the disagreement in results.

Apart from procedural differences, the three studies used certain nonstandard design and analysis methods which may have contributed to some of the disaccord in results. All three had observers underline on typed lists which member of the consonant pair was harder to say or required the most effort. The consequences of this procedure were that (1) the order of the pairs was the same for all observers or for groups of observers, (2) there was no systematic control of the space effect—a consonant was always in the same position in a pair, and (3) the observers could review previous judgments. In Locke's study, moreover, the observers performed the task in groups of 11, and there was no check on whether observers actually whispered aloud or made their judgments on some other basis. With respect to the mode of analysis, Locke (1972) and Parnell and Amerman (1977) ranked the consonants by summing judgments across observers; Malecot probably did the same since he appears to refer to Guilford's Composite Standard Method of Scaling (Guilford, 1954, p. 169). A limitation to ranking the consonants by summing across observers is that a rank order can be achieved even when observers cannot perform the task or when observers disagree with each other. None of the studies provided data to show that observers could actually perform the discriminations reliably or that they agreed with each other if they could.

The validity of a construct such as articulation effort needs to be established before it can have any useful explanatory or predictive potential, especially when the construct reflects a perceptual continuum likely to be multidimensional. Determining the physiological or acoustical correlates of such a continuum may be desirable, but to do so requires the prior demonstration that the dimension shows some perceptual reality. I have examined in detail this position in previous articles (Young, 1969a, 1969b, 1975; Young & Downs, 1968). The goals of the present study, therefore, were to repeat the paired-comparison task without the design limitations of the earlier studies, and to comment on the validity or reality of the articulation effort construct.

SOURCE: Young, M. A. (1981). Articulation effort: transitivity and observer agreement. *Journal of Speech and Hearing Research, 24,* 224–232.

Excerpt 6.12 shows the first two paragraphs of an article that compared two methods of measuring vowel formants. The first paragraph describes the importance of vowel formants in the perception of vowels. The second paragraph stresses the importance of the accuracy of the measurement of vowel formants as a rationale for the comparison of two available techniques used in speech research.

EXCERPT 6.12

A widely accepted premise in the field of speech research is that vowel sounds are perceived, or decoded, by locating the frequencies of the formants or by reference to the overall formant pattern. Although the exact process of vowel perception remains a matter of speculation, the importance of vowel formant frequencies has been demonstrated convincingly by studies of perception using synthetic speech (Cooper, Delattre, Liberman, Borst, & Gerstman, 1952; Flanagan, 1955; Fry, Abramson, Eimas, & Liberman, 1962; Liberman, In-gemann, Lisker, Delattre, & Cooper, 1959). It is not surprising that one of the most frequently referenced papers on acoustic phonetics is one containing the most comprehensive measurements of the vowel formants of American English (Peterson & Barney, 1952). It is generally acknowledged that the first two for-mants, and in some cases the first three, are the most important for vowel perception. In addition to the formant frequencies of a vowel, the bandwidths of the formants, the fundamental frequency contour, the relative levels of the formants, formant transitions, and the length of the vowel are secondary factors which play some role in the identity of a particular vowel (Carlson & Granström, 1979; Carlson, Granström, & Klatt, 1979).

Because of the importance of determining formant frequencies, it is neces-sary to pay particular attention to the measurement technique and to the degree of accuracy which can be achieved through it. Although formant frequencies have been measured for a variety of different studies (cf. Angelocci, Kopp, & Holbrook, 1964; Eguchi & Hirsh, 1969; Monsen, 1976; Peterson & Barney, 1952), the accuracy of these measurements is still a matter of some conjecture. Most of the studies have used spectrographic techniques. Lindblom (1962) estimated the accuracy of spectrographic measurement to be approximately equal to the fundamental frequency divided by 4. A quite different and more recent technique for measuring formant frequencies is linear prediction analy-sis (Atal & Hanauer, 1971; Atal & Schroeder, 1978; Wakita, 1973). Since this technique is potentially of great use in speech research, it is important to assess its accuracy.

SOURCE: Monsen, R. B., & Engebretson, A. M. (1983). The accuracy of formant frequency measurements: A comparison of spectrographic analysis and linear prediction. *Journal of Speech and Hearing Research, 26,* 89–97.

The rationale shown in Excerpt 6.13 takes a somewhat different approach. This argument is not based so much on a review of discrepant results or the need to compare measurements for accuracy but rather on a logical develop-ment of the implications of the nature of different relationships among vari-ables. The relationships among acoustic variables and fluency enhancement have both theoretical implications regarding the process of speech motor control and practical implications regarding the enhancement of fluency through therapy. Notice how the article introduces these notions with a brief literature review in the first paragraph and then develops the argument logically in the next two paragraphs.

EXCERPT 6.13

In the decade following Wingate's seminal articles (1969, 1970) on artificially induced fluency, considerable research effort was directed toward identifying underlying conditions related to fluency enhancement among stutterers. The emphasis of much of this research was on isolating acoustic speech parameters of stutterers' fluent speech that varied concomitantly with stuttering frequency. For example, the relationships among changes in vocal sound pressure level (Adams & Hutchinson, 1974; Adams & Moore, 1972; Conture, 1974), vocal fundamental frequency, and vowel duration and the growth of fluency associated with stutterers' speaking in the presence of loud noise and speaking in accordance with a rhythmic stimulus (Brayton & Conture, 1978) were investigated. Attention was paid to the relationships among changes in vowel duration, continuity of phonation, and vocal sound pressure level and the growth of fluency associated with stutterers' singing (Colcord & Adams, 1979; Healey, Mallard, & Adams, 1976) and choral speaking (Adams & Ramig, 1980). Additionally, it is clear from both perceptual (Runyan & Adams, 1978) and acoustic studies (Metz, Onufrak, & Ogburn, 1979) that stuttering therapy can alter certain acoustic properties of the stutterer's fluent speech.

　These and other related studies have advanced our knowledge regarding which acoustic variables associated with the fluent speech of stutterers change concomitantly with the growth of fluency. However, these studies are based on group data and consequently provide limited information about the nature of the relationships between acoustic variable changes and fluency enhancement. Furthermore, there is no a priori reason to assume that all systematic changes in the acoustic properties of stutterers' speech are necessarily related to fluency enhancement. Some of these alterations may reflect changes in the operation of the motor control processes that underlie fluency enhancement, whereas others may be systematic by-products of the particular fluency-enhancing condition. That is, a given fluency-enhancing condition (or therapy procedure) may have two types of effects on a stutterer's speech: (a) one that imposes changes in speech that directly enhance fluency, and which are reflected in certain acoustic changes and whose occurrence is probably common, to greater or lesser degrees, to all fluency-enhancing conditions; and (b) one that imposes changes in speech that do not directly enhance fluency, and which are also reflected in certain acoustic changes but whose occurrence is probably an idiosyncratic result of ancillary aspects of the particular fluency-enhancing condition. By examining the relationship between stuttering frequency and various acoustic features of stutterers' speech across individuals (in addition to examining group data), we may obtain some clues regarding those variables that are most closely related to changes in stuttering frequency. Although correlation does not necessarily imply causation, acoustic variables closely related to stuttering frequency more likely reflect control processes underlying fluency than variables that are statistically independent of the stuttering frequency dimension within the population of stutterers.

In the present study we explored such relationships in more detail. Specifically, we examined several acoustic variables measured from a single group of stutterers. These measurements included both traditional and previously unexplored acoustic properties of stutterers' fluent speech production. Furthermore, we examined the relationship between these acoustic variables and fluency within a group of mild-to-severe stutterers both prior to and after a concentrated program of stuttering therapy.

SOURCE: Metz, D. E., Samar, V. J., & Sacco, P. R. (1983). Acoustic analysis of stutterers' fluent speech before and after therapy. *Journal of Speech and Hearing Research, 26,* 531–536.

As these examples have shown, a major part of the introduction to a research article spells out the reasons for doing the particular study. The rationale describes the need for the research. The logic of the arguments presented, with appropriate citations from the literature, should convince the reader of the value of the investigation. The rationale may take different forms, depending on the nature of study. Some introductions stress the practical nature of a study such as the need to assess the accuracy of a measurement. Others stress the need to resolve conflicting results or conclusions from previous studies. Many studies develop their rationales on the basis of the importance of the research for theoretical or practical applications. In any case, the rationale for the study is an important component of the text of the introduction.

Review of the Literature

The third component of the text of an introduction is the review of literature. The literature review is not really a separate part of an introduction, but it is the fabric from which the statement of the problem and rationale are woven. The literature citations not only serve to document the need for the study but they also help to put the research into context or historical perspective. Through the use of appropriate references, the researcher identifies how the investigation reported fits into the general theme of research in the same problem area. In a sense, the literature citations pay tribute to those who have gone before. In another sense, the literature citations allow the reader to examine the sources used by the author to make the case for the study. Thus, the reader has an opportunity to evaluate directly the adequacy of the literature citations and to determine whether, in fact, the citations used justify the research reported.

The literature review, then, should be evaluated in regard to (1) the degree to which it helps to place the general problem into perspective and (2) the degree to which it helps to develop the rationale for the study. Different authors have different styles and preferences for the way they use the literature review in relation to the other components of the text of the introduction. For example, Colburn and Mysak in Excerpt 6.8 use the literature review mainly to place the general problem in perspective, whereas Young, in Excerpt 6.11, uses the literature review to develop his rationale. Whitehead and Barefoot in Excerpt 6.10 use the literature review throughout the introduction to develop the general problem and the rationale for the study. Also, some authors cite a string of references and then summarize their general results as Wilson did in Excerpt 6.7. In other cases, authors cite each reference and briefly summarize the findings of each one, as was done by Humes and Ochs in Excerpt 6.9.

Sometimes the literature review does stand on its own, especially if the author's intent is to review new literature or literature from areas that are probably unfamiliar to most readers of a particular journal. An example of this can be seen in Excerpt 6.14 where literature from the areas of gerontology and nursing is briefly reviewed. This literature is likely to be unfamiliar to most speech pathologists and audiologists and needs to be summarized on its own prior to the development of a general problem statement and rationale.

EXCERPT 6.14

The fastest growing age group in the United States are those persons 65 years of age and older (Brotman,1977), and thus, by the year 2000, 12% of our population will be elderly. As we age, our special needs multiply. Many of the elderly require supportive services to meet their housing, food, health care, financial and social needs. While a majority of the aged can function independently or with community support, at least 5% become institutionalized. In 1975 there were over one million people 65 years old and above residing in 23,000 long-term care settings (Health Resources Statistics, 1976). This number represents a dramatic increase from the previous decade, and we can expect even more elderly people will become institutionalized in the next 25 years.

Relocation to a long-term care setting, such as a nursing home or chronic disease hospital, generates a series of personal and social problems for the older person. Social gerontologists have investigated the effects of institutionalization on the elderly (Ainsworth, 1977; Bennett, 1963; Kahana, 1971; Lieberman & Lakin, 1963; Wessen, 1964), the criteria for adjustment to long-term care (Bennett & Nahemow, 1965; Havighurst, 1968; Lowenthal & Haven, 1968), and the social interaction and organization of such settings (Lawton, 1968; Rosow, 1967; Weinstock & Bennett, 1968). An underlying and recurrent theme in this literature is that *communication* is a factor in the integration and adjustment of older people to institutional life. Similarly, the nursing literature emphasizes the strong relationship between staff-patient communication and effective nursing care (Collins, 1977; Lewis, 1973; Meyers, 1964; Shipper & Leonard,

1965). Collins (1977) states that communication is the core of the nurse-patient relationship.

SOURCE: Lubinski, R., Morrison, E. B., & Rigrodsky, S. (1981). Perception of spoken communication by elderly chronically ill patients in an institutional setting. *Journal of Speech and Hearing Disorders, 46*, 405–412.

There are several important questions for the critical evaluator of research to ask about the review of literature in the introduction to a research article. Most of these questions assume some knowledge of the topic on the part of the reader of the article.

First, how thorough is the literature review? Are there important omissions that might change the nature of the rationale or the perspective of the problem? Space limitations in a journal obviously place some constraints on the scope of any literature review. It is simply impossible to cite all the pertinent literature without running into objections by a journal editor who is interested in conserving valuable space. Nonetheless, the key references should be cited to substantiate the need for the study. Despite the apparent thoroughness of a particular literature review, the reader must still determine if key references have been omitted. It is here that the reader's background and expertise in the particular topic of an article play a crucial role in the evaluation process. It is extremely difficult to judge the thoroughness of the literature review without familiarity with the relevant literature.

How recent are the literature citations? Has the author overlooked recent work in reviewing the literature? This does not mean that older references should not be cited. Some older references are classics in a field and have had such a germinal influence on so many studies since their publication that they are constantly referred to. See, for example, Excerpt 6.12 where Monsen and Engebretson comment on the classic work of Peterson and Barney that was published in 1952 and state that it is not surprising that this reference is so often cited. The point is that the author has an obligation to cite the relevant work, new and old, that is necessary to place the problem in perspective and develop a convincing rationale. It may be that there is no recent literature on a given topic because the article represents renewed interest in a topic that received considerable attention 20 or 30 years ago but little attention in the last 5 or 10 years. Here the researcher may be justified in citing only older studies to make the case for a new study. In all instances, when recent literature on a particular topic does exist and is relevant, it should be cited.

A third point is whether the review is critical of previous literature and whether the criticism is objective, unbiased, and justified. Have the data of the previous studies been accurately reported and interpreted? Were the conclusions of the previous research criticized fairly? These are not easy questions to answer because they require the reader to refer to the original studies to determine if the criticisms were justified.

The next question is whether the literature citations are relevant to the purpose and to the need for the study. Once again, the ideal way to evaluate the relevancy of the literature review is to be knowledgeable about the subject matter under investigation. We raise the question of relevancy but we cannot answer it for the reader. There is no easy way of evaluating relevancy without some in-depth familiarity with the topic.

Finally, the careful evaluator of research should be alert to the overuse of unpublished research, to citations from obscure references, to frequent reference to materials appearing in publications that are inaccessible. The major problem is that the reader cannot consult the original sources to determine if the researcher has cited them correctly, drawn appropriate conclusions from them, and so forth. The researcher's use of these citations may also suggest research that is out of the mainstream, idiosyncratic, or unimportant.

In summary, the literature review is at the heart of the introduction to the research report. It is of fundamental importance for the critical reader of research to evaluate carefully the adequacy of the literature citations. Special attention should be given to the extent and thoroughness of the review, the recency and relevance of the citations, the objectivity and accuracy of the criticism of previous research. In the final analysis, the reader of the research report must bring expertise, experience, and knowledge to the evaluation of the literature citations. And, if need be, the reader must return to the cited sources to fully appreciate, understand, and evaluate this aspect of the introduction.

Statement of Purpose, Research Questions, and Hypotheses

The introduction of a research article usually concludes with a specific statement of the purpose of the research, with one or more research questions, or with testable hypotheses. Whichever form is used, this section represents the logical culmination of the general problem statement and rationale. As such, the specific purpose, question, or hypothesis should relate directly to what has preceded it. It is important that the statement be clear and precise. If possible, the statement should allow the reader to identify the independent and dependent variables and the type of research strategy used to study them.

Excerpt 6.15 shows the statement of purpose from a study that compared normal and apraxic speakers on a number of acoustical measures. The statement is broken down into five specific objectives for description of segmental and prosodic characteristics of apraxia. These specific objectives followed quite naturally from the literature review that stressed the need to define and quantify terms used to describe apraxia of speech. The results of the study are later presented in an orderly fashion that follows the outline shown in this statement of specific objectives.

EXCERPT 6.15

This study sought to determine:

1. if the utterances of apraxic subjects are lengthened in comparison to the utterances of normal-speaking subjects

and, if so:

2. whether differential lengthening effects exist as a function of the segmental properties or the syllabic length of utterances

3. whether apraxic and normal speech are distinguished by nondurational aspects of prosody, such as relative syllable intensity or F_0-frequency contour

4. if spectrograms show evidence of phonetic (subphonemic) errors in apraxic speech

5. the degree to which acoustic patterns of apraxic speech confirm perceptually based descriptions of the disorder.

These five objectives were selected because they are within the scope of an acoustic study and because they should lead to a refined description of the segmental and prosodic features of the disorder.

SOURCE: Kent, R. D., & Rosenbek, J. C. (1983). Acoustic patterns of apraxia of speech. *Journal of Speech and Hearing Research, 26,* 231–249.

The statement of purpose and specific research questions shown in Excerpt 6.16 come from a longitudinal study of the language development of hearing children of deaf parents. The two specific purposes of the study are stated first, and then the specific questions and subquestions to be answered are spelled out in detail. The reader can see from the purposes that the study is developmental in nature and that it also includes a comparison of the children's language when talking with their deaf mothers and with a hearing adult. The dependent variables to be examined developmentally are clearly identified. The purposes of the study stem quite naturally from the rationale developed in the introduction and the results section of the article is broken down according to the sequence of the research questions listed in the excerpt. Readers should have no problem in following the presentation of the results, given the outlining of the specific research questions in the introduction.

EXCERPT 6.16

The purpose of this study was (1) to compare the language development of five two-year-old hearing children of deaf parents with the language development of normal children reported in the developmental literature described above;

and (2) to study the discourse interactions of these children with their mothers and with a hearing adult to determine the effect of the mothers' defective speech on the children's ability to process and learn from the mothers' oral language. The specific questions to be answered by this study are as follows:

(1), Is the proportional distribution of the semantic-syntactic relations encoded in these children's utterances similar to that found in the messages of children from hearing environments?

(2), Are the forms these children use to code the semantic relations different from those used by children from hearing environments in terms of the following:
- the ordering of subject-verb-object relationships?
- the sequence of development of Brown's 14 grammatical morphemes?
- the predominant use of pronominal or nominal references for linguistic representation?

(3), Are the oral discourse patterns of these children similar to those of children from hearing environments, and do they vary according to whether the recipient is hearing or deaf in terms of the following:
- imitations?
- categories of contingent speech?

(4), Does the mothers' speech contain grammatical morphemes and systematic ordering of constituents?

SOURCE: Schiff, N. B. (1979). The influence of deviant maternal input on the development of language during the preschool years. *Journal of Speech and Hearing Research*, 22, 581–603.

The example shown in Excerpt 6.17 shows the statement of the specific research question and hypothesis from a study of the effects of hearing-aid use on speech discrimination and listening effort. The statement makes it obvious that the independent variable is hearing-aid use and the dependent variables are speech discrimination and listening effort. The specific procedure used is identified as the double stimulation procedure. Because this is a relatively novel method in speech and hearing research, the author defined the procedure and explained its use in the introduction. Also note that the author advanced a specific hypothesis about what might be expected as a result of hearing-aid use. It should be pointed out that this is *not* the null hypothesis tested by a statistical significance test. Although it used to be common for authors to list the various null hypotheses tested, this is relatively uncommon now because the null hypothesis is usually implied by the statement of a specific purpose or question.

EXCERPT 6.17

In this investigation, a double stimulation procedure was employed to measure effects of hearing aid use on speech discrimination and listening effort. Speech discrimination scores provided the primary task measure. Listening effort devoted to performance of the speech discrimination task was assessed with probe reaction times providing the secondary task measure. The question asked was, "How does use of amplification affect speech discrimination and listening effort of hearing-impaired individuals?" The research hypothesis was that with hearing aid use hearing-impaired individuals would have improved speech discrimination with reduced listening effort.

SOURCE: Downs, D. W. (1982). Effects of hearing aid use on speech discrimination and listening effort. *Journal of Speech and Hearing Disorders, 47,* 189–193.

Excerpt 6.18 shows the statement of the specific purpose from an experiment on the effect of segment and pause manipulations on the identification of treated stutterers. The statement begins with a brief rationale for the particular manipulations used to change tape-recorded speech samples for presentation to listeners and, then, states what effect will be studied. It is clear that rate is the independent variable to be manipulated and that labelling behavior of listeners is the dependent variable that may change as a result of manipulation of the independent variable. The rationale for this specific purpose is clearly developed in the introduction through a review of previous literature on the speech characteristics of treated stutterers and on the ability of listeners to discriminate between treated stutterers and normal speakers.

EXCERPT 6.18

If listeners use rate as their primary criterion for identifying treated stutterers, it should be possible to demonstrate this experimentally and to alter their judgments by manipulating rate. Specifically, if the difference in rate between a pair of talkers can be changed instrumentally from a substantial value to a minimum value, then the labelling behavior of listeners who judge both the original and altered samples should change. The purpose of the present study was to match instrumentally the rates used by a sample of nonstutterers and treated stutterers who were known to be perceptually distinguishable in order to determine the effect of this manipulation on listener judgments.

SOURCE: Prosek, R. A., & Runyan, C. M. (1983). Effects of segment and pause manipulations on the identification of treated stutterers. *Journal of Speech and Hearing Research, 26,* 510–516.

The final example, shown in Excerpt 6.19, is from a study of vocal fundamental frequency of hearing-impaired speakers. The author first explains briefly why vocal fundamental frequency (F_0) should be compared for oral reading vs. spontaneous speech in hearing-impaired speakers and then states what will be studied. Two independent variables will be examined: normal hearing vs. hard-of-hearing (classification variable) and oral reading vs. spontaneous speech. The dependent variable is fundamental frequency.

The results that follow show the means and standard deviations of the fundamental frequencies specifically broken down according to the two independent variables. Again, the author has clearly stated his purpose so that the reader will know exactly what to expect in examining the results of the study.

EXCERPT 6.19

Voice characteristics of deaf and hard-of-hearing individuals during spontaneous or impromptu speech need to be investigated because spontaneous speech is a speaking condition of primary interest. In addition, knowledge of differences (or lack of them) in voice characteristics between oral reading and spontaneous speech should be useful in estimating spontaneous oral performance of hard-of-hearing individuals from their oral reading performance. For normal-hearing individuals, there is some evidence that f_0 distributional characteristics are different between oral reading and spontaneous speech. Snidecor (1943), for example, found that oral reading conditions produced both greater means and standard deviations of fundamental frequency. It was the purpose of the present study to investigate f_0 distributional characteristics of hard-of-hearing individuals during spontaneous speech and oral reading, and to test whether or not f_0 relationships, similar to those found in normal-hearing individuals, exist between the two speaking conditions.

SOURCE: Horii, Y. (1982). Some voice fundamental frequency characteristics of oral reading and spontaneous speech in hard-of-hearing young women. *Journal of Speech and Hearing Research, 25*, 608–610.

A number of factors lead researchers to use one form or another to state the specific purpose of a study. The specific manner of stating the purpose or question or hypothesis is not as important as the clarity with which it is stated. The important point is that the author should capture the nature of the study in a brief paragraph or so and specify the independent and dependent variables. The reader should move from the statement of specific purpose with a clear idea of what to expect in the results section of the article. Whichever form is used, the statement should be well written, explicit, and related to the preceding rationale.

Miscellaneous Considerations

Two final issues need to be addressed with respect to the introduction. First, the reader should be alert to the need for, or the use of, definitions of terms that the author employs throughout the study. Many terms have different meaning for different people. The author has the responsibility of indicating, in the introduction, how those terms are defined in the article. This is accomplished by either defining the term in the introduction or, more commonly, by appropriate citation of other sources that have already defined the term. The reader must remember, however, that the researcher frequently writes for a specific audience, that is, for other researchers working in the same area or for clinicians who presumably are familiar with the subject (and the terminology) under investigation. Thus, terms that the naive reader would like to see defined may not be. Nonetheless, idiosyncratic usage or the use of terms about which there may be differences of opinion as to their meaning do require the specific attention of the author and should be defined in the introduction.

Second, the researcher may spell out some of the limitations of the study about to be reported. There are two types of limitations that might be noted. The first is a limitation that is beyond the investigator's control. An example of this extrinsic limitation is the situation in which a researcher may want to include both males and females in a study but must collect data in a setting in which males predominate. The second type of limitation is an intrinsic one, that is, a limitation self-imposed by the investigator in recognition of the fact that all aspects of a problem area simply cannot be investigated in a single study. Longitudinal studies have to end, despite the researcher's desire to continue to study a child's language development beyond the data-collection period. The investigator who is studying hearing loss in a geriatric population may want to include a number of auditory tests but, because of the nature of the population, limits the study to a selected few procedures.

The limitations of the study, as expressed by the researcher, are important and deserve careful consideration by the reader. Because of the limitations, a study may turn out to be of no consequence. The limitations may suggest that the author should have, at the very least, delayed submitting the research report until the limitations were overcome. The fact that an author recognizes and states the limitations in the introduction does not necessarily relieve the author of the responsibility of dealing with these limitations later in the Discussion section. Because most limitations are, in fact, detailed in the final section of the article, we will have more to say about evaluating author-stated limitations in Chapter 9.

Finally, it goes without saying that the introduction should be well written, clear, and logically organized.

Summary

This chapter has dealt with the introduction to the research article. It is in this introductory section that the researcher describes the problem to be studied, documents the need for the study, and poses the specific purpose, question, or hypothesis to be investigated. The critical evaluator must pay particular attention to the logic and strength of the rationale, to the nature and scope of the literature citations, and to the clarity and specificity of the research questions or hypotheses. The importance of the introduction is underscored by recalling that the introduction serves as the foundation on which the remainder of the article is built. A serious flaw in the foundation can undermine the entire structure.

The Evaluation Checklist that follows summarizes the important points made in the chapter and is designed to facilitate the critical evaluation of the Introduction section of the article.

EVALUATION CHECKLIST

Instructions: The four-category scale at the end of this checklist may be used to rate the Introduction section of an article. The *Evaluation Items* help identify those topics that should be considered in arriving at the rating. Comments on these topics entered as *Evaluation Notes* should serve as the basis for the overall rating.

Evaluation Items   *Evaluation Notes*

1. Title identified target population and variables under study.

2. Purpose, procedures, important findings, and implications were summarized in the abstract.

3. A clear statement of the general problem was given.

4. There was a logical and convincing rationale.

5. There was a current, thorough, and accurate review of literature.

6. The purpose, questions, or hypotheses were logical extensions of the rationale.

7. The introduction was clearly written and well organized.

8. Miscellaneous.

Overall Rating (Introduction):   _____ _____ _____ _____
                                        Poor   Fair   Good   Excellent

Reference

American Psychological Association. (1983). *Publication manual of the American Psychological Association* (3rd ed.). Washington, DC: Author.

7
The Method Section

Introduction

If the Introduction section can be considered the foundation of the research article, then the Method section can be considered its structural framework. Understanding this framework is crucial to the critical evaluation of the Results and Discussion sections that follow. It is in the Method section that the author describes the subjects used in the study, the materials employed, and how those materials are used with the subjects; that is, the procedures. In addition, the Method section helps the reader to identify the type of research being reported as well as the specific research design incorporated in the study. Finally, it is in the Method section that the careful reader can identify how the author dealt with threats to internal and external validity.

The Method section stems directly from the rationale and the purpose of the study stated in the introduction. As such, the first major concern of the critical evaluator is whether the Method section, viewed in its entirety, is related to what has preceded and whether the methods chosen are appropriate to the problem posed in the introduction. We will address this issue in the sample evaluations of complete articles in Chapters 10 and 11. The second concern, and one that we seek to answer in this chapter, is whether the methods chosen by the investigator are adequate in and of themselves.

Subjects

We have noted in Chapter 3 that subject selection can pose a threat to the internal and external validity of both experimental and descriptive research.

The careful reader of a research article must determine, therefore, if the subject-selection procedure reported as well as the type of subjects used compromise the adequacy of the reserach. Before we present some evaluative guidelines, one general guideline needs to be emphasized with respect to the description of the subjects (as well as the description of materials and procedures). This guideline is simply, but importantly, that sufficient description be provided to allow the reader to *replicate* the study reported, at least in its important aspects. Researchers must resist the blue pencil of the cost-conscious editor and the reader must insist on adequate detail or, at the very least, references to previous research that contain the detailed description of procedures. The important point, again, is that the description of methods must be sufficiently complete to allow for replication.

Sample Size

The diversity of research in speech pathology and audiology is reflected, in a sense, in the different sample sizes employed in different studies. Sample sizes range from $N = 1$ to $N =$ thousands. Thus, one of the first questions that must be asked by readers (and doers) of research is whether the size of the sample is adequate for the purposes of the study. Unfortunately, there is no simple answer to this question. Christensen (1977), for example, points out that "the primary guide used by most investigators is the number of subjects used by other investigators within an area" (p. 244). Wood (1974) concurs by suggesting that the would-be researcher consult the literature to determine how many subjects have been used previously. "The issue of how many subjects to test," Wood states, "boils down to a question of belief" (p. 121). This may be overstating the case somewhat. The purpose of the investigation, previous research, the concern about generalizability, the variability found for the attribute under study, statistical considerations, and the research design itself all play a role in deciding if the number of subjects used is appropriate. For instance, in within-subjects designs, in which there are many repeated observations and many data points, small samples have been used and are quite adequate. This type of small sample study is found, for example, in the language-acquisition literature as well as in the psychoacoustic literature. Test standardization and survey research require large samples of subjects. Between-subject designs usually require larger samples than within-subject designs. If one wishes to generalize data to the majority of children who have articulatory disorders, then, a large number of subjects will have to be used. If the experimental treatment is expected to produce only small group differences, then, large samples may have to be employed to demonstrate statistically significant differences. It has to be acknowledged, of course, that small statistically significant differences obtained on a large sample of subjects may have little clinical meaning or value. On the other hand, if large treatment differences are anticipated, on the basis of either pilot data or previous research, then a small sample may be adequate.

Excerpts 7.1 through 7.4 illustrate the broad range of sample sizes found in the speech pathology and audiology literature. The four articles from which the excerpts were selected reflect different purposes, previous sample-size traditions, different research designs, expected variability of the data, and statistical analysis. Each of these considerations may have been more or less responsible for the sample sizes chosen.

Excerpt 7.1 illustrates the use of a large sample of randomly selected subjects. We have mentioned previously that consumers of research can have more confidence in the generalization of results when a large number of subjects have been randomly selected from the population of interest. Most studies, however, do not incorporate random selection of subjects from the total population of interest. The most common reasons are that the universe of subjects of interest is not available to the researcher and the cost of such random sampling procedures may be prohibitive. For practical reasons, then, most studies in speech pathology and audiology do not use large random samples of subjects. The exceptions are usually large-scale descriptive studies such as the one by Quigley, Smith, and Wilbur (Excerpt 7.1). Great care was taken to randomly select a large sample of subjects stratified according to the type of school, age, sex, and geographical region. As the authors noted in the reference to external validity in the last sentence, the generalization of the results of this study should be remarkably good.

EXCERPT 7.1

SUBJECTS

Subjects for the total research program were 450 prelingually and profoundly deaf students, 25 males and 25 females in each of nine age groups ranging from 10 to 18 years, selected from 10 residential and six day programs for deaf students in the United States. All educational programs with 100 or more deaf students were stratified on the basis of geographical region (as categorized by the U.S. Bureau of the Census) and type of program (day or residential). One day and one residential program were then selected randomly from each of the nine geographical regions. Only six day programs were included since three of the geographical regions, New England, East South Central, and Mountain, did not contain day programs with 100 or more deaf students. A 10th residential school was added to provide a sampling of residential students from an oral school. When the 16 educational programs had been selected, 25 male and 25 female subjects were chosen at random from each of the nine age levels, with the number of subjects selected in each geographical region being proportionate to the total number of deaf students in the region and to their distribution in day and residential programs. Also, subjects were selected only from among those students who (1) had sensorineural hearing impairment of not less than

90 dB (ANSI, 1969) at 500, 1000, and 2000 Hz; (2) had suffered hearing impairment before the age of two years; (3) had an IQ of at least 80 on the performance scale of the WISC or WAIS, or some comparable test; and (4) had (in the judgment of school personnel) no apparent disability other than hearing impairment. The stratified, random sampling procedures used for the total research program permit generalization of the results to all deaf students in the United States meeting the criteria established for the study.

SOURCE: Quigley, S. P., Smith, N. L., & Wilbur, R. B. (1974). Comprehension of relativized sentences by deaf students. *Journal of Speech and Hearing Research, 17,* 325–341.

The next excerpt (7.2) describes the selection and group assignment of 84 subjects in a study of fricative discrimination in infants. Although this sample is not as large as the one reported previously and was not randomly selected, it still represents a relatively large sample of subjects. Also, the purpose and design of this study are different from the Quigley et al. study. The more important point in the Eilers and Minifie study is that subjects were randomly *assigned* to experimental and control groups in this between-subjects experiment, a procedure that we indicated earlier is the best method for equating experimental and control groups. In other words, method of group assignment is more important than random selection and sample size in this study. More will be said about procedures for group assignment later in this chapter when we present excerpts dealing with procedures in between-subjects experiments.

EXCERPT 7.2

SUBJECTS

The subjects were 84 infants between four and 17 weeks old identified by parental response to mail solicitation. Twenty-four infants completed Experiment I (16 in the experimental group where order of stimulus presentation was counterbalanced and eight in the control group where no change in stimulus occurred following habituation) and 30 infants each completed Experiments II and III (20 in each experimental group and 10 in each control). Infants were excluded if they failed to suck (chewed on nipple), failed to suck following the second habituation minute, cried persistently, or if termination was requested by the parent. Approximately 60% of the infant subjects completed the session in each of the three experiments. Infants were randomly assigned to either experimental or control groups. Approximately equal numbers of infants were excluded from the experimental and control groups in Experiments I, II, and III because they failed one or more of the inclusion criteria. The age range and median age, respectively of the subjects for each experiment was as follows:

Experiment I, 4 to 15 weeks and 8.3 weeks; Experiment II, 4 to 17 weeks and 10 weeks; and Experiment III, 8 to 17 weeks and 12.4 weeks.

SOURCE: Eilers, R. E., & Minifie, F. D. (1975). Fricative discrimination in early infancy. *Journal of Speech and Hearing Research, 18,* 158–167.

Excerpt 7.3 presents an example from a study of verbal reaction time in which 30 graduate students were randomly assigned to three groups of 10 subjects each. This is a fairly typical sample size for a study of this nature, and most critical evaluators of research would again be more concerned with the random assignment of subjects to the three conditions than with the absolute size of the sample. Because the variability of the data shown in the results section of this article was relatively small, increases in sample size would probably not significantly improve the study.

EXCERPT 7.3

SUBJECTS

Thirty graduate students in the Department of Communication Disorders, University of Oklahoma Health Sciences Center, were randomly assigned into three subject groups of 10 subjects each. All subjects were experienced in phonetic transcription and had normal speech, normal hearing, and normal or corrected to normal vision.

SOURCE: Brennan, D. G., & Cullinan, W. L. (1976). The effects of word length and visual complexity on verbal reaction times. *Journal of Speech and Hearing Research, 19,* 141–155.

In some speech and hearing studies, the sample size and method of subject selection are less important than the instrumentation and procedures and, thus, become almost incidental. This is often true in basic physiologic and psychoacoustic research where the variability of the data is quite small and numerous repeated measurements are made in a within-subjects design. Take, for example, the study by Folkins and Abbs on the effect of resistive loading of the jaw on lip and jaw motor control during speech. The subject-selection section is reprinted in its entirety in Excerpt 7.4. Is this an adequate description of the subjects? How were they selected? Does it matter? Simply put, the nature and purpose of the research were such that any other three adult normal speakers could probably have been used without significantly affecting the data or modifying the conclusions. In this study, then, the instrumentation and the procedures used to measure the effect of jaw loading were more important than the subjects used. Similar examples could easily be cited. Once again, the adequacy of the size of the subject sample and the way subjects are selected depend to a very large extent on the basic purpose of the study, the nature of the research design, and the variability of the data.

EXCERPT 7.4

Three normal adult speakers, two females and one male, were subjects in this experiment.

SOURCE: Folkins, J. W., & Abbs, J. H. (1975). Lip and jaw motor control during speech responses to resistive loading of the jaw. *Journal of Speech and Hearing Research, 18,* 207–220.

Criteria for Subject Selection

As we have mentioned throughout, much of the descriptive research in speech pathology and audiology deals with differences and attempts to answer such questions as: Are stutterers different from nonstutterers? Do people with Ménière's disease differ from people with noise-induced hearing loss? Is test A more sensitive than test B in differentiating aphasics from other brain-injured people? In any study involving group differences (between-subject designs), it is absolutely essential that the researcher describe and perhaps even defend the criteria used in forming the groups. Inadequate group composition, overlapping groups, indefensible selection criteria all pose important threats to the internal and external validity of both experimental and descriptive research.

The lengthy example shown in Excerpt 7.5 is taken from an article by Duffy, Duffy, and Pearson (1975) on pantomime recognition in aphasics. The two basic questions asked in this research were: (1) Do aphasics show a distinctive impairment in pantomime recognition when compared to other brain-injured and nonbrain-injured subjects? and (2) Is there a relationship between severity of language impairment and severity of pantomime impairment in aphasics?

The first part of the subject-selection procedures clearly describes the four groups used in the study. The concern about possible overlap between groups is expressed in the section on subjects with right-hemisphere damage. The authors point out that none of these subjects had any aphasic symptoms on the basis of history or observation. To further document the absence of aphasic symptoms, the authors could have screened these subjects but decided that this was not necessary.

Next, the authors describe where the subjects came from, but, more important, they describe the *exclusion* criteria that eliminated patients whose data might have been confounded by, for example, foreign dialect.

Table 1 in the excerpt and the associated narrative attempt to demonstrate that the four groups were comparable on the extraneous variables of age, years of education, sex, etiology, time postonset, and hemiplegia. This was done to rule out any interaction between these variables and scores on the pantomime test. In a sense, the groups were matched overall on those extraneous critical variables that could affect intergroup comparisons. The authors also point out that statistical tests failed to demonstrate significant intergroup differences on these variables.

The subject-selection section is concluded with the authors' assertion that the aphasic subjects included in the study are similar, at least on the PICA, to a larger random sample of aphasics used in the development of the PICA. The assertion deals directly with the subject-selection threat to external validity and sets the stage for possible subsequent generalizations to many aphasic patients.

EXCERPT 7.5

SUBJECTS

Four groups of subjects were used in the studies. One group consisted of aphasics and three, nonaphasics. Of the three nonaphasic groups, one had no evidence of neurological impairment (control); one had neurological impairment of the subcortical motor system (subcortical); and one had cerebral damage with resultant motor or sensory deficits or both and possibly the general effects of brain damage (right-hemisphere-damaged). The four groups were selected as follows.

Aphasics

Patients with medical evidence of left-hemisphere damage indicated by right-sided motor or sensory impairment or both and who scored below the ninety-fifth percentile on the Porch Index of Communicative Ability and who exhibited a PICA score profile consistent with the diagnosis of aphasia were classified as aphasics. An aphasiologist experienced with PICA scoring independently reviewed all profiles and eliminated those suggestive of nonaphasic test performances (N = 44).

Right-Hemisphere-Damaged

Patients with medical evidence of right-hemisphere damage indicated by left-sided motor or sensory impairment or both were included in the right-hemisphere-damaged group (N = 30). Those with evidence of bilateral motor or sensory deficit were excluded. Although some of the patients in this group could have had lesions that also produced some mild aphasic symptoms, there were none reported in the medical record, by any clinical staff member, or noted by the examiner during any of the testing and interviews. It was, therefore, presumed that as a group these subjects represented a nonaphasic population and no specific test of aphasic language impairment was used to screen them.

Subcortical Damage

The subcortical-damaged group included patients with medical diagnoses of conditions and diseases consistent with primary subcortical motor impairment, for example, parkinsonism, multiple sclerosis, and cerebellar damage (*N* = 26).

Controls

Patients with no history or medical evidence of neurological damage comprised the control group (*N* = 30).

TABLE 1.   DATA DESCRIPTIVE OF THE AGE, EDUCATION, AND SEX OF APHASIC, RIGHT-HEMISPHERE-DAMAGED, SUBCORTICAL, AND CONTROL GROUPS OF SUBJECTS. ALSO PRESENTED ARE DATA DESCRIPTIVE OF THE ETIOLOGY, TIME POSTONSET, AND INCIDENCE OF FRANK HEMIPLEGIA FOR THE APHASIC AND RIGHT-HEMISPHERE-DAMAGED GROUPS

Subjects	Age in Years			Years of Education			Sex	
	N	Mean	SD	*N*	Mean	SD	Male	Female
Aphasic	44	61.8	13.1	34*	9.8	2.7	35	9
Right hemisphere	30	65.7	9.0	27*	10.0	3.0	20	10
Subcortical	26	67.7	8.9	22*	10.5	3.6	21	5
Control	30	62.3	9.8	25*	8.8	2.9	26	4

	Etiology			Weeks Postonset			Hemiplegic	
	CVA	Neoplasm	Trauma	*N*	Mean	SD	Yes	No
Aphasic	40	2	2	40*	22.4	40.2	36	8
Right hemisphere	29	1	0	20*	39.8	65.9	23	7

*Information not available on all subjects.

All groups were drawn from the same five hospitals in Connecticut using all available patients. Any patient whose medical diagnosis was unclear, with multiple problems or evidence of bilateral cerebral damage, was excluded from the study. Also excluded were patients with gross indications of different cultural backgrounds (that is, foreign birth or foreign dialect) because of the influence of cultural background on gestural and pantomimic behavior.

Data descriptive of the four subject groups are presented in Table 1. Perusal of the data reveals strong similarity among the groups. In addition, statistical tests of critical differences failed to reach the 0.05 level of significance for all variables of age, education, sex, etiology, time postonset, and presence of frank hemiplegia. The hypothesis of no differences among the groups is, therefore, supported.

Based on the distribution of the overall scores of the Porch Index of Communicative Ability, the aphasic subjects may be considered to be a representative
sample of a general population of aphasics. The mean (10.03), median (10.5),
standard deviation (2.81), and range (2.9 to 14.0) of the overall PICA scores
obtained by the aphasic group closely parallel the original PICA scores obtained by Porch (1967), which were based on a random sample of 150 aphasic
subjects.

SOURCE: Duffy, R. J., Duffy, J. R., & Pearson, K. L. (1975). Pantomime recognition in
aphasics. *Journal of Speech and Hearing Research, 18,* 115–132.

Because subject selection procedures are so important in between-group
studies in speech pathology and audiology, we have chosen another illustration, this time from the audiology literature. Excerpt 7.6 presents the description of subjects from a descriptive between-groups study by Owens
(1971). The purpose of this clinical research was to assess the value of a
variety of audiometric tests or constellation of tests in identifying the site of
lesion of aural pathology in adults. The subject classification format is similar to that found in audiological research designed to evaluate the sensitivity of tests used in differential diagnosis.

EXCERPT 7.6

SUBJECTS

Patients with sensorineural hearing loss, who had been referred for special
audiologic testing to help in localization of lesion, were divided into groups as
shown in Table 1: Ménière's Disease (N = 147); Other Cochlear Lesion (N =
77); Retrocochlear Lesion (N = 88); and Sudden Loss (N = 100).

Ménière's disease

The subjects in this group all had the symptom-triad of hearing loss, tinnitus,
and episodic "spinning" vertigo that defines Ménière's disease, and the three
symptoms were clearly interrelated. This triad of symptoms has been associated consistently with a hydrops of the labyrinth (Hallpike & Cairns, 1938;
Lindsay, 1942; Schuknecht, 1963; Altmann & Kornfeld, 1965; Lindsay, Kohut,
& Sciarra, 1967). All patients were diagnosed by otolaryngologists on the staff at
the University of California, San Francisco, who were highly alert to the possibility of retrocochlear involvement. X-ray studies of the internal auditory
meati (all normal) were obtained for 76 of the patients. Neurologic consultation
was arranged for all patients when there was suspicion of retrocochlear lesion.
In two patients, the presence of the hearing loss-tinnitus-vertigo triad was
deceptive. One patient was eventually found to have a cyst in the cerebellopon-
tine angle, and the other, a glomus tumor invading the labyrinth. The first
patient was included in the *Retrocochlear Lesion* group; the second was excluded from the survey because involvement of the VIIIth nerve, although
strongly suspected, could not be verified. Golding-Wood (1960) described a

patient whose symptoms simulated Ménière's disease despite the presence of an acoustic neurinoma, but stressed the infrequency of such a case.

Other cochlear lesion

In these patients, vestibular symptoms differed from the episodic, spinning vertigo of Ménière's disease or were absent. About one-third of the group had symptoms and signs suggesting hydrops; often-heard complaints, for example, were "roaring" tinnitus, fluctuating hearing loss, sensitivity to loud sounds, and a feeling of fullness. The most common diagnoses were "atypical Ménière's disease" and "labyrinthine hydrops." The remaining two-thirds of the group had hearing losses thought to be associated with such factors as vascular disorders, lues, allergy, and diabetes. Most often, the diagnosis was "end-organ lesion, etiology unknown." Patients with hearing loss primarily related to prolonged noise exposure, ototoxic drugs, or old age were excluded.

All patients in the *Other Cochlear Lesion* group had X-ray studies of the internal auditory meati and petrous pyramids, including tomograms in many instances. Over half of this group had also been examined by a neurologist. All neurologic studies and examinations were normal. According to published observations (Crabtree & House, 1964; Valvassori, 1969), retrocochlear lesions are sometimes missed by radiography in the absence of iophendylate studies. Such studies were obtained on only a few patients in our group. It can only be said that patients were excluded from the *Other Cochlear Lesion* group at the slightest suspicion of retrocochlear lesion expressed by the otolaryngologist, neurologists, and neurosurgeons involved.

TABLE 1. PATIENTS WHO HAD BEEN REFERRED FOR SPECIAL AUDIOLOGIC TESTING IN LOCALIZATION OF LESION

Classification	Number
Ménière's Disease	147
Other Cochlear Lesion	77
Retrocochlear Lesion	88
Sudden Loss	100

Retrocochlear lesion

Eighty-three of the 88 patients in the *Retrocochlear Lesion* group had surgically identified neoplasms, four had multiple sclerosis, and one had an internal carotid aneurysm shown by vertebral arteriograms to be pressing against the VIIIth nerve in much the same manner as a tumor. Classification of neoplasms was difficult because of different terminology used by individual neurologists, neurosurgeons, otolaryngologists, and histopathologists, but the following classifications seemed appropriate for this survey: (a) sheath tumors, (b) meningiomas, (c) cysts, (d) brainstem gliomas, and (e) other. Sheath tumors included those labeled neuroma, neurinoma, perineural fibroblastoma, neurilemmoma, schwannoma, and acoustic (VIIIth nerve) tumor. Among the cysts were epidermoid, arachnoid, and those referred as "type unknown." The brainstem glioma classification included astrocytomas. Diagnoses are listed in Table 2. Insofar as could be determined from operative reports, the neoplasm was ipsilateral to the hearing impairment in all instances.

TABLE 2. DIAGNOSES FOR THE
RETROCOCHLEAR LESION GROUP

Diagnosis	Number
Sheath tumor	49
Meningioma	8
Cyst	11
Brainstem glioma	6
Other[a]	14
	88

[a]Includes multiple sclerosis (4), malignant tumor of the posterior fossa (2), cholesteotoma (2), chondroma (1), hemangioendotheloma (1), aneurysm acting as a tumor (1), neurofibroma with von Recklinghausen's disease (1), granulomatous meningitis (1), and hemangioblastoma (1).

Sudden loss

All of these patients had had dramatic onset of hearing loss, usually severe. Descriptions of the onset were vivid and detailed, in contrast to those given by the other patients in the survey. Tinnitus, vestibular symptoms, or both had sometimes occurred simultaneously with the hearing loss. While the tinnitus, if occurring, tended to persist, the vestibular symptoms, although sometimes lasting for several days, typically failed to recur after subsiding. In short, the onset of sudden loss, with or without tinnitus and vestibular symptoms, was related to a single episode. Obscure etiology is inherent in the definition of sudden loss employed here. Loss of hearing due to head injury or mumps, for example (see Welsh & Welsh, 1963), is not included in the definition.

All patients in the *Sudden Loss* group were examined and diagnosed by staff otolaryngologists. Neurologic consultation and X-rays of the internal auditory meati and petrous pyramids (all normal) were obtained for most of these patients and several in the group were referred for complete medical and neurologic studies to rule out retrocochlear involvement. The literature suggests, however, that retrocochlear lesion in the form of a neoplasm is rarely found in hearing loss of sudden onset as defined above. Sheehy (1960) reported three patients with retrocochlear lesion in a series of 247 patients with sudden loss; Hallberg (1956) reported two in a series of 178 patients. None were found among our *Sudden Loss* patients. Of our 88 *Retrocochlear Lesion* patients, only one, a patient with a meningioma, reported a sudden onset of hearing loss. She described her loss as beginning with a "pop." However, she presented with other, nonauditory, symptoms of retrocochlear involvement.

SOURCE: Owens, E. (1971). Audiologic evaluation in cochlear versus retrocochlear lesions. *Acta Otolaryngologica* (Supplement 283).

Several points should be noted. First, and the most important, is that the medical criteria used for subject classification are clearly specified for the four groups. In addition, the specific diagnoses for the 88 subjects in the retrocochlear group are identified. It is essential to recognize that the several audiometric tests evaluated by Owens were *not* used to identify subjects as having Ménière's disease, other cochlear lesions, and so on. Next, subjects were excluded if definitive medical data could not be obtained. Note, for example, the statement that ". . . patients were excluded from the *Other Cochlear Lesion* group at the slightest suspicion of retrocochlear lesion expressed by the otolaryngologists, neurologists, and neurosurgeons involved." Subjects were also excluded from the Other Cochlear Lesion category if they had hearing loss primarily related to extensive noise exposure, ototoxicity, or old age. It would have been helpful for Owens to have indicated why noise-exposed subjects were eliminated because the type of hearing loss caused by noise is usually cochlear in nature. Because the site of lesion in presbycusis is less certain, it is clear why older subjects were excluded. Finally, a question remains about how the subjects were selected. This information is contained in a brief procedure section, which is shown in Excerpt 7.7. Note, here, Owens's concern about the sampling procedures used and the fact that although the sample was probably unbiased, it was not selected randomly. Here, again, Owens refers to the effect of the exclusion criteria and also emphasizes that a number of subjects were excluded because they had not been given the special audiometric tests. The selection procedures employed by Owens resulted in a large N for this type of study. The size of the sample and the care taken in choosing the sample reduce the threat to external validity. One final and rather subtle point should be stressed. Owens indicates that the tests were done when the patients were referred, ". . . *and then, at a later date, their records were checked for the final diagnosis*" (our italics). This means, in essence, that the audiologist's test data and test procedures were uncontaminated by knowledge of the patient's final diagnostic category. Although this is primarily a procedural issue, it is an issue that can have an important effect on the objectivity of the data reported subsequently.

EXCERPT 7.7

PROCEDURE

The audiologic records for all of these groups were obtained over a period of approximately 6 years. The tests were done when the patients were referred to us and then at a later date, their records were checked for the final diagnosis. Although the patients forming the *Retrocochlear Lesion* group were unselected, a number of patients with Ménière's disease and some who had experienced sudden loss were omitted because they had not been given the special tests.

The special requirements already outlined for the *Other Cochlear Lesion* group served to exclude as many as 50 patients, most of whom had symptoms suggesting hydrops. Thus, the sampling, although believed to be unbiased, was not truly random; neither did it represent a critical incidence. At several points throughout the survey, analyses were undertaken on pertinent questions. The Ns for these analyses differed according to the number of patients on whom data were available at the time.

The audiologic evaluations were done in one clinic by audiologists employing essentially the same test methods. In the majority of cases the writer either did the evaluation or participated as an observer.

SOURCE: Owens, E. (1971). Audiologic evaluation in cochlear versus retrocochlear lesions. *Acta Otolaryngologica* (Supplement 283).

Another aspect of subject selection that directly affects internal validity is whether or not subjects were selected on the basis of extreme scores. We pointed out in Chapter 3 that selecting subjects because of their extreme scores may produce regression effects. That is, apparent changes in post-treatment scores may merely reflect the tendency for extreme scores to become less extreme (regress toward the mean) rather than reflecting true treatment effects. The critical reader should be especially alert to regression effects in studies of therapy programs.

Excerpt 7.8 is taken from the Discussion section of a study by Andrews and Harvey of regression to the mean in stuttering measures. They measured regression during a pretreatment waiting period and compared their findings to previous studies. Although the amount of regression they found was small, note their suggestions for incorporating a correction for regression in pretest-posttest studies of the effects of stuttering treatment. Note their comments about measures of speech attitude and reaction to speech situations as well as the actual speech measures of fluency. Similar studies with other speech disorders would help to improve the design of therapy experiments.

EXCERPT 7.8

The six studies in the literature that have measured stutterers at two or three points in time prior to treatment have all reported a statistically nonsignificant improvement trend. This improvement may be evidence that stutterers come for treatment when their stuttering is worst and spontaneously improve a little with time. Although it is difficult to aggregate data from this small set of studies, examination of the time of the improvement, as reflected by the effect-size statistic, shows that the improvement can be evident as early as three months after initial contact.

The present study of 132 subjects showed that many stutterers waiting for treatment did improve significantly. This may be evidence of regression in the severity of their stuttering to a previously established mean level. Analysis of the present data by the time subjects spent on the waiting list showed that the improvement occurred within the first three months and that no further improvement occurred thereafter.

Regression to the mean appears an effect that could confound estimates of the improvement due to therapy in pre-post treatment outcome designs. There are two ways of allowing for the effect. First, stutterers could be held on a waiting list for three months or until a stable baseline is demonstrated so that the effects of treatment will not be confounded by regression to the mean. Second, if subjects receive treatment immediately after they apply for treatment, a small but definable part of the improvement following treatment will be due to spontaneous regression to the mean, and the treatment results should be corrected accordingly.

Aggregating the data from the six reports in the literature and from the present study suggests that the magnitude of this effect is small; mean effect size = 0.21 (SE 0.04). Subtracting this amount from the pre-post effect size would approximate the actual treatment-related improvement. In practical terms, a group of adult stutterers of mean severity 17%SS when first seen will spontaneously improve to a mean of 14%SS three months later, and improvement beyond this point following treatment is likely to be due to the effects of treatment.

Self-report measures of speech attitude and reaction to speech situations also showed improvement trends, but in both Gregory (1972) and the present study, the changes were of much smaller magnitude than those of speech measures. This improvement trend is so small that it can be disregarded when using self-report measures to calculate the improvement produced by therapy.

SOURCE: Andrews, G., & Harvey, R. (1981). Regression to the mean in pretreatment measures of stuttering. *Journal of Speech and Hearing Disorders, 46,* 204–207.

The relevant questions about subject-selection criteria that need to be asked for between-group studies can be summarized as follows: (1) Are the criteria for group composition clearly defined and defensible? (2) Is there overlap between groups on the variable that distinguishes the groups? (3) Are exclusion criteria defined and defensible? (4) Are the groups comparable on important extraneous variables? and (5) Have subjects been selected on the basis of extreme scores? These questions deal primarily with the issue of internal validity. Regarding external validity, the question is: Are the subjects comparable, on important dimensions, to the population to which the author wishes to generalize?

One final point deserves brief attention. The author of a research article should indicate if subjects were volunteers and whether they were paid (or unpaid) to participate in the study. A complete discussion of the effects of the volunteer subject on the outcomes of research is beyond the scope of this book. (The interested reader should consult Rosenthal and Rosnow [1975].) Suffice it to say that volunteer subjects, whether paid or unpaid, may be different in important respects from the population to whom the investigator wishes to generalize, thus affecting external validity.

Materials

The materials part of the research article is a key component of the Method section. The reason for its importance is that it is in this section that researchers identify the materials that have been used to measure or generate the variables under study, and it is here that the critical consumer of research can identify instrumentation threats to internal validity. Underscoring the importance of such threats is the fact emphasized in Chapter 3 that instrumentation threats to internal validity transcend type of research or research design.

There are two basic evaluation questions that need to be asked by the consumer: (1) Was there adequate selection and measurement of the independent (classification, predictor) variable? and (2) Was there adequate selection and measurement of the dependent (criterion, predicted) variable? Although the researcher's rationale for the selection of variables may appear either in the Introduction or the Method section (and this rationale requires careful scrutiny on the part of the reader), the measurement of variables will almost always be described either in the Materials or Procedures section. Our purpose here, then, is to lay down some general guidelines that can be used by the critical reader to evaluate possible instrumentation (i.e., materials) threats to the internal validity of both experimental and descriptive research.

Hardware Instrumentation and Calibration

Instrumentation. Hardware instrumentation plays an important role in research in speech pathology and audiology, especially in speech and hearing science. Much of what we know about normal (and disordered) processes is due, in large part, to technological advances that have made possible the measuring, recording, and analyzing systems that are found in speech and hearing laboratories throughout the country. This is not to say that all research is dependent on or requires sophisticated electronic instrumentation. The exciting advances made in understanding how children acquire language have not required much more than an audiotape recorder or a relatively simple videotape recording system. It is to say, however, that the critical reader of research is often required to read research articles that are heavily weighted in instrumentation. The critical evaluation of such material can be an exceedingly difficult task, especially for the student who has minimal course work or experience in electronics or instrumentation.

Although instrumentation can be complex, the purposes to which the instruments are put are reasonably straightforward. Instruments are used to produce signals (e.g., an audio-frequency oscillator), to measure the signal (e.g., a sound-level meter), to store the signal (e.g., a tape recorder), to control the signal (e.g., an electronic switch), to modify the signal (e.g., a band-pass filter), and to analyze the signal (e.g., a sound spectrograph). The reasons for using an instrument are equally straightforward. The researcher (or clinician) uses an instrument to standardize data-acquisition procedures, to help acquire data under known conditions, and to provide a permanent record of the data. Most important, instruments allow the measurement of events that are not directly observable by the senses (Plutchik, 1974). There is nothing inherently mysterious about instrumentation. What is mysterious, perhaps, is why so little attention is paid to laboratory instrumentation in most master's-level speech pathology and audiology training programs. This may very well be the reason that many consumers of research approach the apparatus section of an article with fear and trepidation. Another point to keep in mind is that instruments, like statistics, are tools. The instrument itself, with few exceptions, is not the reason for the research. Thus, again like statistics, a sophisticated instrumental array cannot improve an inadequate research problem and cannot modify a poor research design.

Several guidelines can be used by the practitioner or student while reading the instrumentation section of an article. First, and at the very least, the principal components of the system should be identified by manufacturer and model number. This enables the interested reader to duplicate the system using the same or comparable equipment. It also allows the reader to determine if the components are reasonably standard pieces that have been manufactured by reputable companies. If a new instrument has been developed for a particular study, enough information should be provided to allow the reader to reconstruct the piece. Circuit diagrams, photographs, line drawings, and the like, should be included for this purpose. The point here is that there should be sufficient detail for replication purposes and to permit the reader to determine if the components are standard pieces of equipment likely to be found in a well-equipped speech and hearing laboratory. A block diagram showing the interrelationships among components is a useful device for describing the instrumentation array.

Another criterion is whether the same or a similar instrumental array has been used by the investigator in a previously reported study or has been used by other investigators studying the same phenomenon. References to previous research can be of considerable value in assessing the adequacy of instrumentation. The absence of such references, especially when confronted with a custom-built instrument, should alert the reader to the possibility of instrumental error.

Some basic characteristics of the instrumentation used may also be reported in the instrumentation section and may be of value to the reader in helping to assess whether the instrumentation was appropriate to the task at hand. The frequency response characteristics of the earphones, the linearity of attenuators, and the intensity range of an amplifier are just three examples of the kind of descriptive information that might be provided in the instrumentation section.

If there is controversy or differences of opinion about the value or appropriateness of a given piece of equipment used to measure a given phenomenon, then, the differences of opinion should be identified fairly and the reasons for the author's use of the instrument should be provided.

The final criterion, one which probably cannot be used until the reader delves into the Results or Discussion section, is whether the data reported are reasonably consistent with data previously reported on the same phenomenon. If the results are grossly at odds with previous data or with theoretical expectations, then one possible reason for the discrepancy may lie with instrumentation.

Excerpts 7.9 and 7.10 represent two somewhat different instrumentation descriptions. In the first, Raffin, Lilly, and Thornton (1976) provide all the information the reader would need in replicating this study of time-intensity trading relationships for speech. Each piece of equipment is identified by manufacturer and model number. In a later section (not shown here), there is an equally precise description of how the speech stimuli were recorded, including considerable detail about how the system was calibrated.

EXCERPT 7.9

APPARATUS AND CALIBRATION

A speech audiometer (Grason-Stadler, Model 162) was used to determine the SRT for each subject and to control the signal levels in the main experiment. The output of a magnetic tape recorder (Magnecord, Model 1020) was fed to the auxiliary input of the audiometer. All of the data for this experiment were gathered with the subject seated in a double-walled sound-insulated test room (Industrial Acoustics, Model 1204–A). The magnetic tape recorder was calibrated to conform with specifications promulgated by the National Association of Broadcasters (NAB, 1965). One channel of the speech audiometer was fed directly to a dynamic earphone (Telephonics, TDH-39) mounted in a neoprene cushion (Telephonics, MX-41/AR). This channel was designated as the "lagging" channel in the main experiment. The second channel of the speech audiometer was fed to an impedance-matching transformer (United Transformer, LS-33),through the experimenter's attenuator, through the subject's attenuator, through a second impedance-matching transformer (United Transformer, LS-33), and then to a second (matched) earphone (Telephonics, TDH-39) mounted in a cushion (Telephonics, MX-41/AR). All of the attenuators used in this experiment were found to be linear ±0.2 dB) within the range of attenuation values required for the study. A remote monitoring circuit, that was part of a method-of-adjustment system, was used to determine the setting on the subject's attenuator.

SOURCE: Raffin, M. J. M., Lilly, D. J., & Thornton, A. R. (1976). Time-intensity trade for speech: A temporal speech-Stenger effect. *Journal of Speech and Hearing Research, 19,* 749–766.

Compare the next excerpt taken from a study of chest-wall kinematics during speech production. Certainly the description provided by the authors would permit replication. However, the *adequacy* of the equipment array could probably best be evaluated by individuals who are familiar with equipment used to measure respiratory phenomena. Most speech pathologists and audiologists will simply not have the background to allow a critical evaluation of this section of the Hixon, Goldman, and Mead article.

EXCERPT 7.10

Equipment

Figure 2 is a schematic diagram of the electronic equipment used. Changes in anteroposterior diameters of the rib cage and abdomen were sensed with electromagnetic transducers (that is, magnetometers). The devices used were somewhat smaller (coils 2 cm in length and about 0.5 cm in diameter), but basically of the same design as prototype units whose specifications are reported in detail elsewhere (Mead et al., 1967). Only the important functional features of the system will be discussed here. The basic principle of diameter measurements with magnetometers in that of sensing with one coil, the strength of a magnetic field generated by a coil mate. Two generator-sensor pairs were used, one pair to sense rib cage diameter changes and the other pair to sense abdominal diameter changes. (For coil placements, see the following section.) Each generating coil was driven sinusoidally at its resonant frequency, and its respective coil mate sensed the magnetic field produced. At the driving frequencies used (1.53 k Hz for the rib cage and 0.69 k Hz for the abdomen), body tissues and air have negligible effects on the strengths of the magnetic fields produced, a fact of crucial importance to biological applications of the devices. With the long axes of a generator-sensor coil pair oriented parallel, the voltage induced in the sensor is inversely proportional to the cube of the distance between the two mates. As the devices were used in this investigation, distance changes between the generating and sensing coils were small, relative to the absolute distance between the coils, so that the relationship between voltage change and distance change was essentially linear over nearly the entire range of motion of both the rib cage and the abdomen.

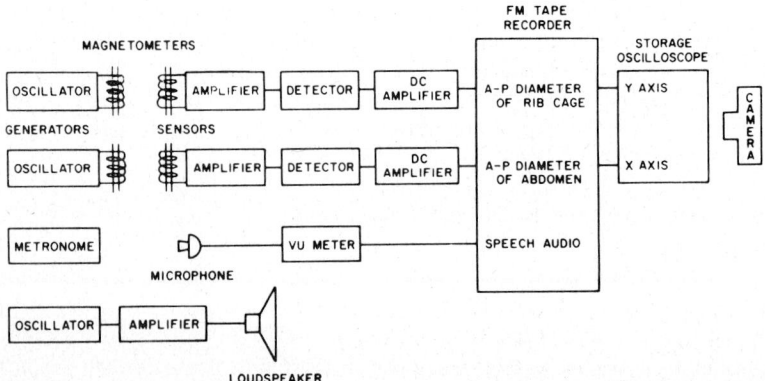

Figure 2.   Block Diagram of electronic equipment used in this investigation.

Processing of each magnetometer signal involved amplification of the amplitude-modulated output from the sensor, half-wave rectification, filtering (to prevent crosstalk between the two pairs of coils), and passage of the signal through a DC amplifier. The voltage related to the absolute distance between coil mates was zero suppressed at the DC amplifier, and only the voltage equivalent of intercoil distance change was amplified. With both the generating and sensing coils movable, the output of the sensing coil indicates changes in distance between it and the generator, whether there is movement of one or both coils. If one coil in a pair is relatively stable, as was the case for the back coils in the measurements made here, then the output of a sensor may be thought of as providing a continuous measurement of the unidimensional change in the position of a point in reference to a fixed point (that is, the coil on the back.)

The processed signals from the magnetometers were fed to two channels of a FM tape-recording system where they were stored for subsequent playback into a storage oscilloscope. During playback, the diameter signals for the rib cage and abdomen were displayed against one another on the oscilloscope, rib cage on the Y-axis and abdomen on the X-axis (for details, see results section on "Data Displays: Orientation and Interpretation"). Data displays on the screen of the oscilloscope were stored and then recorded permanently by photographing the screen with a Polaroid camera.

Three portions of the electronic equipment arrangement provided information to the subjects to guide them in certain of their utterances. Acoustic signals were sensed by a unidirectional microphone and fed through a VU meter to a direct record channel of the FM tape recorder. The VU meter served as an index of speech intensity. A loudspeaker, driven by a power amplifier and controlled by an oscillator, provided pure tone frequency standards against which the subjects could match their vocal fundamental frequency. Finally, an electronic metronome was used for certain conditions to pace each subject in his rate of speech utterance.

SOURCE: Hixon, T. J., Goldman, M. D., & Mead, J. (1973). Kinematics of the chest wall during speech production: Volume displacements of the rib cage, abdomen, and lung. *Journal of Speech and Hearing Research, 16,* 78–115.

With the increasing impact of rapid technological developments on the field of communication disorders, however, consumers of research will find it more and more difficult to evaluate the research in the field without some background in instrumentation. It is obviously beyond the scope of this book to attempt to teach principles of instrumentation to clinicians and students. Recent attempts have been made to make professionals aware of the need to understand instrumentation in speech and hearing. Levitt (1983) addressed this issue at the 1983 ASHA National Conference on Undergraduate, Graduate, and Continuing Education. He concisely summarized the problem when he said (Levitt, 1983, p. 88):

In short, modern technology is transforming virtually every aspect of our profession (and of every other profession as well). It is imperative that a concerted effort be made to train porfessionals in our field to function effectively in this new environment.

Levitt outlined several issues to be considered in developing guidelines for future incorporation of technological instruction in the education of speech pathologists and audiologists and made several suggestions to help professionals to understand and use the advancing technology in future clinical and research activities. Levitt (1983, p. 88) emphasized the importance of making technological innovations meaningful and useful to our service-oriented profession, stating:

> It is wholly unrealistic to develop preservice and in-service training programs that will cover all aspects of modern technology. There is a need to be selective. For example, one need not understand the principles of xerography in order to use a xerox machine effectively. On the other hand, the characteristics and inherent limitations of acoustic amplifiers need to be understood in order to prescribe hearing aids properly.

Students and clinicians must also accept some responsibility for updating their knowledge of technicological innovations in the field. Many state and national conventions now offer continuing education activities that deal with the use of technical innovations, computers, and various kinds of instrumentation. Also, many recent articles have appeared in the clinical and research literature that attempt to provide knowledge about instrumentation that is geared to clinicians. Hixon and his associates, for example, have tried to make some of their research instrumentation more clinically available and useful to clinicians with the publication of several recent articles on the application of instrumentation in clinical speech measurement (Hixon, Bless, & Netsell, 1976; Hixon, Hawley, & Wilson, 1982; Netsell & Hixon, 1978; Smitheran & Hixon, 1981). The "Research Notes" of the *Journal of Speech and Hearing Research* often present information on instrumentation that may help clinicians update their knowledge and skills (e.g., see Barlow, Cole, & Abbs, 1983; Guillemin & Nguyen, 1984). As technological advances progress, speech pathologists and audiologists need to take advantage of courses and continuing education in instrumentation to keep current in their clinical work and prepare themselves to evaluate the research in the field that relies more and more on electronic instrumentation. The time has come when knowledge of instrumentation is as important a tool to speech pathologists and audiologists as traditional tools such as knowledge of phonetic transcription, anatomy and physiology, or linguistics have been in the past.

The next example (Excerpt 7.11) shows how Schwartz and Sanders complement the block diagram with a narrative description of the equipment employed. Again, manufacturer and model numbers are provided, and there is a reference to the previous study after which their instrumentation was patterned. The section on apparatus is followed by a brief section on calibration.

EXCERPT 7.11

Pure-tone threshold testing was done in a sound-isolated test room having a suitable acoustic environment for threshold measurements. The test signal was delivered by a portable audiometer (Beltone, Model 10D) and transduced in a set of TDH-39 earphones mounted in MX 41/AR cushions.

Pressure-compliance functions (tympanograms) and stapedial reflex threshold measurements were obtained with an electroacoustic impedance bridge (American Electromedics, Model 83). This instrument also provided the pure tone, broadband noise, and bandpass filtered noise stimuli necessary for carrying out the SPAR test.

The instrumentation used for determining the critical bandwidth in the acoustic reflex was patterned after that described by Djupesland and Zwislocki (1973) and is shown schematically in Figure 1. The stapedius reflex was elicited by means of a two-tone complex geometrically distributed around center

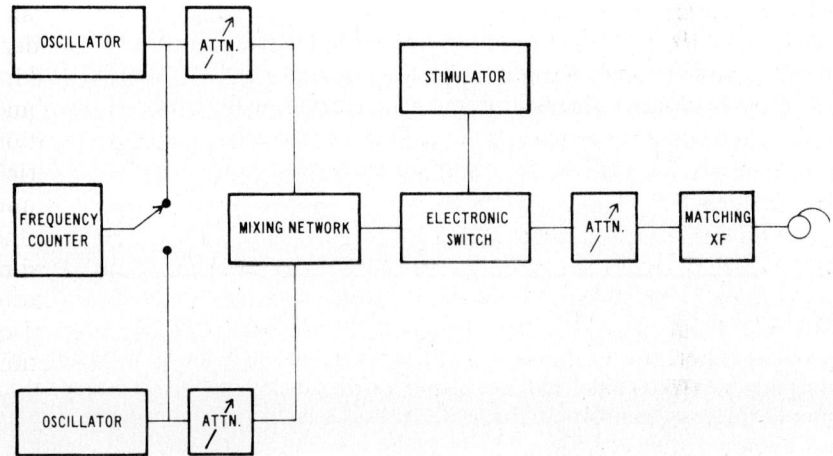

Figure 1. Schematic diagram of the apparatus for producing a complex of two pure tones.

frequencies of 1000 and 2000 Hz and was monitored with the impedance bridge. Each component of the pure-tone complex originated from a variable frequency oscillator and was attenuated by means of a precision attenuator. Frequency settings were made with an electronic frequency counter. The two individual sinusoids were then made with an electronic frequency counter. The two individual sinusoids were then mixed in a resistive network and passed through an electronic switch set for a rise-decay time of 10 msec. The switch was triggered by a stimulator set for a signal duration of 500 msec and permitting single-pulse presentations. From the electronic switch the signal was routed through a third attenuator and an impedance matching transformer and then delivered to a TDH-39 earphone.

SOURCE: Schwartz, D. M., & Sanders, J. W. (1976). Critical bandwidth and sensitivity prediction in the acoustic stapedial reflex. *Journal of Speech and Hearing Disorders, 41*, 244–255.

Calibration.   Adequate calibration of instruments used in a given study is absolutely essential to the reduction of a possible threat to internal validity posed by instrumentation. Faulty calibration must lead to faulty data, either in the laboratory or in the clinic. Unfortunately, calibration procedures are sometimes given short shrift in a journal article. Thus, it is difficult to assess the adequacy of the calibration procedures employed. As a result, the reader may have to rely on the integrity and honesty of the researcher in judging the adequacy of calibration.

The three major questions that the reader must ask about calibration of equipment are: (1) What was calibrated? (2) What equipment was used for calibration purposes? and (3) When was calibration performed? Excerpt 7.12 is taken from a study on the effect of increment size on Short Increment Sensitivity Index (SISI) Scores. Note that in this brief paragraph, Sanders and Simpson idenfity the equipment used for acoustic calibration, specify when calibration took place, and emphasize the reason special care was taken to ensure the absence of transient distortion at the onset of the stimulus increment.

EXCERPT 7.12

Acoustic calibration of the equipment was carried out with an artificial ear assembly (Allison, Model 300) just before testing, during the testing period, and after testing was completed. The artificial ear assembly was monitored with a noise source (Bruel and Kjaer, Model 4240). In addition to the acoustic calibration, an acoustic analysis was made of the SISI stimulus with an oscilloscope (Tektronix, Type 532) to ensure accuracy in rise-decay and duration and to ensure that transient distortion was not present at the onset of the increment. This latter procedure was considered of extreme importance because the presence of transient energy in the onset of the increment might easily result in spuriously high SISI scores, even in normal ears.

SOURCE: Sanders, J. W., & Simpson, M. E. (1966). The effect of increment size on short increment sensitivity index scores. *Journal of Speech and Hearing Research, 9*, 297–304.

Another example (Excerpt 7.13) is taken from a study of laryngeal valving actions of normal and hearing-impaired speakers. The equipment for high-speed filming of the larynx is described briefly and reference is made to a previous study that included a more detailed description of the apparatus and procedure. The details of calibration of the filming system are described and the authors also include a description of the expected error of measurement with the optical system. In addition, the linking of the acoustical data with the film data is described and the temporal resolution of the timing code for linking film and acoustic data is indicated. Another significant aspect of their method section is the description of the interjudge and intrajudge reliability in making the glottal area measurements from the film data.

EXCERPT 7.13

Equipment

High-speed laryngeal films (4000 frames/s) were made of each subject using the equipment and procedures described by Metz, Whitehead, and Peterson (1980). Briefly, the equipment and procedures permit making high-speed laryngeal films and obtaining noise-free high-quality acoustic recordings simultaneously. Two adjacent sound attenuating rooms isolate the subject from the camera (Redlake Hycam, 40–004) and from all noise-producing equipment. Laryngeal filming is accomplished by projecting two high-intensity light beams (Skanmart Xenon Illuminator, XEN–300F–141) at paraxial angles to the camera lens (230mm Century Tele-Anthenar with Angenieux reflex viewfinder) through an optically flat sound attenuating window. These two light beams intersect on a specially constructed oval laryngeal mirror, which is permanently fixed in the optical path 107 cm from the focal plane of the lens. The mirror has two degrees of freedom which permit separate vertical and horizontal adjustments without changing the absolute 107-cm working distance. This optical configuration results in a 0.25 image/object ratio (lens reduction factor) if the plane of focus on the vocal folds is 114 cm. If the plane of focus on the vocal folds is 112 cm, the image object ratio is 0.2571. Because all film data were collected with a focus range between 112 and 114 cm, a standard image/object ratio of 0.2535 was used in all subsequent glottal area calculations. Establishing this standard was necessary because of small focusing adjustments that are required during actual filming. The resulting calibration error is negligible compared with the glottal area variations associated with phonation. For example, if the maximum glottal area was 5 mm², one would expect a calibration error $\pm .0035/5 = \pm .0007$ mm².

Acoustic data were recorded with a microphone (Electro-Voice), which was attached to the laryngeal mirror shaft 5 cm from the subject's mouth. Acoustic data were transmitted from the subject room to the equipment room via a patch panel and recorded on magnetic tape (Ampex, ATR–100). A Redlake Crystal TLG/LED Driver (13–0003) applied a timing code to the film border and a separate channel of the magnetic tape. This timing code was used to temporally synchronize the film and acoustic data with a resolution of 1 ms.

Intra- and Interjudge Glottal Area Measurement Reliability

The research assistant remeasured 10% of the frames from each film. Intrajudge agreement coefficients (Pearson r's) ranged from .76 to 1.00 with an overall average agreement coefficient of .90 and a maximum measurement error of 1.07 mm²($\bar{x}$ = .93 mm²).

These same frames were remeasured by the senior author. Interjudge agreement coefficients ranged from .68 to .91 with an average agreement coefficient of .82 and a maximum measurement error of 2.33 mm²($\bar{x}$ = 1.72 mm²).

SOURCE: Metz, D. E., Whitehead, R. L., & Whitehead, B. H. (1984). Mechanics of vocal fold vibration and laryngeal articulatory gestures produced by hearing-impaired speakers. *Journal of Speech and Hearing Research, 27,* 62–69.

The last example in this section is taken from an article by Shipp and McGlone and is shown in Excerpt 7.14. The interesting point here is that not only was there calibration of the instruments used but a physiologic calibration procedure was also employed. The need for this latter calibration procedure is described as well.

EXCERPT 7.14

INSTRUMENTAL CALIBRATION

Calibration signals for the six physiologic data channels were recorded prior to subject preparation. To calibrate the four EMG channels, a custom-built input simulator was used that generated single pulse signals at 50, 100, 200, and 500 microvolts. The subglottal pressure channel was calibrated using a U-tube manometer, so that pressures from zero to 24 cm of water could be recorded. Calibration of the air-flow channel was conducted using a direct connection between the pneumotachograph and a Brooks flow meter attached to an air supply cylinder. Air-flow rates were recorded in 100 cc/sec steps, from zero to 1000 cc/sec.

PHYSIOLOGIC CALIBRATION

No intersubject muscle comparisons could be made from absolute EMG microvolt values, since the magnitude of the EMG signal is a function of the distance between the recording electrodes and their location within the muscle. These positions could not be replicated between subjects; therefore, a physiologic calibration measure was incorporated to normalize the data and permit intersubject comparisons. Immediately before the first experimental task, subjects performed the calibration maneuver of inspiring air, then phonating the vowel /a/ in diatonic steps from the middle to the top of their modal registers. At different points in the performance of this calibration task, high levels of activity were picked up from each of the four muscles. From the EMG data obtained during the calibration maneuver, a metric of muscle activity was established from 100, representing each muscle's maximum activity generated during the calibration maneuver, to zero, the average baseline noise level in that channel.

SOURCE: Shipp, T., & McGlone, R. E. (1971). Laryngeal dynamics associated with voice frequency change. *Journal of Speech and Hearing Research, 14,* 761–768.

Reliability and Validity of Behavioral Instruments

Under behavioral instruments, we include the enormous array of standardized and nonstandardized tests such as paper-and-pencil tests of various types, articulation tests, language tests, speech-discrimination tests, hearing tests, attitude measures, and the like. Any of these kinds of materials may be used by researchers to make measurements of independent or dependent variables. Major problems with such instruments can pose significant threats to internal or external validity. Thus, the critical reader needs to assess carefully the adequacy of behavioral instruments used in research. Most speech pathologists and audiologists have had a reasonable amount of exposure to behavioral instruments through academic and practicum courses and clinical work. Also, there are some sources that interested readers can consult for specific information on various behavioral instruments such as Darley (1979) or Buros (1972). In this section, we will show some examples to illustrate some of the concepts of reliability and validity of measures that were discussed in Chapter 3.

Standardized Instruments. Many research articles in speech pathology and audiology report the use of standardized tests for the measurement of variables in their method section. In some cases, the researcher provides citations to the test manual that contains data on standardization or reference to previous research on the reliability and validity of the instrument used. If a standardized test was modified in administration or scoring, the author should identify the modification and explain the reason for the change. Significant modification may raise a question about whether the test as standardized has been compromised in some important way. That is: Have its reliability and validity been affected by the modification?

Several of these points are illustrated in Excerpt 7.15. In this study of basic concepts in hearing-impaired children, Davis used the Boehm Test of Basic Concepts. In the first paragraph, the author cites the test manual published by Psychological Corporation and provides a brief description of the instrument. The next two paragraphs provide an explanation for two changes in the procedure: the test was administered individually rather than as a group test; test directions were simplified to take into account the hearing impairment of the subjects.

Is the Boehm Test of Basic Concepts valid and reliable? If the reader is unfamiliar with this test, the test manual would have to be consulted to determine how the test was validated and what reliability data are provided. Another valuable source is Buros (1972) because the Boehm test is reviewed there (p. 335). The second question is whether the test modifications made by the researcher compromised the test instrument. Because the modifications, in this instance, seem relatively minor, it is unlikely (but not impossible) that they had an effect on the adequacy of the tool or the outcome of the study.

EXCERPT 7.15

PROCEDURES

The Boehm Test of Basic Concepts (Boehm, 1971) was administered individually to each child. The Boehm Test consists of 50 picture displays which represent concepts selected from basic kindergarten, first, and second grade curriculum materials, and which are considered necessary for understanding instructions and verbal directions issued by teachers in these grades (Boehm, 1971). The concepts tested consist of 23 space concepts, four time concepts, 18 quantity concepts, and five miscellaneous concepts, such as *different, other,* and *matches.* Test items begin with simple and progress toward more difficult concepts. Each picture display consists of three items from which to choose an answer.

Although the Boehm Test is designed as a group test in which children mark the appropriate answer in an individual test booklet, we decided to administer the test individually to the hearing-impaired children in order to maximize their chances of hearing and understanding the stimuli involved. Directions were simplified by this procedure, since the examiner could indicate the array of pictures from which the child was to choose an answer without using the complicated directions given in the test manual, for example:

> *Look for the gray box like this one on your page. Put your finger on the gray box with the book in it. Now take your finger off the box and pick up your pencil. Look at the circles and boxes. Mark the box that is at the center of the circle. . . . Mark the box that is at the center of the circle.* (Boehm, 1971).

Because of the importance of being able to follow directions in context, however, only the instructions regarding page descriptions were omitted. Instructions for the item given above were "Look at the circles and the boxes. Show me the box that is at the center of the circle. Put your finger on the box that is at the center of the circle." Each child was asked to look at the picture array, watch the face of the examiner as the stimuli were presented, and put his finger on the appropriate item.

Since the children attended several different schools in a fairly wide geographic area, they were tested in rooms provided by the school systems. In every case, the rooms were carpeted, quiet, and free from excessive auditory and visual distractions. These circumstances were considered optimal so that the children's errors were less likely to reflect poor listening conditions than actual lack of knowledge of the concepts being tested. None of the children exhibited an inability to perceive the stimulus materials, and many of them repeated portions of the directions before responding. The same procedures were employed for the children with normal hearing.

SOURCE: Davis, J. (1974). Performance of young hearing-impaired children on a test of basic concepts. *Journal of Speech and Hearing Research*, *17*, 342–351.

In a study of divergent semantic behavior in aphasics, Chapey, Rigrodsky and Morrison (1976) used seven tasks (tests) to measure divergence. Note in Excerpt 7.16 the literature citations to the original sources of the tests and the specific attention devoted to their reliability and validity.

EXCERPT 7.16

All of the experimental materials used in the present study were semantic tasks intended to elicit responses which could be measured in terms of their divergence. Seven tasks were used in the present study. Three were developed by Guilford (1967), two by Torrance (1966), and two by Felsenstein (1971). The validity and reliability of the measures have been established (Guilford and Hoepfner, 1971; Torrance, 1966).

SOURCE: Chapey, R., Rigrodsky, S., & Morrison, E. B. (1976). Divergent semantic behavior in aphasia. *Journal of Speech and Hearing Research*, *19*, 664–677.

A more extensive discussion of reliability and validity is illustrated in Excerpt 7.17. Here Woods deals directly with both issues and actually reports additional data in an attempt to demonstrate both the validity and reliability of the Ohio Social Acceptance Scale.

EXCERPT 7.17

It should be noted that a sociometric test does not indicate who a child's friends are, but who he wishes his friends were. Therefore, traditional tests of validity or reliability are somewhat inappropriate for evaluating any sociometric test. Jennings (1950) stated that sociometric choices have "face validity" because they are direct measures of the phenomenon under investigation. Thus, the validity of a child's response that he would like to have another child as a friend can hardly be questioned. Also, test–retest reliability studies will be affected by memory of previous responses if given too close together and affected by actual changes in group structure if too much time elapses between administrations (Remmers, 1963). Other data can corroborate or cast doubt on these ratings, however.

The validity of both the modified Ohio Social Acceptance Scale and the speaking competence scale (described below) was evaluated by comparing the assigned numerical ratings with the reasons the children reported for the ratings they gave. Reasons were available for practically all self-estimates and No. 4 ratings. The agreement between ratings and reasons obtained in a pilot study and in the present data indicated that the children knew what the numerical ratings meant and assigned them appropriately. Likewise, the accuracy with which a classroom teacher could predict how the class ratings would rank order the boys in her class on social position or speaking competence dimensions was partial evidence of the reliability of these measures. Mean Kendall's Tau coefficients (Siegel, 1956) indicated that the teachers' predicted rank orderings were significantly associated ($p < 0.05$) with those obtained from the class data for 74% of the classrooms on social position and 85% of the classrooms on speaking competence. Also, none of the differences between the mean percentile rankings obtained from the teachers' predictions and from the children's ratings of the stuttering boys was significant ($p > 0.05$) for either social position or speaking competence. These comparisons suggest that it would not be unreasonable to assume that the children's ratings were sufficiently reliable.

SOURCE: Woods, C. L. (1974). Social position and speaking competence of stuttering and normally fluent boys. *Journal of Speech and Hearing Research, 17,* 740–747.

Just because a standardized test is well known or widely used does not necessarily mean that its reliability and validity are adequate. McCauley and Swisher (1984) recently reviewed the psychometric characteristics of 30 language and articulation tests intended for use with preschool children. They applied 10 criteria in evaluating the 30 test manuals to assess the documentation of the reliability and validity of the tests as well as the documentation of other factors such as size and description of the normative samples, description of test procedure, qualifications of examiners, and statistical analysis of test scores of normative sample subgroups. Their analysis found many of the tests lacking in basic documentation of factors such as reliability and validity and concluded (McCauley & Swisher, 1984, p. 41):

> Most failures of tests to meet individual criteria occurred as a result of an absence of sought-after information rather than as a result of reported poor performance on them. The tests were not shown to be either well developed or poorly developed. This fact may falsely comfort some readers who may assume that, if collected, the data on their favorite test would be favorable. However, when given no information about a psychometric characteristic, the test user is realistically left to wonder whether or not a test is invalid and unreliable for his or her purposes. Stated differently, no news is bad news.

The lesson for the consumer of research is to look for evidence of reliability and validity of standardized tests used in research and not to assume that a test is reliable and valid just because it is popular.

Nonstandardized Instruments. Many studies make behavioral measurements with instruments that have not been standardized or published commercially. It is important for researchers using such behavioral instruments to indicate the reliability and validity of measurements made with such materials. Excerpt 7.18 illustrates the use of a nonstandardized behavioral instrument for measuring children's perception of vocal cues of emotional meaning. Notice how the authors describe the development of the measuring instrument and the attempts to assess its content validity. A careful rationale for the development of the instrument is presented and testing of the degree to which the items matched the intended representation is reported. Although the instrument is not a standardized test, information is reported that documents its content validity for the intended use.

EXCERPT 7.18

Development and Pretest of Instrument

The instrument used to measure the children's sensitivity to the vocal cues of emotion was developed and pretested in two stages. It is referred to subsequently as the *Measurement of Vocalic Sensitivity* (MOVS) instrument. For this initial study, only male voices were used. Even though Dimitrovsky employed both male and female voices on her stimulus tape, her findings indicated that the sex of the speaker interacted in complex ways with the emotion being presented. Because our primary interest was the exploration of differences in the interpretative skills of language-disordered and normal children, the potentially confounding influence of having both male and female speakers was not introduced.

In accordance with the recommendations of Beldoch (1964), a complete sentence containing neutral content was selected. The phrase was "Would you bring that to me." In the first stage of development, three professional actors recorded this phrase, supplying vocal cues corresponding to the emotions of happiness, anger, love, and sadness. Each actor provided numerous "takes" of each emotion, until he felt he could not improve upon his performance.

Subsequently, each take for each actor was evaluated by undergraduate students (N = 135). They were told the emotion each actor was portraying and were asked to rate the quality of each take. Based on these ratings, one performance of each emotion for each actor was selected as the most representative. This procedure produced a single stimulus tape containing 12 versions of the same sentence—three distinct male voices producing each of the four emotions. Both the actors' voices and the emotions were randomized on the tape to guard against order effects.

The second stage consisted of developing a method by which the children could express their recognition of these emotions. Because many of the children could not be expected to verbalize the various emotional labels, it was decided that all children would respond by pointing to the picture which matched the recorded emotional expressions. Although Dimitrovsky (1964) employed stick figures for this purpose, it was felt that pictures of actual people would be more realistic and valid. Three photographs developed for training people in "recognizing emotions from facial expressions" were selected to portray the emotions of happiness, anger, and sadness (Ekman & Friesen, 1975). These photographs contained only three male faces. A fourth picture, representing loving, depicted a father hugging his child. This final picture was selected from a magazine and contained the shoulders, necks, and faces of these characters; no commercial product or trademark was visible. All photographs were enlarged to 8 × 10 inches (approx. 20 × 25 cm) in black and white and were displayed on a plain background.

To test the content validity of the MOVS instrument, a second group of undergraduate students (N = 367) was employed to pretest the MOVS instrument. This group was composed of adult, native English speakers, who were judged to be normal in all aspects of speech and language production. As a group, these students successfully matched the vocal stimuli with their intended visual representations 96% of the time. Moreover, there was no indication of the tendency to select negative labels as reported by Dimitrovsky. These data, therefore, provided additional evidence that the task represented a valid indicant of the ability to interpret vocal cues of emotion.

SOURCE: Courtright, J. A., & Courtright, I. C. (1983). The perception of nonverbal vocal cues of emotional meaning by language-disordered and normal children. *Journal of Speech and Hearing Research, 26,* 412–417.

Excerpt 7.19 shows a portion of the Method section of a study of language development and symbolic play of normal and mentally retarded children. This section documents the authors' extensive analysis of the reliability of a number of measures of both language development and symbolic play that they employed. Their documentation of reliability of the measures is more extensive than the documentation to be found in some of the manuals of the standardized tests reviewed by McCauley and Swisher (1984)!

EXCERPT 7.19

Reliability

Several different types of reliability measures were taken. For assessing the reliability of MLU Stage placement, additional observers collected separate language samples (minimum of 50 utterances) from randomly selected children. Their MLU Stage placement of the children based on this independently collected sample was compared to the children's initial MLU Stage placement. The second language samples were gathered within a maximum of 14 days following the original language sample. This was performed for a total of 12 children, 5 normal (3 PI, 2 MLU I) and 7 mentally retarded children (3 PI, 4 MLU I). The experimenter and observers agreed on four of the five normal children's MLU Stage placement and on all seven of the mentally retarded children's MLU Stage placement.

Two methods were utilized to collect interjudge measures of scoring the children's symbolic play responses. First, observer reliability was based upon several independent and naive judges' examinations of a prepared videotape of randomly selected experimental trial symbolic play responses from several children. The 112 samples on this videotape were positive instances of symbolic play (i.e., the child's response previously was judged to represent typical conventional usage comparable to typical usage of the standard object). The judges viewed this reliability tape, and for each of the 112 samples they indicated which standard object was represented in the children's behavior. The audio portion of the reliability videotape was not presented. The comparison was point to point with the experimenter's initial scoring of the children's responses. Five judges viewed this prepared reliability videotape. The proportion of interjudge reliability ranged from .94 to .95, with a mean of .95. Intrajudge reliability for this procedure was 1.00.

Additional interjudge reliability measures in which two observers independently viewed randomly selected videotapes of several children's entire experimental sessions were collected. Here the judge observed the videotape of the entire session and scored the children's responses. A point-to-point comparison was made with the experimenter's initial scoring of the children's symbolic play responses and proportions of agreement calculated. A total of 11 children's individual experimental sessions were viewed. The breakdown of the 11 children were as follows: 6 normal children (3 PI, 3 MLU I) and 5 mentally retarded children (2 PI, 3 MLU I). The range of interjudge agreement for the normal children was .93–1.00, with a mean of .95. The range of interjudge agreement for the mentally retarded children was .87–1.00, with a mean of .946. Intrajudge reliability for the normal children ranged from .93 to 1.00, with a mean of .96, while the range was .93–1.00, with a mean of .98 for the mentally retarded children.

Temporal reliability of the children's responding to the experimental task was assessed by presenting the experimental task a second time to several children selected at random. The children's responses from the second administration were compared to their initial responses and the proportion of agreement calculated. The second administration occurred within 5 days of the initial experimental session. Temporal reliability of 11 children, 5 normal (2 PI, 3 MLU I) and 6 mentally retarded children (3 PI, 3 MLU I) was calculated. The range of temporal reliability for the normal children was .92–.96, with a mean of .94. The mentally retarded children's temporal reliability ranged from .94 to .96, with a mean of .95.

SOURCE: Casby, M. W., & Ruder, K. F. (1983). Symbolic play and early language development in normal and mentally retarded children. *Journal of Speech and Hearing Research*, 26, 404–411.

Excerpt 7.20 shows a portion of the Method section of a study by Campbell and Shriberg of pragmatic functions, linguistic stress, and natural phonological processes in speech-delayed children. Three different procedures for measuring these three variables are described in the method section. The description of each procedure includes a rationale for the measurements and appropriate literature citations to help document the development of valid procedures for measuring what the authors intended to measure. The description of the measurement of linguistic stress that is shown in Excerpt 7.20 illustrates the use of training procedure for ensuring that the judges would actually determine the type of stress correctly. Judges were provided with definitions and examples and extensive practice in the use of the procedure. Also described in the excerpt is an assessment of the intrajudge and interjudge reliability in identifying the stress types. The description of the phonological process analysis and the pragmatic function analysis in this Method section shows similar attempts to document the reliability and validity of those measures as well.

EXCERPT 7.20

STRESS TYPE ANALYSIS

To obtain ratings of linguistic stress, a tape containing 71 topics and 305 comments was constructed from 20 original tapes. Topics and comments were embedded in utterances ranging from two to nine words in length. All the words in the pragmatic analysis were included in this second (stress) analysis, with the exception of 36 single word utterances. Dubbing and editing of utterances containing these topics and comments from the original 20 tapes onto the experimental tape was accomplished by feeding the output of a Sony TC–270 audiotape recorder into a Crown 800 audiotape recorder.

Training Session.   Two speech-language pathologists with experience in listening studies were trained to determine the type of stress used during production of topics and comments. During a 1-hour training session, definitions and examples of two types of stress were presented to each judge. The two stress classifications used were primary stress and nonprimary stress. *Primary stress* was defined as the strongest word in a spoken utterance. Words produced with primary stress differed from words produced with nonprimary stress in one or all of the following suprasegmental characteristics: greater loudness, higher pitch, and increased length. *Nonprimary stress* was defined as any stress type that is not primary, including secondary, tertiary, and minimal stress types. A training tape consisting of 12 utterances, totaling 67 words, was presented individually to each judge. Judges were instructed to categorize each word in the 12 utterances as having primary or nonprimary stress. A word-by-word analysis of the 67 words judged for stress type by both judges yielded an interjudge agreement of 87%.·

Listening session.   Seven days following the training session, a listening session for both judges was held in a listening laboratory. The experimental tape was presented via a Sony ER-740 tape recorder that fed two listening booths equipped with Koss Pro 20 headphones. There were 376 utterances randomized and put into two groups. A written list of 188 utterances was prepared for each judge and served as a scoring sheet. Judgments were made individually, and each judge could listen to a given utterance up to three times before making a final decision.

Reliability assessment. During the listening session 50 utterances were presented twice to both judges to determine interjudge and intrajudge agreement for stress adjustments. These 50 utterances had been selected randomly from the total sample and placed in random order on the tape. Utterances consisted of 15 topics and 59 comments, respectively 21% and 19% of the utterances representing each pragmatic function. Intrajudge agreements were 94% and 96%. Interjudge agreement was 86%.

SOURCE: Campbell, T. F., & Shriberg, L. D. (1982). Associations among pragmatic functions, linguistic stress, and natural phonological processes in speech-delayed children. *Journal of Speech and Hearing Research, 25,* 547–553.

To summarize, the basic task in evaluating the adequacy of behavioral instruments in the Method section of a research article is to identify threats to internal validity posed by unreliable or invalid instruments. The task may be simplified if standardized tests are reported because reliability and validity information may be available for these instruments. The task may be more difficult if nonstandardized instruments are used. Here the consumer of research must evaluate the manner in which the instrument was constructed and used in order to determine its adequacy. The description of behavioral instruments used should be clear and comprehensive enough to allow the reader to determine if the instruments can yield valid and reliable results.

Other Measurement Considerations

In addition to concern about the calibration of hardware and the reliability and validity of behavioral instruments, several other miscellaneous aspects of the measurement process should be discussed in evaluating the materials described in the Method section. These include the appropriateness of measurements made, the role of the experimenter in making the measurements, the test environment, and the test instructions.

Appropriateness of Measurements. Assuming that the instruments used provide reliable and valid measurements of the variables of interest, the reader should be concerned about the appropriateness of the measurements for fulfilling the specific purpose of the study. In other words, the Method section should be evaluated in light of the purpose and rationale spelled out in the introduction to the article. Excerpt 7.21 includes material from both the introduction and method sections of an article on the use of pretreatment measures to predict outcomes of stuttering therapy. The first part of the excerpt shows the author's development of a rationale for the use of measures of stuttering severity, personality, and attitudes toward stuttering as pretreatment predictors of therapy outcome in the introduction to the article. The second part of the excerpt is from the Method section and shows how the author selected instruments for measuring each of these three general variables.

EXCERPT 7.21

In all the recent studies, the only high correlation between a pretreatment measure and outcome is the finding by Gregory (1969) that pretreatment severity rating was positively correlated (r = 0.78) with change in severity rating from before to immediately after treatment. This result is not surprising, however, since severe stutterers enter therapy with higher levels on the severity scale and thus have a greater range to travel during treatment. Moreover, this correlation is dependent on when outcome is measured. When the nine-month posttreatment changes in severity were correlated with pretreatment severity, the correlation dropped from 0.78 to 0.48.

Changes in stuttering severity from immediately after to many months after treatment, such as shown by Gregory's subjects, are not unusual. Data are now available to support the long-standing clinical impression that many stutterers regress considerably after treatment (Ingham & Andrews, 1973; Perkins, 1973). In fact, those who improve most in treatment may show the greatest regression later (Prins, 1970). Thus, studies which measure stuttering immediately after treatment, such as those of Lanyon (1965, 1966), Prins (1968), and Gregory (1969), may not have assessed the most clinically important outcome of treatment. Long-term outcome is a more accurate assessment of how treatment has affected a stutterer. Of the studies cited here, only Perkins (1973) used longer term outcome in attempting to find predictors of treatment effects.

The lack of useful predictors of long-term outcome of stuttering treatment suggests a need for further investigation. Although personality measures by themselves have not been effective predictors, they might well be combined with overt measures of pretreatment stuttering for prognosis. Besides measures of personality and level of stuttering, some assessment of attitudes might also be helpful in forecasting outcome. This seems particularly possible in light of recent evidence that cognitive variables are important in determining overt behaviors (Kimble, 1973).

The present study was designed to evaluate a combination of pretreatment measures of stuttering, attitudes toward stuttering, and personality factors, as predictors of long-term outcome of treatment.

. . . .

The basic design of the study was to obtain pretreatment measures from subjects in Group 1 and then evaluate their fluency a year after treatment. Following this, multiple regression analyses were carried out to determine the degree to which pretreatment measures predicted the subjects' outcomes. Equations derived from the regressions were then used to predict the outcomes for subjects in Group 2 on the basis of their pretreatment measures. Correlations between the predicted and actual outcomes for subjects in Group 2 provided cross-validation of the findings for subjects in Group 1.

Pretreatment Measures. The pretreatment data, which included measures of personality, attitudes about stuttering, and amount of stuttering, were obtained when subjects entered the hospital.

Personality was assessed by the extroversion and neuroticism scales of the Eysenck Personality Inventory (Eysenck & Eysenck, 1963). Neuroticism and extroversion have been shown previously to be associated with success and failure on stuttering therapy programs (Brandon & Harris, 1967).

Attitudes toward stuttering were measured by the short form of the Erickson Scale of Communication Attitudes (Erickson, 1969; Andrews & Cutler, 1974) and by an abbreviated version of the Stutterer's Self-Rating of Reactions to Speech Situations (Johnson, Darley, & Spriestersbach, 1963; Cutler, 1973). Only the avoidance and reaction responses of the Stutterer's Self-Rating form were used because these appeared to be most related to attitudes.Clinical experience suggested that those stutterers who scored high on the avoidance and reaction parts of this assessment were more likely to be emotionally affected by their stuttering, regardless of their actual level of stuttering.

In addition to the above assessments, amount of stuttering was measured when the subjects entered treatment. Stuttering was measured during conversational speech in percentage syllables stuttered (pre%SS) and syllables per minute (preSPM). These measures have been shown to correlate highly with listener judgments of severity and to be reliable (Young, 1961; Andrews & Ingham, 1971). Stuttering scores used for the multiple regression analyses were %SS and "alpha" score, a measure which combines frequency of stuttering and speech rate. The alpha score was developed because speech rate has been considered an important adjunct in the assessment of fluency (Ingham, 1972; Perkins, 1975).

Posttreatment Measures. Twelve to 18 months after the subjects completed the three-week treatment program, they were contacted by a management consultant who was unknown to them, and a meeting was arranged in his office in a different part of the city from the place of treatment. A five-minute sample of conversational speech was recorded and later scored by the experimenter. Measures of outcome were percentage of syllables stuttered (post%SS), alpha score (postalpha), and percent change in frequency of stuttering (%change). This last score, %change, was calculated by the following formula:

$$\frac{\text{pre\%SS} - \text{post\%SS}}{\text{pre\%SS}}$$

SOURCE: Guitar, B. (1976). Pretreatment factors associated with the outcome of stuttering therapy. *Journal of Speech and Hearing Research, 19,* 590–600.

Another aspect of appropriateness is whether the researcher has selected the most appropriate kind of measurement from among the various options available. Different kinds of measurements are more or less appropriate for answering different kinds of questions. Many different kinds of measurements may be applied in the study of a particular problem to investigate different aspects of the problem. In the brief introduction shown in Excerpt 7.22, Kent and LaPointe justify the appropriateness of acoustic measurement of the speech of a patient with palilalia as a follow-up to a previous description of the characteristics of this patient's speech.

EXCERPT 7.22

An earlier report (LaPointe & Horner, 1981) described a patient with palilalia, which is described in the literature as an acquired disorder characterized by reiteration of utterances in a context of increasing rate and decreasing loudness. The patient, J.L.B., was a 29-year-old man with palilalia of 4 years' duration. The LaPointe and Horner report is apparently the first detailed description of the nature and severity of palilalic reiteration. The subject of the case study generated a large quantity of reiterative samples, as about 38% of a total speech sample of 5,489 words was reiterated.

LaPointe and Horner reported several characteristics of the pathological reiterative utterances, including reiteration types, frequency of reiteration for seven speech tasks, and consistency and adaptation effects. However, their report did not attempt to verify the acoustic properties that usually are mentioned as characteristic of palilalia, namely, increasing rate (accelerando) and decreasing loudness (decrescendo) over a reiteration series. The present report describes the acoustic properties of reiterated utterances and attempts to answer the general question: What is the systematic acoustic variation, if any, from item to item in a repetition series?

SOURCE: Kent, R. D., & LaPointe, L. L. (1982). Acoustic properties of pathologic reiterative utterances: A case study of palilalia. *Journal of Speech and Hearing Research, 25*, 95–99.

The final concern deals with the appropriateness of the instrument for the subjects studied. A test standardized on adults may be ill suited for use with children. A test developed on children from one socioeconomic group may not be valid when administered to children from a different socioeconomic level. Arndt (1977), for instance, recently criticized the Northwestern Syntax Screening Test (NSST) on several grounds, one of which was that the test may have limited applicability because of the nature of the sample used for standardization, namely middle- to upper middle-class children from one geographical area. In addition, the norms do not extend beyond age 6 to 11 (Lee 1977). Both the researcher *and* the clinician must recognize the limitations of the test and use the test accordingly. To reiterate, the point is simply that the critical reader of a research article must determine if the instruments used are appropriate to the sample investigated.

Experimenter Bias in Research Measurement. Another measurement consideration is the problem of experimenter bias, or the Rosenthal effect in the making of research measurements (Rosenthal, 1966; Rosenthal & Rosnow, 1969). As discussed in Chapter 3, the Rosenthal effect can be of two types: (1) experimenter attributes that can interact with an independent variable to influence subjects' behavior or (2) experimenter expectancies that bias an observer's measurement of the behavior of subjects. The first type actually changes subjects' behavior, whereas the second type does not change the subject's behavior but changes the way it is measured. It is important to note that expectancy effects have been identified in a wide variety of areas, including learning studies, reaction-time studies, psychophysical studies, and animal research (Christensen, 1977).[1]

There are several different methods that an experimenter can use to reduce or control experimenter bias. The critical reader of research should be alert to these methods and attempt to identify them *somewhere* in the Method section. One way of controlling experimenter expectancy is to use a blind technique whereby the experimenter knows the hypothesis but does not know which treatment condition the subject is in. Barber (1976) makes a distinction between an investigator (designs, supervises, analyzes, and reports the study) and an experimenter (tests subjects and collects data) and urges, as another way of controlling experimenter bias, that the investigator and experimenter *not* be the same person. Still another method is to automate procedures and, where possible, to record and analyze responses by mechanical or electrical devices. Experimenter bias can also be reduced, according to Barber (1976), by the use of strict experimental protocols and by frequent checks to determine if the protocol, designed by the investigator, is being followed by the experimenter. To control for experimenter attributes, different experimenters, with different attributes, could be used in a given study. Or a study could be replicated using a different experimenter, especially if experimenter attributes were believed to have confounded the data of the first study.

Surprisingly little attention has been paid to the problem of experimenter bias in speech pathology and audiology research. One study (Hipskind & Rintelmann, 1969) did investigate the effect of experimenter bias on puretone and speech audiometry and found no influence of attempts to bias experienced or inexperienced testers with true or false information about prior audiometric results. No systematic research has been published to identify areas of speech and hearing research that are more or less susceptible to experimenter bias, however. A few studies may be found in the speech pathology and audiology literature that have introduced some control procedures to attempt to reduce or eliminate problems of experimenter bias.

The examples shown in the next three excerpts may help readers to identify how researchers have tried to reduce experimenter bias threats to internal validity. Excerpt 7.23 shows two portions of the Method section taken from a multidiscipline study of functional hearing loss, an area where testor or investigator bias has long intruded. The last sentence of the first part of the

---

[1]There is some controversy over the existence and magnitude of experimenter-expectancy effects. For a detailed discussion of this issue, the reader is urged to see Barber and Silver (1968) and Barber (1976).

excerpt is the key one and indicates that of the several investigators involved in the evaluation of subjects (including a psychologist and a psychiatrist),

---

EXCERPT 7.23

SUBJECT SELECTION

Methodological and procedural inadequacies of subject selection in previous studies have been fully discussed (Chaiklin & Ventry, 1963). In this study an effort was made to develop precise sampling procedures, objective general and medical eligibility criteria, and specific audiometric criteria.

A monthly schedule of appointments (covering a 25-mo period) was established specifying the random order in which subjects for the two major groups would be hospitalized for evaluation. The appointment designations referred not to individual subjects but only to the order in which subjects for the two groups would be evaluated. Twice as many functional as nonfunctional subjects were included in the schedule. The order in which subjects were scheduled was known only to the project audiologists. Thus all research evaluations, except the audiological evaluation, were performed without examiners knowing to which group a subject was assigned.

. . . .

All inpatient examinations for both groups were conducted in the suite containing the I.A.C. 1201 booth. In addition, this suite contained a Grason-Stadler Békésy audiometer Model E 800, and an accessory Random Variable Attenuator (RVA) that allowed six different values of attenuation (0 to 25 dB in 5-dB steps) to be introduced into the earphone line before each repeat measurement.

The face of the RVA is blank but there is provision for quick read-out of the amount of attenuation introduced into the line. The six attenuation values are arranged randomly on the RVA's selector switch. Before a repeat measurement the experimenter rotated the dial to introduce one of the attenuation values. After the repeat measurement the RVA value was determined and then subtracted from the hearing level dial reading to produce the correct measurement figure. The use of the RVA made test–retest measurements relatively free from tester bias. The RVA was designed and constructed by Mr. L. G. Pew, Electro-Acoustic Co., San Carlos, California.

SOURCE: Chaiklin, J. B., & Ventry, I. M. (1965). Introduction and research plan. *Journal of Auditory Research, 5,* 179–190.

---

only the audiologists knew what subjects were in the control (nonfunctional) group or in the experimental (functional) group. The other experimenters did "blind" evaluations. How did the audiologists control for their bias? Because they knew which subjects were in which group, experimenter expectancy could not be totally controlled. However, expectancies with regard to certain aspects of the data were controlled, in part, as shown in Excerpt 7.23. Test-retest measurements constituted an important part of the audiologic evaluation and the RVA controlled, to some extent, experimenter bias from influencing the test-retest measurements. In addition, a rigid test protocol was followed by the entire research staff.

The next example, shown in Excerpt 7.24, is from a study of stuttering in monozygotic and dizygotic twins. Note that two diagnoses had to be made: one for zygosity and one for stuttering. In both instances "blind" judges were used who had no knowledge of the other diagnosis while making the diagnosis for which they were responsible. Also note the use of two judges for zygosity, one of whom had contact with the twins and one of whom did not in order to have no information available to that judge about stuttering concordance.

EXCERPT 7.24

Diagnosis of Zygosity

Twin pairs were classified as either monozygotic (MZ) or dizygotic (DZ), based on the following four criteria: (a) blood grouping for nine systems: ABO, Rhesus, MNSs, P, Lutheran, Kell, Lewis, Duffy, Kidd (Race & Sanger, 1968). Permission for blood tests was granted by 22 pairs, six of whose HLA tissue typing was also available; (b) total ridge counts and maximal palmar ATD angle (Holt, 1968); (c) cephalic index (Weiner & Lourie, 1969); and (d) height.

In seven pairs, DZ classification was certain because of the presence of at least one blood type difference. For each remaining pair, the probability of dizygosity was calculated, given the observed intrapair differences and similarities on the four criteria (Maynard-Smith & Penrose, 1955; Race & Sanger, 1968). The calculated probability of dizygosity was less than .05 in all but three of the pairs classified as MZ and greater than .95 in all but four of the pairs classified as DZ. Final classification was based on the probabilities examined in conjunction with intrapair differences in iris color, hair color and form, earlobe attachment, and finger ridge patterns. Zygosity was assessed by two judges, one of whom had direct contact with the twins, while the other made the diagnosis on the basis of profile and full-face photographs and all the relevant data. Thus, the second judge had no information about stuttering concordance. The zygosity classifications of the two judges agreed in every case.

Speech Samples and Diagnosis of Stuttering

For each subject, two 500-word speech samples were recorded: a monologue with standard instructions ("Tell the story of a book or film"); and a conversation with the experimenter on standardized topics. The recordings of the 60 subjects were arranged on audiotape in random order, and stuttering was diagnosed by a speech pathologist who had never met the twins and had no knowledge of twin pair membership or zygosity, thus ensuring independence of stuttering diagnosis and zygosity classification.

SOURCE: Howie, P. M. (1981). Concordance for stuttering in monozygotic and dizygotic twin pairs. *Journal of Speech and Hearing Research, 24,* 317–321.

The third example is from a study of sign and verbal language training with retarded children. The first section of Excerpt 7.25 briefly describes the assembling of the three groups for the experiment. The second section of the excerpt describes the trainers who were used with the three groups. Note that several different trainers were used; that all of them expected some gain, regardless of the group with which they worked; and that none of the trainers knew the specific hypotheses of the study, although they were aware of the general purpose of the study and group assignment. Although the trainers were not totally "blind", they were all reasonably homogeneous with respect to the influence of expectations, and they were unaware of the specific hypotheses and sensorimotor data on the subjects. It would be difficult to use trainers in a study like this who were totally "blind" as to all aspects of the research throughout the course of the entire study.

EXCERPT 7.25

The matched subjects were randomly assigned to one of three groups in a stratified manner so that each group contained two subjects living at home and two subjects living in the residential facility. The three groups consisted of a group receiving speech training using the program developed by Bricker, Dennison, and Bricker (1976); a group receiving training in sign language using a program adapted from the Bricker et al. program (this was done to keep the two language training programs as similar as possible); and a placebo group receiving instruction in an area other than communication.

. . . .

Each of the two trainers worked with two children from each of the three groups. In addition, the trainers were at different training sites and had no opportunity to observe each other. During the 33 months of this project, there were six trainers, three at each site. This was due to the trainers, who were also graduate students, completing their coursework and getting full-time jobs. Thus, the trainers were changed each summer at each site. The trainers were told which subjects were in each group and the overall purpose of the study. They were told that all of the subjects, even the placebos, were expected to show gains. They were unaware of the sensorimotor assessment data and of the hypotheses of the study.

SOURCE: Kahn, J. V. (1981). A comparison of sign and verbal language training with nonverbal retarded children. *Journal of Speech and Hearing Research, 24,* 113–119.

The problem of experimenter bias is basically a problem in determining the *validity* of the measures made by an experimenter. The more free of bias an experimenter is, the more valid are the measurements made by that experimenter. An issue that is closely related to experimenter bias, then, is the *reliability* of the experimenter in making these measurements. Researchers can check an experimenter's reliability in one of two ways. *Inter-experimenter* reliability is the consistency among two or more experimenters in making a measurement. *Intra-experimenter* reliability is the consistency of one experimenter in remaking a particular measurement a second time. Excerpt 7.26 shows information on experimenter reliability taken from the method section of an article on laryngeal behavior during the production of voiced and voiceless consonants. Both intrajudge and interjudge reliability are assessed for both the laryngeal behavior judgments and the phonetic transcriptions of the voiced and voiceless consonants.

EXCERPT 7.26

Intra- and Interjudge Reliability

To assess the intrajudge and interjudge reliability of the laryngeal behavior judgments, 52 randomly selected consonantal utterances (9% of the total) were selected for remeasurement. From four to eight productions were selected from each of the eight speakers, so that the sample consisted of 28 plosives (15 voiced and 13 voiceless) and 24 fricatives (13 voiced and 11 voiceless).

The first author rejudged the vocal fold behavior associated with the 52 consonantal productions while the second author separately analyzed the same subset of samples. Analysis of intrajudge agreement of laryngeal behavior determined for the 52 samples (agreement/disagreement + agreement, after Sander, 1961) revealed considerable agreement (.98), ranging from .84 to 1.00 for individual subjects. Interjudge agreement was .87 for all subjects combined (range = .66–1.00 for individual subjects' productions).

To assess the intratranscriber reliability of phonetic transcription, a subset of 64 randomly selected samples (8 productions from each speaker for 13% of the total) were retranscribed by the first author. Of the 64 test words, 35 were word-initial plosives (19 voiced and 16 voiceless) and 29 were word-initial fricatives (18 voiced and 11 voiceless). Comparison of the first author's original and second transcription revealed intratranscriber agreement of .97 (range = .87–1.00).

Intertranscriber reliability of phonetic transcription was assessed by having two judges (R1 and R2) transcribe each speaker's second production of the entire stimulus set. Interjudge agreement (Sander, 1961) between the first author and R1 was .91 (range = .70–1.00 for transcriptions of individual speakers), whereas intertranscriber agreement between the first author and R2 was .93 (range = .83–1.00).

SOURCE: Mahshie, J. J., & Conture, E. G. (1983). Deaf speakers' laryngeal behavior. *Journal of Speech and Hearing Research, 26,* 550–559.

One final example should suffice. Toler and Bankson explored the efficacy and reliability of an interrogative model as a means of studying parental questions and children's responses to various interrogative forms. Excerpt 7.27 provides a detailed description of both intrajudge and interjudge reliability. Note that a technique commonly employed to produce high rater reliability was not employed in this study, to wit, a rater training program. The substantial interjudge agreements shown in Table 3 of Excerpt 7.27 might have been even higher if a formal training program had been employed by the researchers.

EXCERPT 7.27

SCORER RELIABILITY

One form of support for Leach's classification and analysis system was obtained through the high degree of inter- and intrajudge reliability obtained for the category placements. Item-by-item interjudge reliability comparisons of the language measures were made between judgments of the first investigator and two other speech pathologists. Each judge was familiar with Leach's model (Leach, 1972) and was informed of the modification made in Leach's classification system for this investigation. No formal training program relating to the use of the model in judging sample questions and responses was afforded the judges, however. Using a transcript of the interactions, the three judges independently assigned an interrogative category number for each of the mother's questions and judged the child's responses from the mother-child interaction as appropriate or inappropriate.

Decisions of Judge 1 were those utilized in the analysis of data. While variation existed in the percentage of agreement between Judge 1 and the other two

TABLE 3. PERCENTAGE OF INTERJUDGE AGREEMENT BETWEEN THE INVESTIGATOR (JUDGE 1) AND TWO JUDGES OF THE MOTHERS' INTERROGATIVES AND CHILDREN'S RESPONSES IN THE MOTHER-CHILD INTERACTIONS

| | Judge Pairs | | |
Subject	1 and 2	1 and 3	2 and 3
1. Interrogatives	0.94	0.96	0.90
Responses	0.90	0.94	0.92
2. Interrogatives	0.92	0.86	0.82
Responses	0.92	0.92	0.92
3. Interrogatives	0.74	0.86	0.77
Responses	0.86	0.96	0.82
Overall interrogatives	0.87	0.89	0.83
Responses	0.89	0.94	0.88

judges regarding the types of interrogatives used by mothers and the appropriateness of the children's responses, in no instance was this agreement lower than 86% between Judge 1 and at least one of the other judges (Table 3). The highest overall interjudge reliability was achieved for Subject 1, while the lowest occurred for Subject 3. It appeared that the lower reliability scores for Subject 3 were in part a result of the *wh-* interrogative questions being judged as interrogating for a nominal segment by one of the judges. For example, "What color is it?" was incorrectly categorized as a Category 9 (*wh-* interrogative nominal segment) question.

Interjudge reliability comparisons were also made for the children's responses to the interrogative probe. Interjudge item-by-item reliability between each pair of judges ranged from 93 to 100%.

Intrajudge reliabilty measures were made of Judge 1's classification of mothers' interrogatives and children's responses six weeks after the initial judgments were made. Item-by-item percentages of agreement ranged from 90 to 100%.

SOURCE: Toler, S. A., & Bankson, N. W. (1976). Utilization of an interrogative model to evaluate mother's use and children's comprehension of question forms. *Journal of Speech and Hearing Disorders, 41,* 301–314.

Test Environment.   The environment within which research measurements are made may be an important aspect of measurement in many studies. Test environment may affect both internal and external validity. With regard to internal validity, test environment should be specified if measurements could vary from one environment to another. Also, the constancy of environments across all measures should be ascertained if measurements need to be made in different environments. If environmental variables need to be controlled, sufficient detail should be provided to allow the environment to be replicated in future research. Excerpt 7.28 shows a description of the test environment from a study of speechreading and visual evoked-responses. Sufficient description of the environment is necessary for replication and for allowing readers to evaluate the adequacy of the environment for making the kind of measures reported. Note, for example, the isolation of the subjects from the "characteristically audible 'pop' of the photostimulator flash tube."

EXCERPT 7.28

Each subject was tested individually in a double-walled, electrically shielded, sound-attenuating IAC chamber. The photostimulator was situated in an adjacent IAC chamber facing the subject on the other side of a 6-paneled window which separated the two rooms. This arrangement produced an effective isolation of the subject from the characteristically audible "pop" of the photostimulator flash tube.

During the session, subjects sat in a comfortable, high-backed, padded chair equipped with a head rest. They were instructed to keep their eyes closed during each condition, to remain in a comfortably still and relaxed position, and to keep their heads oriented toward the flash source. During each condition, the lights in the subjects' room were extinguished. Subjects were given a 2-min rest period between conditions during which the room lights, which produced a relatively dim illumination, were turned on. Between conditions, subjects were instructed to open their eyes and relax until the start of the next condition.

SOURCE: Samar, V. J., & Sims, D. G. (1984). Visual evoked-response components related to speechreading and spatial skills in hearing and hearing-impaired adults. *Journal of Speech and Hearing Research, 27,* 162–172.

Research studies in audiology or in speech science report the kind of test room used and the background noise levels because of the importance of maintaining an adequately low background noise level to eliminate masking in audiology studies and to yield noise-free recordings for speech analysis. Studies of lipreading often report the illumination characteristics of the room because of the importance of lighting for lipreading. Anytime environmental variables can affect measurements taken in a given research study, they should be specified.

With respect to external validity, the environment may serve as a "reactive arrangement" so that generalizations may be limited to individuals functioning only in that particular environment. The question facing the critical reader is whether the test environment is so different from environments to which the reader wishes to generalize as to preclude such generalization. An adequate description of the environment in which testing or treatment took place can help the reader judge the possible reactivity of the environment. It would be even better for the researcher to discuss the possible threat to external validity of reactive arrangements or to test the generality of results to other environments with a systematic replication.

Excerpt 7.29 is from a study by Andrews and Ingham that addresses the issue of generalization of the results of stuttering therapy to other environments. The first part of Excerpt 7.29 is from their Introduction section, the second part is from their Results section. We have italicized a portion of the excerpt to highlight the authors' concern about external validity of stuttering-treatment effects. Note the authors' expression of concern regarding the lack of information about generalization in the reporting of results of many treatments and the unique feature of a generalization probe to test the degree to which their results were "laboratory-bound."

EXCERPT 7.29

This paper is addressed to the problem of evaluating the effects, or outcome, resulting from the treatment of stuttering. It will be argued that a satisfactory procedure for evaluating the outcome of treatment must establish a method of measuring stuttering behavior, *must show that changes occurring in the treat-ment situation carry over into the outside world,* and must be capable of es-timating the degree to which the results achieved prove stable over time. The stuttering therapy literature is generally bereft of reports which fulfill these suggested criteria. Genuine therapeutic success in individual cases is probably not uncommon and apparently occurs with many of the currently used therap-ies. But lack of preparedness to systematically measure progress and assess outcome of treatment may have led to the present crisis in confidence over the efficacy of treatments for stuttering (Van Riper, 1970; Wingate, 1971).

. . . .

One strangely neglected feature of many treatments is the absence of a design which ensures that improvements attained within the laboratory generalize to the outside world, or are not "laboratory-bound." In the present program, gen-eralization of treatment gains was assessed by the use of a "probe" measure of speech performance during treatment. Each evening the subjects were assessed in conditions which were independent of most stimuli associated with the laboratory. From this measure it was found, for example, that subjects who were treated by a regular contingent token-system schedule displayed im-proved performance in both the probe and laboratory situations. However, when subjects were treated with a mixed noncontingent and contingent token-system schedule, they did not show significant improvement in the probe measure, despite concurrent laboratory improvement. Thus the contingent token-system schedule, as used in this therapy program, was demonstrated to produce treatment and token control effects over stuttering (Ingham, 1972).

SOURCE: Andrews, G., & Ingham, R. J. (1972). An approach to the evaluation of stuttering therapy. *Journal of Speech and Hearing Research, 15,* 296–302.

In summary, the test environment is an important part of the materials section of an article for two reasons. First, the environment may be impor-tant in determining the internal validity of the study by assessing the degree to which the environment affects the measurements made. Second, the nature of the research environment is important in determining the external validity of the results with regard to generalizing to other settings.

Instructions.   The final consideration in this section has to do with instruc-tions. Instructions to subjects can be thought of as part of instrumentation because instructions are the tools by which the researcher attempts to elicit the desired response or behavior and to maintain a consistent response set across subjects. Inadequate, inappropriate, poorly worded instructions thus pose an instrumentation threat to internal validity. In many circumstances, instructions are rather straightforward and, in fact, are specified in the ad-ministration of standardized test instruments. In other instances, the re-searcher may have to develop a set of instructions. The intent of the instruc-tions, the thrust of the instructions, if not the instructions themselves, need to be specified by the researcher. The critical evaluator needs to ask two questions: (1) Are the instructions appropriate to the task at hand? and (2) Is sufficient detail provided to allow for replication or for clinical application?

An illustration here may be instructive. One of us (IMV) was involved in a series of studies dealing with the measurement of most comfortable loudness (MCL), a measure that is highly subjective and, thus, prone to different interpretations by researcher and subject alike. In the first article of the series (Ventry, Woods, Rubin, & Hill, 1971), three appendices detailed the instructions that were employed. Because of the length of the manuscript, the editor suggested that the instructions be either condensed or omitted entirely. Our response, in correspondence with the editor, was as follows:

> We would prefer to present the instructions in toto because instructions for MCL measurement are critical. The exact instructions might be useful for subsequent studies of MCL or for replication studies or even for clinical use. It may be that the instructions can appear within the text rather than as Appendices. This would be perfectly acceptable to us.

The editor acceded to our request and the instructions were printed in their entirety. That the editor's final decision was correct is attested to by the fact that the same instructions or the instructions with minor modifications have been used by investigators in subsequent studies of comfortable loudness. If nothing else, the use of similar or identical instructions across studies reduces the confounding influence of instructions when making interstudy comparisons.

Earlier in this chapter, we reprinted a rather lengthy excerpt from the study by Duffy et al. (1975) on pantomime recognition in aphasics (see Excerpt 7.5). Excerpt 7.30 is taken from the same study and shows how the researchers used nonverbal training techniques to instruct subjects in the task of responding to a pantomime act. The specific procedures used to train (instruct) subjects are detailed in an appendix. Because instructions are so critical to the pantomime test, the authors identify the number and type of subjects who could not understand the instructions (paragraph 2) as well as the time required to instruct each group of subjects (paragraph 3). Certainly the nonverbal instructions were appropriate to the task and sufficient detail was provided to allow for replication.

EXCERPT 7.30

Task Instruction by Nonverbal Training

To circumvent the effects of impaired verbal comprehension among the aphasic subjects, nonverbal training procedures were developed to instruct subjects in the task of pointing to a picture in response to the pantomimic act of the examiner. The specific procedures used are described in Appendix B.

Of the 134 subjects who were given the nonverbal training procedures only four could not be satisfactorily conditioned. Of these, none were from the aphasic group, two were right-hemisphere-damaged, and two were from the subcortical group. These four were generally confused and disoriented and although two of them met the initial conditioning criterion they had to be frequently reinstructed in the task. These results demonstrate that even the most severely impaired aphasic subjects can quickly and easily learn the required response without concern that their responses are contaminated by a misunderstanding of verbal instruction.

Completion Time for Training

Not only was the nonverbal training process highly successful but it required a relatively brief time even for aphasic subjects. The mean time (in minutes) for the four groups of subjects was aphasics, 1.6; right-hemisphere-damaged, 1.2; subcortical, 1.3; and control, 1.4. The differences among the four groups were not significant ($F = 0.74$; df = 3, 126; $p > 0.05$). The control group had the largest standard deviation (1.6 minutes) and widest range (0.6 to 9.2 minutes). For the aphasic group the range was 0.4 to 6.5 minutes with a standard deviation of 1.4. There was a tendency for the more severely impaired aphasics to take longer than those with milder impairments as indicated by the correlation between conditioning time and overall PICA score (Pearson $r = -0.41$; $p < 0.01$).

Completion Time for the Test

Extensive training of the examiners was undertaken to insure that each of the 50 stimuli was pantomimed in exactly the same manner by each of the three examiners. The pace and manner of the presentation of stimuli and the recording procedures were carefully controlled among the examiners. Since the pace and procedures of the examiners were carefully standardized, differences in completion time on the test among the four groups of subjects can be attributed to differences in the subjects' performances.

SOURCE: Duffy, R. J., Duffy, J. R., & Pearson, K. L. (1975). Pantomime recognition in aphasics. *Journal of Speech and Hearing Research, 18,* 115–132.

The example shown in Excerpt 7.31 is from a study of vocal characteristics of stutterers and normal speakers during choral reading. The authors not only describe their instructions to the subjects but also provide a detailed rationale for the specific instructions used relative to the purpose of the study. The instructions are presented in sufficient detail for another investigator to replicate the procedure.

EXCERPT 7.31

Subjects were tested individually in a sound-treated room. The conditions were presented in a counterbalanced order with at least a 20-minute rest period between them to minimize adaptation (Jamison, 1955).

Each condition began with a subject receiving a standard set of instructions. In the experimental condition, these directions included the statement, "If you experience a disfluency, stumble over or misread a word as you are reading in unison, don't try to rush to catch up. Just skip ahead in the reading to the word you hear the model speaker producing." These instructions were given for the following reasons: It was assumed that a subject who experienced any of the speech production lapses mentioned above, would as a result, fall behind and out of unison with the model speaker. Consequently, the subject might be tempted to shorten his subsequent vowel durations in an effort to speed up, catch the model and get back in unison with him. We wanted to discourage such a reaction. Had we failed to do this, the subject could have modified his vowel durations for reasons that had nothing to do with any effect that the independent variable might have had on them. When signalled to begin, the subject read aloud into a microphone (Sony ECM 50) that was positioned and maintained a set distance from his mouth. During the experimental condition only, the subject wore earphones in order to hear the tape of the speaker with whom he was instructed to read in unison. This taped signal was presented to subjects at a comfortable loudness level with the playback volume setting fixed. Subjects' oral readings were audio-taped (Ampex AG 350).

SOURCE: Adams, M. R., & Ramig, P. (1980). Vocal characteristics of normal speakers and stutterers during choral reading. *Journal of Speech and Hearing Research, 23,* 457–469.

In conclusion, the major emphasis of this section on materials has been to identity instrumentation threats to internal validify. Inadequate instrumentation and inadequate materials can vitiate the value of an elegant design, but, to reiterate, a poor problem cannot be salvaged with even the most sophisticated instrumental array. Thus, the need for the enlightened consumer of research to put the Materials section of the research article into proper perspective. The Materials section is important but it constitutes only one portion of the research article.

Procedures

The Procedure section of the research article usually concludes the Method section. It is here that the researcher describes what is done to the subjects with the materials. It must be recognized that for convenience and simplicity, we have divided the present chapter into the three *typical* parts of a Method section. Reading just a few issues of journals such as *JSHD* and *JSHR* will quickly reveal that there may be considerable overlap among parts; some procedures may be described in the Materials section, subject-selection procedures might be handled in the Procedures section, and so on. Despite the variety of formats used, the critical reader's responsibility is to identify how the researcher has dealt with the threats to internal and external validity detailed in Chapter 3. Because the preceding sections of this chapter have dealt primarily with the threats to validity posed by subject-selection procedures and instrumentation (materials), this section will deal with the remaining threats to validity.

It should be apparent by now that prinicpal ways to reduce threats to validity are through the use of an appropriate experimental design or through the use of special precautions when employing a descriptive design. For example, the one group pretest–posttest design is far weaker than the randomized pretest–posttest control-group design. A between-subjects design with faulty subject-selection criteria is far less adequate than a within-subjects design where appropriate attention has been given to counter-balancing or randomizing test conditions. However, a within-subjects design can be faulted if, for example, randomization or counterbalancing has not been employed. The point, then, is for the critical evaluator to identify the type of design employed by the researcher and to assess the adequacy of the design, keeping in mind the advantages and disadvantages of the various designs described in Chapters 2 and 4. To help develop this critical skill, the remainder of the chapter includes some rather lengthy excerpts from the research literature. Our accompanying narrative shows how the reader can identify the type of research design employed and how the researcher has dealt with threats to validity.

Within-Subjects Experimental Design

Excerpt 7.32 is taken from the Method section of a study by Conture on the effects of loudness and frequency spectrum (two independent variables) on stuttering frequency, reading rate, and vocal level (three dependent variables). The design is within-subjects because all the stutterers were exposed to all levels of the independent variables and there was only one group of subjects. Each subject participated in all four sessions in this experiment and several important design strategies were used to reduce threats to internal validity. Note first, that a measure of TTS was used each day to ensure that no threshold shifts would contaminate the data with a carry-over effect from the previous day's noise exposure. Also note that rest periods were used to reduce short-term maturation (fatigue) and an adjustment period was used before the preexposure period to stabilize subjects' speaking behavior. The sequences of conditions and passages read during each condition were both randomized to control for sequencing effects. This within-subjects experimental design, then, shows several concerted attempts to minimize threats to internal validity.

EXCERPT 7.32

SUBJECTS

The subjects were nine adult male stutterers who were receiving speech therapy at the Wendell Johnson Speech and Hearing Center at the University of

Iowa. All nine subjects had hearing threshold levels of better than 15 dB (re ANSI, 1969) at 500, 1000, and 2000 Hz.

STIMULUS MATERIAL

The stimulus material consisted of five prose readings taken from the same level of the *Reader's Digest Reading Skill Builder* series (ninth-grade level, Part 3). A random sample of 100 words was taken from each of the five readings and rated according to Brown's (1945) "word weights." The similarity of the average word weight among the five readings indicated that the five passages were suitably equated with regard to Brown's four linguistic factors (Conture, 1972).

EXPERIMENTAL CONDITIONS

Each subject read during four sessions separated by at least 24 hours. There were two conditions in three sessions and one condition in the fourth. At the beginning of the first session, and at the start of every subsequent session, each subject performed a fixed frequency (4000 Hz) Bekesy tracing for two minutes in each ear. The middle one-minute segment from each ear was used to determine whether a subject's exposure to noise from the previous session might have produced a temporary threshold shift (TTS). If a shift of 5 dB or greater was noted on this task at the beginning of any session, then the subject was asked to leave and to come back another day.

After the TTS check, the subject began to read aloud continuously from the prepared readings while two conditions were presented. The sequence of presentation of the six experimental conditions and one control condition was as follows: the subject read for five minutes (adjustment period), then for another five minutes (preexposure period), followed by a 10-minute rest period. The same sequence was presented after the rest period, except that a different condition was presented during the exposure period. Sessions 2, 3, and 4 were identical to Session 1 except for the type of experimental or control conditions presented during the exposure period. The sequence of conditions and the particular passage that was read during a condition were all determined by chance through the use of a table of random numbers.

SOURCE: Conture, E. G. (1974). Some effects of noise on speaking behavior of stutterers. *Journal of Speech and Hearing Research, 17,* 714–723.

Between-Subjects Experimental Designs

Excerpt 7.33, taken from a study of the effect of speech therapy on language recovery in aphasia, quickly identifies the research as a between-subjects experimental study. In this study, 31 severely impaired aphasic subjects were assigned to three groups; one group received programmed instruction, one group received nonprogrammed speech therapy, and one group received no intervention. Note the authors' implicit recognition of the value of random assignment to treatment groups as well as the reason why this was not possible. At first glance, this design could be diagrammed as follows, maintaining the notation system described in Chapter 4:

$$\underline{O_1 \quad X_{PI} \quad} O_2$$
$$\underline{O_3 \quad X_{NPI} \quad} O_4$$
$$O_5 \qquad\qquad O_6$$

Here X_{PI} represents programmed instruction, X_{NPI} represents nonprogrammed instruction, and the third group received no treatment. The reader should recognize this as the nonequivalent control-group design. Recall that a major shortcoming of this design is the subject-selection factor. That is, because subjects are not selected randomly or randomly assigned to the control or experimental group, subjects may, in fact, be quite different on certain extraneous variables that may interact with the independent variable. Sarno and her associates recognized this problem and determined that the subjects in the three groups were not different on six extraneous variables: age, symptom duration, Functional Communication Profile (FCP), previous speech therapy, time in therapy, and number of treatment sessions. In a sense, the groups were matched on those dimensions that might interact with the treatment.

It should be apparent to the reader that this type of therapy study is exceedingly difficult to design so that all threats to internal and external validity are circumvented. Even with the care taken by Sarno, Silverman, and Sands, history and the reactivity of the measures employed could affect internal validity and pretesting and reactive arrangements could affect external validity. It is interesting to note that the results of this study led the authors (p. 621) to conclude that ". . . severe aphasic stroke patients do not benefit from speech therapy." Recognizing that only two types of therapy

---

EXCERPT 7.33

SUBJECTS

Patients were at least 18 years old, had suffered a CVA with right hemiplegia, were premorbidly right-handed, and spoke fluent American English. There was no upper age limit. All patients exhibited severe aphasic symptomatology of at least three months duration. This cutoff point was chosen to avoid biasing the results with the possible effects of spontaneous recovery (Eisenson, 1964; Lenneberg, 1967). There was no upper limit on duration of symptoms. Severe aphasia was operationally defined as an Overall Functional Communication Profile (see Materials section) score of below 31%. For the most part patients in this category had no speech function and little understanding of speech. At best, some were able to say a few words and understand some simple commands. Despite the severity of their language impairment, the majority of the patients were alert.

Those who did not have adequate motor and sensory function in at least one hand, and vision and hearing adequate for the task requirements were excluded, as were those who were heavily medicated or had a premorbid lan-

TABLE 1. RANGE, MEDIAN, AND MEANS FOR AGE, OVERALL FCP SCORES, DURATION OF SYMPTOMS FOR ALL TREATMENT GROUPS

Treatment group	Age			Duration of Symptoms			FCP Overall Scores		
	Range	Mean	Median	Range	Mean	Median	Range	Mean	Median
Programmed instruction	46–80 $n = 16$	63.81 $n = 16$	63.50 $n = 16$	3–144 months $n = 16$	33.69 $n = 16$	19.50 $n = 16$	5–31 $n = 15$	17.06 $n = 16$	18.00 $n = 16$
Nonprogrammed	54–83 $n = 7$	66.86 $n = 7$	64.00 $n = 7$	3–72 months $n = 7$	27.00 $n = 7$	18.00 $n = 7$	11–27 $n = 7$	16.29 $n = 7$	14.00 $n = 7$
Control	54–70 $n = 7$	63.71 $n = 8$	65.00 $n = 8$	18–72 months $n = 7$	41.14 $n = 8$	45.00 $n = 8$	5–29 $n = 8$	17.75 $n = 8$	20.00 $n = 8$

guage impairment. The presence of a right homonymous hemianopsia was not considered sufficiently incapacitating to preclude participation in the study. All study candidates were examined by a neurologist to exclude patients who showed signs of bilateral brain damage.

Patients with aphasia secondary to brain trauma or tumor were excluded since their recovery process is known to be different from that of the post-CVA patient.

A total of 31 patients were assigned to three groups: programmed instruction, nonprogrammed speech therapy, and an untreated control group. It was virtually impossible to balance the treatment groups by random assignment due to the varied location of patients, limitations in the availability of a programmed-instruction clinician and/or a nonprogrammed clinician. However, all groups were found to be equivalent with regard to age, symptom duration, Functional Communication Profile (FCP) scores, previous speech therapy, total time on program, and number of treatment sessions. (See Tables 1 and 2.)

TABLE 2. COMPARISONS BETWEEN SUBJECTS ASSIGNED TO PROGRAMMED INSTRUCTION, NONPROGRAMMED INSTRUCTION, AND CONTROL GROUPS

Groups	Age		Symptom Duration		FCP		Previous Speech Therapy		Time in Therapy (Weeks)		Therapy Sessions	
	t	df	t	df	t	df	t	df	t	df	t	df
PI-NPI	0.70	21	0.41	21	0.23	20	0.75	19	0.53	20	0.91	19
PI-C	0.03	21	0.47	21	0.19	21	0.90	20	—	—	—	—
NPI-C	0.66	12	1.13	12	0.36	13	0.26	13	—	—	—	—

Note: None of the t-values were significant at the 0.05 level.

SOURCE: Sarno, M. T., Silverman, M., & Sands, E. (1970). Speech therapy and language recovery in severe aphasia. *Journal of Speech and Hearing Research, 13,* 607–623.

were employed for a relatively small group of subjects, they recommend "further studies using other methods of treatment and a larger group of patients. . . ."

Sarno, Silverman, and Sands could not randomly assign subjects to treatment groups; instead, they had to employ an overall matching procedure. Wilson, on the other hand, used a stronger procedure in his 1966 study of speech therapy with educable mentally retarded children (Excerpt 7.34). In this large-scale study, Wilson first drew a sample of 1000 children. Although we do not know if this is a random sample, we do know that it is a large sample and, in fact, may include *all* of the educable mentally retarded children enrolled in the Special District program. The sample size was then reduced to 777 when the three exclusion criteria identified in the first paragraph were applied. Subjects were then divided into two groups, those with speech deviations and those without. The third paragraph of the excerpt is the key in identifying this study as a between-subjects experimental study. Three groups were formed and most important, the speech-deviant subjects were *randomly assigned* to one of the three groups. As we have emphasized previously, random assignment to treatment and control groups is the best way to minimize such threats to internal validity as history, subject selection, and maturation. Although the Wilson study is superior in this respect to the Sarno, Silverman, and Sands study (random assignment vs. overall matching), Wilson's research suffered a mortality problem that did not exist in the Sarno research. Because Wilson's study was 3 years in duration, subjects dropped out and, although random assignment should, in theory, produce a comparable mortality rate across treatment groups, it is apparent that this was not the case here. The mortality rate was 18% for the experimental group, 26% for the control group but 50% for the placebo group. Interestingly enough, Wilson's results did not demonstrate significant group differences in phoneme errors over the 3-year duration of the study. Further investigation would be necessary to assess the influence of the differential mortality rates on the results of the study.

EXCERPT 7.34

METHOD

Subjects

A sample of 777 children between the ages of six and 16 years was drawn from the 90 classes of educable mentally retarded children[1] of the Special District for the Education and Training of Handicapped Children of St. Louis County, Missouri. This sample of 777 children was derived from a larger group of 1000 by eliminating children with hearing disabilities, severe organic problems, and no current intellectual assessments.

The initial classification of children established two basic groups: (1) a group with normal speech, and (2) a speech-deviant group. The classifications were based on the results of the Hejna Articulation Test administered by three speech clinicians. A scale of articulatory severity that had been used by Special District speech clinicians for five years was applied to the speech-deviant group. From the criteria on the scale, a rating from least to most severe was made. The severity scale rating for the speech-deviant group was made by one clinician. Of the 777 children tested, 415 children (53.4%) had speech deviations. The remaining 362 children (46.6%) had normal speech. The median chronological age (CA) of the deviant group was 10.6 years, and the median CA

---

[1]The IQ range of children in classes for educable mentally retarded children in the state of Missouri is 48–78.

of the nondeviant group was 12.5 years. The median mental age (MA) of the speech-deviant group was 6.8 years and the median MA of the nondeviant group was 8.5 years. These scores were based on current psychological evaluations using an individual intelligence test. Based on the intelligence test, the median IQ for the speech-deviant group was 63 and for the nondeviant group 68. There were 461 males, with 251 speech-deviants and 210 normals. There were 316 females, with 164 speech-deviants and 152 normals.

The 415 speech-deviant children were randomly divided into three groups labeled Experimental ($N = 140$), Placebo ($N = 130$), and Control ($N = 145$). The number of children remaining in each category after a three-year program was 115, 65, and 107, respectively. The decrease in number was due primarily to the transient nature of the population.

In this particular project, speech therapy was limited to specific articulation therapy. The program of treatment for each of the three groups was as follows:

Experimental. Children in this group received two half-hour sessions of direct speech therapy per week, as previously defined. Each child had some individual and some group therapy. At no time did group size exceed four. The three clinicians who performed the initial evaluation were assigned to provide therapy. They were not given specific, detailed instructions or therapy lesson plans, but were directed to plan a corrective speech program for each child within the framework suggested by Van Riper (1956).

Placebo. Children in this group received two half-hour sessions of non-phoneme-oriented speech and language stimulation per week. They did not receive specific guidance in correcting individual sound errors. The purpose of the placebo segment of the sample was to offset the possibility that alterations in the speech of the experimental group, either positive or negative, might have resulted primarily from the special attention derived from the therapy situation.

Control. Children in this group were given articulation tests at the same intervals as those in the other groups. No therapy was administered, and the testing situation was their only contact with the speech clinician.

SOURCE: Wilson, F. B. (1966). Efficacy of speech therapy with educable mentally retarded children. *Journal of Speech and Hearing Research, 9,* 423–433.

The two previous examples of between-subjects designs (Excerpts 7.33 and 7.34) are from experimental studies of the effects of therapy that involve rather long-term studies of the subjects. Most short-term experiments, like the one by Conture of the effects of noise on stuttering shown in Excerpt 7.32, use within-subjects designs because allowing subjects to act as their own controls by participating in all experimental conditions eliminates problems of differential subject selection. The example shown in Excerpt 7.35 illustrates a short-term experiment on the effects of practice and instructions on lingual vibrotactile thresholds using a between-subjects design. A between-subjects design was used because of the probability that a permanent carry-over effect could not be eliminated with counterbalancing

EXCERPT 7.35

Procedure

The 30 subjects were divided randomly into three groups of 10 each. Each group was assigned to a condition involving a different instructional set for obtaining their lingual vibrotactile thresholds. A counterbalancing design, although desirable, could not be employed since naiveté was a prerequisite for each subject to be used in the study. Once a subject received an instructional set, that subject would no longer be naive; therefore, it would be difficult to determine whether the instructions previously given interacted with a new instructional set. The instructional sets were as follows:

Condition 1—Strict instructions. Subjects were given simple but relatively strict instructions to raise their hands as soon as they felt the stimulus on their tongue.

Condition 2—Comprehensive instructions. Subjects were given more comprehensive instructions in which the idea of threshold was stressed. This set of instructions told the subjects to raise their hands as soon as they felt the stimulus, no matter how faint it appeared to be. They were encouraged to respond even if they only thought the stimulus was present.

Condition 3—Comprehensive instructions with examiner reinforcement. Subjects were given the same instructions as in the second condition, but appropriate examiner feedback was supplied regarding the accuracy of their responses. If their responses did not conform to what we have experienced as fitting within the range of previously generated normative threshold data, appropriate feedback was provided. The following subject responses and examiner feedback occurred during this experimental condition:

Subject Responses	Examiner Feedback
1. False alarm.	1. Make sure you are feeling the tickling before you raise your hand.
2. Should be responding earlier.	2. You probably feel the stimulus before you raise your hand.
3. Appropriate response.	3. You are responding right about where I would expect you to.

Examiner feedback used in Condition 3 was based on normative lingual vibrotactile threshold data obtained from 110 normal young adults (Telage, Fucci, & Arnst, 1972).

SOURCE: Fucci, D., Small, L. H., & Petrosino, L. (1983). Effects of practice and instructional set on the measurement of lingual vibrotactile thresholds. Journal of Speech and Hearing Research, 26, 289–293.

or randomization of the conditions presented to the subjects. Note the authors' rationale for using the between-subjects design instead of counterbalancing conditions because subjects could not become naive again after having been exposed to the instructions. Thus, a within-subjects design would be exposed to the danger of carryover of the effect of one instruction set onto another subsequent instruction set in later conditions. Note also that the authors dealt with the problem of differential subject selection by randomly assigning subjects to one of the three conditions.

Mixed (Between-Subjects *and* Within-Subjects) Design

The example shown in Excerpt 7.36 illustrates a mixed design in which one independent variable is studied with a between-subjects design and another independent variable is studied with a within-subjects design. This study is also an example of combined experimental–descriptive research because one independent variable is manipulable and the other independent variable is subject classification. The between-subjects independent variable is the subject classification (normal vs. defective articulation), or the non-manipulable, descriptive independent variable. The within-subjects independent variable is the manipulable, experimental independent variable (type of recall stimuli). The dependent variable is performance on the recall task.

The between-subjects component of the study is identified in the Subjects section of Excerpt 7.36. This section describes the subject-classification independent variable and reveals the comparative (descriptive) aspect of the study. Note the care taken to ensure that the two groups of subjects are comparable on important extraneous variables (e.g., chronological age, sex, race, etc.). The exclusion criteria described in the last paragraph of this section (no subjects with hearing loss, stuttering, bilingual background, and so forth) also helped to reduce the threat to internal validity posed by differential selection of subjects. It is clear, then, that the subject-selection procedure employed by Saxman and Miller produced two groups of comparable subjects that differed primarily (if not solely) in articulation skills.

The within-subjects component of the study is described in the Materials and Procedure sections. Three kinds of recall stimuli were presented to the subjects: randomized digits, random-word strings, and active-declarative sentences. The Procedure section reveals two important aspects of the within-subjects design: (1) all subjects received all levels of the experimental independent variable (stimuli) and (2) the three stimuli were presented in random order.

The Saxman and Miller study, then, illustrates both the use of a mixed (between-subjects and within-subjects) design and the use of combined experimental–descriptive research. The study examines the effect of the experimental independent variable on subjects in two different classifications.

Careful attention should be given to this type of research design because it is so commonly encountered in the literature. The analysis of the data from this same study is shown in Chapter 8 in Excerpt 8.27 and serves as an excellent example of the use of the analysis of variance for examining the main effects of two different independent variables and their interaction effect.

EXCERPT 7.36

SUBJECTS

The subjects used in this study were 28 public school kindergarten children with defective articulation and 28 subjects with normal articulation. The group with defective articulation, 17 boys and 11 girls, performed one standard deviation or more below the norms for their age and sex on the Templin-Darley 176-item diagnostic test of articulation. They ranged in age from five years six months to six years seven months, with a mean age of six years.

The group with normal articulation, none of whom had more than one articulation error, were selected and matched with the subjects who had defective articulation. Subjects were matched on the basis of chronological age, sex, race, and father's occupation and level of education.

All subjects were screened for normal hearing (25 dB ISO; 0.25 to 8 kHz) and had no obvious motor disabilities or apparent organic deviation determined by an oral peripheral examination. In addition, no subject was from a bilingual home, was a twin or a stutterer, or was considered by his classroom teacher to have a significant intellectual deficit.

MATERIALS

The materials for the immediate recall tasks consisted of three lists: strings of randomized digits, random-word strings, and active-declarative sentences. The digit strings were constructed by drawing digits from a table of random numbers with replacement resulting in strings from two to nine digits in length. There were two strings at each length level for a total of 16 strings. Fourteen active-declarative sentences were constructed using the controlled vocabulary of Rinsland (1945). The sentences ranged from four to 10 words in length with two sentences at each length. The random-word strings were constructed by numbering consecutively each word in the sentence list. A table of random numbers was used to make word strings of two to nine words in length. There were two word strings at each length for a total of 16 random-word strings. This procedure insured the same vocabulary for both the sentences and random-word strings.

PROCEDURE

Each subject was seen individually for the immediate recall tasks. The subject was instructed to repeat the materials read by the examiner. For example, the examiner would read, "I want you to say exactly what I say. If I say 6–2–3, what do you say?" The child would respond, "6–2–3." Several examples of each of the three types of materials were given as practice items to insure that the subject understood the task. The materials were read by the examiner at a practiced constant rate of approximately one word per 0.75 seconds and with a flat intonational contour.

In presenting each of the three lists, the items were read in the order of shortest to longest items. When the child missed three consecutive items on a list, testing was stopped for that list. The lists were presented in random order. All responses were recorded on a Nagra IV tape recorder for later transcription and analysis.

SOURCE: Saxman, J. H., & Miller, J. F. (1973). Short-term memory and language skills in articulation-deficient children. *Journal of Speech and Hearing Research, 16*, 721–730.

Within-Subjects Time-Series Experiments

The next example is the Procedure section taken from a within-subjects time-series study by Martin and Siegel on the effects of simultaneously punishing stuttering and rewarding fluency. Excerpt 7.37 illustrates the considerable care taken by the authors to establish a stable base rate in a rather straightforward time-series experiment. Note that although the basic design is A–B in nature, the last paragraph indicates the use of an extinction period that resulted in an A–B–A design for some of the experimental sessions. The time-series experiment is easy to identify. But the critical evaluator of such studies must pay very close attention to the manner in which the base rate has been established. As we pointed out in Chapter 4, unstable base rates can easily serve to invalidate a time-series experiment.

Also shown in Excerpt 7.37 are two figures from the Results section that illustrate the data for one of their subjects. These figures are particularly instructive about several aspects of time-series designs. Note that the abscissa of each figure indicates time from the start of each session from left to right and that the ordinate indicates number of stutterings in each 2 minutes from 0 on the bottom to a high value of 80 stutterings-per-2-minutes at the top. Figure 1 in Excerpt 7.37 shows the data for a 40-minute session that is essentially a first baseline segment with no experimental manipulations. Although there is some variation (as would be expected) in the number of stutterings, the baseline is relatively stable within a range of about 10 stutterings-per-2-minutes. The Figure 2 in Excerpt 7.37 shows the second session in which the first 10 minutes served as baseline. The vertical line at 10 minutes separates the baseline (A) segment from the start of the experimental (B) segment and the vertical line at 40 minutes separates the end of the experimental (B) segment from the start of a second baseline (A) segment in which no stimuli were delivered. This figure shows quite clearly the nature of a short-term A–B–A time-series design. Note how stuttering remains high and relatively stable in the first 10 minutes (A segment or baseline) and then drops precipitously as the B (experimental) segment is introduced. At the end of the B segment at 40 minutes, another A (baseline) segment is introduced and stuttering starts to increase toward the level of the first A segment. This indicates a temporary reduction in stuttering due to the experimental treatment and a trend toward reversal to the higher baseline levels of stuttering that were evident in the original baseline.

EXCERPT 7.37

PROCEDURE

Each subject was run for a number of individual sessions separated by at least one week. During all sessions the experimenter observed the subject both visually and auditorally and depressed the hand switch each time the subject stuttered. When appropriate, the experimenter also attached the wrist strap, delivered the specific instructions, delivered the response contingent verbal stimuli, and removed the strap.

During Session 1 the subject read continuously for 40 minutes. No specific instructions or experimental treatments were introduced during this base-rate session. The first few minutes of each subsequent session also served as a base-rate period, and the various experimental manipulations were always withheld until the subject's stuttering frequency had stabilized. Stabilization was considered achieved when the variations in stuttering frequency in three successive two-minute periods did not exceed certain limits. The amount of variation allowed depended on the frequency of stuttering during the first of the three two-minute periods. If a subject stuttered between zero and nine times in a given two-minute period, his performance was defined as stable if he did not deviate from that frequency by more than ± 1 in either of the next two successive periods. Similarly, if the subject stuttered between 10–19, 20–29, 30–39, 40–49, 50–59, or 60–69 times during a given period, his performance was considered stable if, in either of the next two periods, his frequency did not vary by more than 2, 3, 4, 5, 6, or 7, respectively. In addition, the subject must have read for at least 10 minutes in a given session before he was credited with achieving a base rate.

This procedure for defining the base-rate period allowed for considerable flexibility between sessions and between subjects. The determination of base rate was made anew during each session, and was thus anchored to the subject's performance during that session. Consequently, variations in the time required to reach base rate, and the frequency level at which it was achieved, served as a source of comparison from session to session.

When the subject's stuttering rate stabilized, some combination of instructions, discriminative stimulus, and reinforcing and punishing stimuli was introduced. In Sessions 2 and 5, the following specific instructions were given at the end of the base-rate period: "Now I want you to read very carefully. Don't worry about keeping the sentence going. Just say each word fluently." In all other sessions where specific instructions were given, they were identical with the above except for the addition of the sentence, "I am going to put this strap on your wrist as a reminder to say each word as fluently as possible."

An extinction condition was included at the end of some sessions. In this condition no instructions were given, no verbal stimuli were presented, and the strap was not attached.

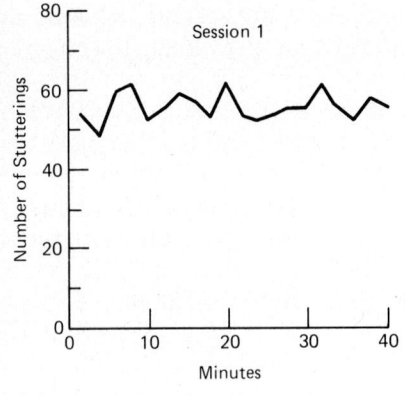

Figure 1.   Number of stutterings emitted by Subject N during Session 1 (40 minutes). No instructions given, no strap attached, and no stimuli delivered during entire session.

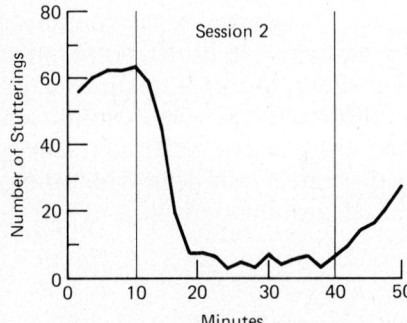

Figure 2.   Number of stutterings emitted by Subject N each two minutes during Session 2 (50 minutes). Base rate for first 10 minutes. Instructions given, "not good" delivered contingent upon each stuttering, and "good" delivered contingent upon each 30 seconds of fluency for next 30 minutes. No stimuli delivered for last 10 minutes.

SOURCE: Martin, R. R., & Siegel, G. M. (1966). The effects of simultaneously punishing stuttering and rewarding fluency. *Journal of Speech and Hearing Research, 9,* 466–475.

Excerpt 7.38 shows portions of the Method and Results sections of an article by Costello and Hurst that used a time-series design in an experiment with three subjects over a longer period of time. The subject for whom the data are shown participated in 27 sessions over a period of about 9 weeks. This particular example illustrates several other points about time-series designs. First, the speaker participated over a longer term for more extended analysis of their behavior. The Experimental Design section explains how the A–B–A–B–A–C time-series design was executed. Second, the design used two reversals of baseline (A) and experimental segment (B), with several sessions included in each segment. Note in the first paragraph of the

Experimental Design section where the authors discuss the reasons for using this repeated reversals design. Third, the authors studied the effects of the experimental manipulations on different dependent variables (two stuttering behaviors for Subject 1 and three behaviors each for Subjects 2 and 3). This allowed them to check the effect of manipulations on "target" behavior as well as generalization to other behaviors. After the second baseline, the manipulation was changed to the nontarget behavior to evaluate the effect on both behaviors.

Figure 1 in Excerpt 7.38 illustrates the data for the first subject. As with the figures in Excerpt 7.37, time is shown on the abscissa and number of stutterings on the ordinate. However, because this is a longer term study, the time is indicated by sessions rather than minutes, with number of disfluencies-per-minute averaged for each session. The two dependent variables (stuttering behaviors) are indicated by the two lines with open and filled circles. Note reasonable stability of both behaviors in the first A segment, a decrease in both behaviors in the first B segment, an increase back toward the first baseline levels in the second A segment, and another decrease in both behaviors in the second B segment. Both behaviors increased again in the third A segment and decreased in the C segment, although tremor disfluencies (which became the nontarget behavior in the C segment) began to increase again when they were no longer punished. Excerpt 7.38 illustrates the many possibilities for variation with multiple baselines, multiple treatments, and multiple dependent variables with time-series designs. One caution that must be entertained in discussing these variations is that multiple-treatment interference is a threat to external validity that can best be dealt with through multiple replications to ferret out individual treatment effects and interactions among treatments.

EXCERPT 7.38

Experimental sessions were approximately 40 minutes in length. Subjects 1 and 3 attended sessions three days per week, while Subject 2 came for sessions four days per week. Subject 1 participated in 27 sessions, Subject 2 in 51, and Subject 3 attended 39 sessions.

Experimental Design

The stuttering behavior of each subject was studied through a within-subject repeated reversals experimental design. For each subject, two or three selected types of stuttering behavior were separately and concurrently measured and one of them was directly manipulated by a punishment procedure. Experimental and baseline/reversal conditions were systematically alternated over several sessions yielding a repeated reversals design, often referred to as an ABAB design (Hersen & Barlow, 1976, p. 185). This design allows repeated observations of the effects of the independent variable on the form of stuttering behavior being manipulated (the target disfluency), as well as on the unmanipulated disfluency types being measured concurrently.

Baseline condition.   During baseline (Condition A) the clinician instructed the subject to speak in monologue or to read for the entire 40 minutes. Noncontingent (never following a moment of stuttering) social reinforcers in the form of smiles and nods from the clinician were provided on the average of every 60 seconds while the subject was speaking. Further, the clinician maintained continuous attention to the subject's speaking throughout each session by maintaining eye contact. During the baseline sessions the experimenter differentially counted the frequency of occurrence of each selected stuttering topography. Baseline sessions were continued until stuttering was stable or was not systematically decreasing. Stability was said to have been achieved when the within-session average disfluency rate of each disfluency type showed variation no greater than plus or minus one disfluency per minute in three consecutive sessions. When the baseline data indicated stability, the experimental condition was introduced. All changes in conditions were introduced within sessions.

Experimental condition.   As in the baseline sessions, subjects continued speaking in monologue or reading during experimental (Condition B) sessions, and the clinician provided continuous social reinforcement in the form of attention as long as the subject was speaking fluently. However, during experimental sessions every occurrence of the target disfluency was consequated by one of two punishment procedures. In one, referred to as time-out from positive reinforcement (Costello, 1975), each occurrence of the target disfluency was immediately followed by the clinician saying, "Stop," and looking away from the subject for ten seconds. The subject was required to stop speaking immediately. After the time interval had elapsed the clinician looked up, smiled, and said, "Begin." In the other punishment procedure each occurrence of the target disfluency was followed by the immediate presentation of a one-second burst of a 90-dB, 4000-Hz tone through headphones, a procedure similar to that described by Flanagan, Goldiamond, and Azrin (1958).

During the experimental condition the experimenter continued counting the frequency of occurrence of all of the selected stuttering behaviors for each subject. The experimental condition was continued until the data were stable or until the direction and nature of change were clear. At this time Condition A was reintroduced in order to assess whether changes produced by the introduction of the independent variable could be reversed by its withdrawal. Following this the experimental condition was reintroduced in order to demonstrate further the control of the independent variable over the dependent variables by replication of the original effect.

Subsequent manipulations.   Following the last reversal session (Condition A) for Subject 1, the target disfluency was changed to the previously nonmanipulated disfluency form. This was continued for three sessions. For Subject 2, during the final experimental condition, all disfluencies regardless of topography became the targets for punishment by time-out. This condition continued until the end of the study.

. . . .

Experimental Findings

The data from each of the three subjects indicate that stuttering behaviors tended to covary directly with one another. When a punishing stimulus was applied to one topography of disfluency, other topographies were seen to decrease in frequency of occurrence, even though they were never directly manipulated.

Subject 1.   Figure 1 shows the session-by-session data collected for Subject 1 across all experimental conditions. The speaking modality for this subject was reading and the two topographies of disfluency selected for measurement were: (1) jaw tremors; and (2) unitary repetitions of phonemes, syllables, and monosyllabic words. Jaw tremors were chosen as the target disfluency for the application of punishment contingencies during experimental conditions.

Condition A (baseline) was conducted for five complete sessions. Jaw tremors averaged 18.20/min while repetitions averaged 4.45/min. After the first ten minutes of Condition A in session 6, Condition B was initiated. A time-out interval of ten seconds was presented contingent upon every instance of tremors. The experimental condition was in effect for seven sessions wherein a decrease in the frequency of occurrence of tremors was noted, as well as a progressive decrease in the frequency of occurrence of untreated repetitions. Condition A was reinstated for five sessions after the first ten minutes of session 12. An immediate increase in the frequency of tremors and of repetitions demonstrated the functionality of the punishing stimulus and the reliability of the direct covariation phenomenon. During session 16 the experimental condition was reinstated for six sessions. Time-out contingencies applied to all tremors once again produced a decrease in the frequency of occurrence of these behaviors and direct covariation of untreated repetitions, thus replicating the effects of the first experimental condition and further verifying the response class relationship between tremor and repetition disfluencies for this subject. During the third session of this condition (session 18), the time-out interval was decreased from ten to five seconds, with no apparent influence on the data. Reversal Condition A was once again instated during session 21 for four sessions, resulting in an immediate increase in the frequency of occurrence of tremors and repetitions to their original baseline levels. It is unlikely that changes in speaking rate (word output) systematically varying across conditions would have accounted for these ABABA results because speaking rate has been shown to remain independent of disfluency rates in studies using procedures similar to those of this study (e.g., Costello, 1975; Martin, 1968).

In Condition C, introduced during session 24 for four sessions, time-out was no longer presented contingent upon tremors, but rather contingent upon repetitions, heretofore untreated. The frequency of occurrence of repetitions was observed to decrease. A corresponding initial decrease in the rate of now untreated tremors was noted, but this was followed by a gradual increase toward the baseline level. Thus the direct covariation observed to occur reliably across behaviors when tremors were treated was not replicated clearly when the treatment target was changed.

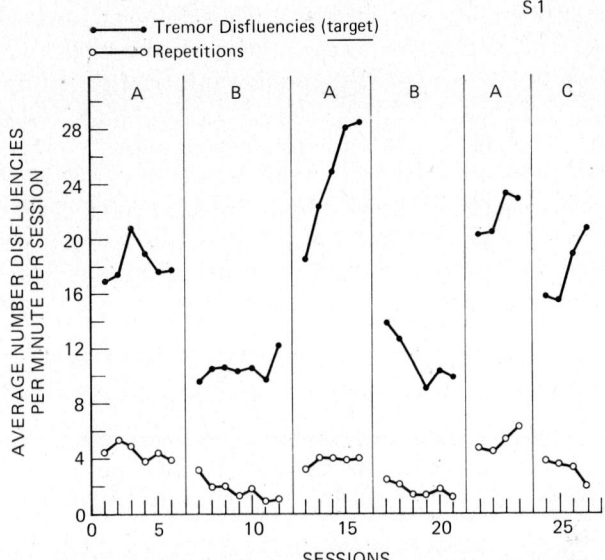

Figure 1. Disfluency data for Subject 1, The ordinate indicates the number of disfluencies per minute averaged across each session; the abcissa represents individual sessions, except where changes in condition occurred. The last data point in each condition is from the same session as the first data point in the subsequent session. Experimental conditions are indicated at the top of the graph and are separated by dark vertical lines. The selected stuttering topographies measured for Subject 1 are defined in the legend at the top of the graph, and the one which served as the target disfluency is also indicated.

SOURCE: Costello, J. M., & Hurst, M. R. (1981). An analysis of the relationship among stuttering behaviors. *Journal of Speech and Hearing Research, 24,* 247–256.

Between-Subjects Comparative Design

The basic structure of a descriptive study employing a comparative design has already been illustrated in the subject selection section of this chapter (see Excerpts 7.5 and 7.6). Because of the frequency with which this type of design has been employed, another brief example is appropriate with respect to procedural considerations. Excerpt 7.39 is from a comparative study of the use of contrastive stress by normal, aphasic, and autistic children. The purpose statement outlines the groups of children to be studied and the dependent variables to be compared for these children. The Subjects part of the

Method section describes the three groups of children, indicates how they were selected, and displays data regarding relevant subject characteristics. Table 1 of Excerpt 7.39 shows comparative information on the central tendency and variability of the three groups regarding three important subject characteristics: language production, language comprehension, and chronological age. The procedure part of the Method section outlines the procedure for eliciting responses from the children. Note the care taken in the pretrial training procedure to ensure that the children were familiar with the words used and were able to produce the type of utterances needed.

EXCERPT 7.39

The purpose of this study was to determine (a) to what extent autistic, aphasic, and normal children with a similar mean length of utterance were able to use contrastive stress to express pragmatic information; and (b) to compare the use of contrastive stress in these groups. In addition to determining the number of possible errors made, the pattern of errors also was of interest. It was hypothesized that differences in performance might occur in different sentence positions.

METHOD

Subjects

The subjects were 7 normal, 7 aphasic, and 7 autistic children. The normal subjects were recruited from a local nursery school. Normal subjects had to exhibit no identified physical or psychiatric defects and have verbal and nonverbal IQs in the normal range as measured by standardized tests. The aphasic subjects were recruited from a classroom for the severely language handicapped in the public school system. They had to exhibit a severe oral language handicap as measured by standardized tests but had to have a nonverbal IQ in the normal range. Various labels have been applied to such children (Bloom & Lahey, 1978) including *aphasic, specific language disordered,* and *language disabled.* (For purposes of simplicity and to distinguish this group clearly from the autistic children who also suffered from a language disability, we have chosen to use the term *aphasic* here.) The autistic subjects were recruited from the Center for the Study of Childhood Psychosis, University of California, Los Angeles, and conformed to the diagnostic criteria of infantile autism as enumerated in the *Diagnostic and Statistical Manual of Mental Disorders* (DSM III, 299.OX). These criteria were (a) onset before 30 months of age; (b) pervasive lack of responsiveness to others; (c) gross deficits in language development; and (d) if speech was present, peculiar speech patterns, such as immediate and delayed echolalia, metaphorical language, and pronominal reversal. All the autistic subjects had been judged on clinical examination to have prosodic deficits.

Mean length of utterance (MLU) for all subjects ranged between 1.9 and 4.1 morphemes, with a mean of about 3.0 morphemes for each group. Thus, the

TABLE 1.   DESCRIPTION OF NORMAL, APHASIC, AND AUTISTIC SUBJECTS

Normal Subjects $n = 7$		Aphasic Subjects $n = 7$		Autistic Subjects $n = 7$	
Language Production					
MLU range	1.98–3.8	MLU range	2.43–4.11	MLU range	1.9–4.0
mean:	3.07	mean:	3.00	mean:	2.78
SD:	0.60	*SD*:	0.59	*SD*:	0.75
Language Comprehension					
PPVT,[a] Form A		PPVT, Form A		PPVT, Form A	
range:	101–140	range:	74–108	range:	59–87
mean:	113.00	mean:	83.71	mean:	67.16
SD:	13.25	*SD*:	12.68	*SD*:	11.03
Chronological Age					
CA in months:		CA in months:		CA in months:	
range:	29–48	range:	44–130	range:	52–146
mean:	39.70	mean:	86.70	mean:	87.42
SD:	7.80	*SD*:	33.90	*SD*:	35.16

[a]PPVT, Form A, was used as a measure of vocabulary comprehension for the above subjects.

subjects within each group were at similar language production levels, based on MLU. The ranges in chronological age were 2:9–3:11 for the normal group, 3:8–10:9 for the aphasic group, and 4:4–12:2 for the autistic group. Table 1 gives the ranges, means, and standard deviations for each group's MLU, Peabody Vocabulary scores, and chronological ages.

Procedure

A contrastive stress task was designed using toy manipulation and yes-no questions as elicitation techniques. The contrastive stress task required that each subject assess the presupposition of a yes-no question which was counterfactual to an actual situation. Responses were judged on the basis of correct contrastive stress placement on the element placed into counterfactual context. For example, to elicit contrastive stress on subject position, toy manipulation showed a girl named Pat sitting in a chair. The subject was then asked, "Is Mike sitting in the chair?" The truth value of the presupposition of the yes-no question was contradicted by the actual situation. New information, and hence contrastive stress, therefore was expected to mark subject position in the expected response, "No, Pat is sitting in the chair."

The contrastively stressed utterances were elicited in a structured play situation using eight easily manipulable toys. Their labels were easily identifiable nouns. Four high-frequency activity verbs were also selected. The nouns and verbs in various combinations were used to make up 16 simple neutral, noncontrastive declarative utterances consisting of subject-verb-object sequences. A neutral, noncontrastive declarative utterance is here defined as one in which all the information transmitted is new or in which all stressable elements carry an equal information load (Schmerling, 1976). These neutral utterances formed the basis of the contrastive stress condition. The selection of neutral utterances as the base for the contrastive stress paradigm was based on Stockwell (1971). Contrastive stress was elicited for subject, verb, and object positions for each of the 16 utterances. Each subject was thus required to respond to a total of 48 stimulus queries. (See Appendix for a list of nouns, verbs, and sample sentences.)

Testing and pretrial training procedures established each subject's familiarity with the nouns and verbs used and the ability to produce utterances of the type to be elicited in the present task. The investigator followed a protocol containing all the desired contrasts for a subject, verb, and object positions for each of the 16 base utterances, which had been randomized in advance.

Each subject was seen individually by the examiner in a playroom, equipped with a table and two chairs. An omnidirectional microphone was suspended two feet above the table in front of the subject, who was seated in a chair at the table. The investigator manipulated the objects on the table in front of each subject to elicit the desired utterances containing the individual contrasts. The examiner's accompanying queries contained a lexical item which conflicted with the reality of the situation. This was the lexical element that was to be placed in contrastive stress position (e.g., "What's happening? Is the baby drinking milk?" Expected answer: "No, the baby is drinking *coke*," with toy manipulation shwoing the baby drinking coke accompanying the query). No specific additional instructions were given to the subjects regarding the type of responses they should make. Thus, contrasts were elicited for subject, verb, and object positions. If the subject did not respond the first time, the procedure was repeated once. If there still was no response, the expected response was modeled twice for the subject, and the subject was required to imitate the modeled response. This imitation procedure was employed both in order to ensure a response from the children and because imitative abilities have been correlated with level of language production (Fraser, Bellugi, & Brown, 1963).

Each of the queries and responses was tape-recorded using an Ampex 440G tape recorder and transcribed using gross phonemic transcription. Two evaluators with advanced degrees in linguistics then listened to the recordings, which had been transcribed earlier, and independently marked a duplicate set of transcripts as to the occurrence of contrastive stress. The transcripts had not been identified as belonging to specific subject groups. Interrater agreement, based on marking of transcripts for stress assignment, was computed at 95%.

SOURCE: Baltaxe, C. A. M. (1984). Use of contrastive stress in normal, aphasic, and autistic children. *Journal of Speech and Hearing Research, 27,* 97–105.

Developmental Research Designs

The characteristics of developmental research were discussed in Chapter 2. Three basic designs for developmental research were discussed: cross-sectional (between-subjects design), longitudinal (within-subjects design), and semilongitudinal (mixed design). In this section, we will present excerpts from each of these three different types of developmental studies to illustrate the way subjects were selected and procedures were outlined for studying the development of their behavior. Note that two of the studies are concerned with the development of young children and one of them concerns the geriatric population. As mentioned earlier, these are the two age ranges of greatest concern in developmental research because the greatest maturation occurs in the younger and older years.

Excerpt 7.40 is taken from a developmental study of voice onset time in a normal-aged population. As stated in the purpose shown in the excerpt, the authors wished to extend the developmental model of speech timing to older subjects. The study was cross-sectional, in that it used a between-subjects design to compare the behavior of a group of 25-to-39-year-old adults, a group of 65-to-74-year-old adults, and a group of adults over 75. In other words, three *different* groups of subjects representing three different levels of maturation were compared with each other to examine developmental trends. The excerpted material shows a brief statement of the specific purpose of the study followed by a portion of the Method section that describes the three groups of subjects who were compared in this cross-sectional developmental study. Note the selection criteria that were used to ensure that adults were selected who were normal with respect to various health measures and the use of a physician to examine the older subjects. The subjects' ages are shown in the excerpted table (along with their sex and vital-capacity data). Inspection of the table shows that the groups represent three well-separated age groups with no overlapping among the ages of the three groups and that males and females are equally represented in all three groups.

EXCERPT 7.40

The purpose of this descriptive study, therefore, was to obtain measures of VOT and vowel duration in healthy older subjects as a necessary first step in the extension of a developmental model of speech timing control to the later years. Results relating to voice onset time are reported in this paper.

METHOD

Subjects

Three groups of 10 subjects were used. The control group, Group 1, was composed of subjects between 25 and 39 years of age. Groups 2 and 3 subjects were 65–74 years and over 75, respectively. Subject characteristics are summarized in Table 1.

All subjects were living independently, were considered to be embedded in the social structure of the community, were free of any chronic or debilitating disease, had measured vital capacities within the normal range, and presented

TABLE 1.   CHARACTERISTICS OF THE 30 SUBJECTS

Subjects by Group	Age	Sex	Vital Capacity (liters)
Group 1			
Age 25–40			
1-1	39	M	4.5
1-2	38	F	3.1
1-3	29	F	2.8
1-4	38	F	2.9
1-5	30	M	4.7
1-6	32	F	3.1
1-7	28	M	6.4
1-8	30	F	2.5
1-9	30	M	4.6
1-10	36	M	4.4
Mean age	33		
Group 2			
Age 65–74			
2-1	71	M	3.0
2-2	71	M	2.8
2-3	73	M	3.3
2-4	66	F	2.0
2-5	66	M	4.4
2-6	69	F	1.9
2-7	69	F	1.8
2-8	66	F	3.0
2-9	67	F	2.2
2-10	68	M	3.7
Mean age	68.6		
Group 3			
Age 75 and over			
3-1	88	M	1.9
3-2	77	M	3.1
3-3	75	F	2.1
3-4	77	F	2.3
3-5	81	F	2.0
3-6	76	F	2.5
3-7	91	M	1.9
3-8	87	F	1.9
3-9	79	M	3.2
3-10	82	M	1.8
Mean age	81.3		

negative histories for hearing problems, cardiovascular, respiratory, neurological and laryngeal disorders. All were native speakers of English and had been raised in homes in which only English had been spoken. Within 15 days of testing, each of the Groups 2 and 3 subjects was seen by a physician who was aware of the subject criteria of the study and who certified that the heart and lungs were normal on auscultation and percussion, that blood pressure was within normal limits, and that there was no apparent neuropathology.

SOURCE: Sweeting, P. M., & Baken, R. J. (1982). Voice onset time in a normal-aged population. *Journal of Speech and Hearing Research, 25,* 129–134.

Portions of a longitudinal developmental study are shown in Excerpt 7.41. This study examined the concept of agent in the emerging language of three children as they developed from about age 11 months to age 2 years. The first part of the excerpt shows the research questions posed. This is followed by a description of the three subjects who were studied and the method of observing them. Note that the children were observed 10 times over a 12-month period of development. The observation sessions and the children's ages at each session are detailed in Table 2 shown in Excerpt 7.41. Whereas the cross-sectional study shown in Excerpt 7.40 used a between-subjects design, this longitudinal study used a within-subjects design to observe the children repeatedly over the developmental span and to watch their behavior change directly. Note that a larger number of subjects was employed in the cross-sectional study ($N = 30$) and a smaller number of subjects was used in the longitudinal study ($N = 3$) as is usually the case.

EXCERPT 7.41

The research that follows examines the emergence of the cognitive concept of agent as hypothesized in Table 1. This was done by observing those overt, nonverbal behaviors (i.e., gestures) assumed to be indicative of the cognitive notion of agent, and subsequently describing the evolution of these behaviors over time in three children. Specifically the following questions were addressed: What gestural behavioral sequences indicate the child's nonverbal concept of agent? To what extent does actual development of the cognitive notion of agent match the hypothesized 5-level developmental sequence proposed in Table 1?

METHOD

To discover behavioral changes which emerge over the course of a child's early development, a descriptive, longitudinal study was conducted. The methodology used a modification of the traditional observation approach (Bloom, 1970, 1973; Bloom, Lightbown, & Hood, 1975; Bowerman, 1973; Brown, 1973; Carter, 1974; Greenfield & Smith, 1976). Rather than using only diary-like observations of free unstructured sessions in which no specific activities are scheduled for administration and observation, this study included several activities having a high probability of eliciting the behaviors hypothesized in Table 1, depending on the child's current concept of agent (Edwards, 1974; Ingram, 1971; Lock, 1976; Piaget, 1952, 1954; Snyder, 1975; Sugarman, 1973).

Subjects

The three subjects were selected on the basis of a normal prenatal and perinatal history, meeting developmental milestones as determined by the *Bayley Scales of Infant Development* (Bayley, 1969) and the Uzgiris and Hunt scales (Uzgiris & Hunt 1975), and by a normal medical history. At the beginning of the study, all three children were 11 months old, and according to the author's interpretation of the Uzgiris and Hunt scales their performance was most characteristic of Piaget's sensorimotor Stage IV (see Appendix A). The subjects, two boys and one girl, were from upper-middle-class families; the mothers of all three children either worked or attended school, resulting in the children spending at least part of the day with babysitters. One boy had an older sibling, whereas the other two subjects had none. At the beginning of the study, all three subjects were producing prelinguistic vocalizations (i.e., consonant-vowel combinations, fussing, whining); according to the parents, none of the children had used any consistent phonetic forms to label people, objects, events, or activities. All three children were using crawling as their predominant means of locomotion during the first observation session, and walking during the second.

Procedures

The children were videotaped in their respective homes 10 times over 12 months at approximately 1-month intervals; each session lasted 1 hour. Table 2 indicates the age of the children at each videotaping session. The observations for two children extended from the prelinguistic vocalization period (11 months) to their beginning use of 2-word utterances, particularly agent + action, agent + object, action + object constructions. The observations for one of the children extended from his use of vocalization (11 months) to his use of successive single-word utterances. During each session the mother-child pair and the investigator were present.

The children were observed during each hour-long videotaping session under two conditions: a free-play situation and an elicitation situation. The tasks in the elicitation situation were designed to supplement the data obtained in the free-play situation by providing specific opportunities for agentive behaviors to occur. They are described in detail in Appendix B. The basic structure of these agentive elicitation tasks remained the same over the 12-month period whereas specific objects within a task frequently changed from session to session. This provided some degree of structure and continuity across taping sessions and across subjects; it also allowed for more reliable observations of changes in agentive behavior (Greenfield & Smith, 1976; Schlesinger, 1974). During each session a minimum of 10 agentive elicitation tasks were presented—2 tasks for each of the 5 levels of behavior described below. These agentive elicitation tasks were interspersed throughout the free-play session. This for-

TABLE 2. VIDEOTAPED SESSIONS PER CHILD; GIVEN
ARE TYPICAL AGE (MONTHS) VERSUS ACTUAL AGE
(MONTHS:DAYS)

Session	Typical Age	Actual Age		
		Denise	Michael	Christopher
1	11	10:24	10:23	11:6
2	12	11:26	11:23	11:30
3	13	12:29	12:28	13:3
4	14	13:28	13:27	14:1
5	15	14:24	14:22	15:12
6	16	15:30	15:28	16:11
7	17	17:10	16:24	17:20
8	18	18:22	17:27	18:20
9	20	20:16	19:17	20:8
10	22	22:4	22:1	22:20

mat allowed for both freeplay by the children, as well as their elicited responses to particular tasks.

SOURCE: Olswang, L. B., & Carpenter, R. L. (1982). The ontogenesis of agent: cognitive
notion. *Journal of Speech and Hearing Research, 25,* 297–306.

The final example of a developmental study (Excerpt 7.42) is taken from a
study by Wilder and Baken of respiratory patterns in infants and illustrates
the use of a semilongitudinal design. The first paragraph of the excerpt
provides a description of the 10 subjects and serves to emphasize the point
that the infants were developmentally normal and had normal hearing sensitivity. The second paragraph and Figure A in Excerpt 7.42 capture the
essence of the semilongitudinal design. For instance, the measurement of
Subject 1 began at 2 days of age and continued at various intervals until the
child was about 80 days old. Subject 9, on the other hand, entered the study
at 161 days of age and measurements ended when the child was 255 days
old. Each subject was followed for about the same length of time (the longitudinal, within-subjects aspect), but subjects had different ages at the time of
participation in the study (the cross-sectional, between-subjects aspect).
Thus, the semilongitudinal design is a compromise between the cross-sectional and longitudinal designs that incorporates aspects of each one. Note,
for example, that the number of subjects studied is neither as high as the
cross-sectional example in Excerpt 7.40 nor as low as the longitudinal example shown in Excerpt 7.41. The semilongitudinal design tries to maximize
the advantages of both the cross-sectional design and the longitudinal design
while minimizing their disadvantages.

EXCERPT 7.42

METHOD: SUBJECTS

The population for this study was composed of 4 male and 6 female infants who presented unremarkable pre-, peri-, and postnatal histories, and who had 5-minute Apgar scores of 8 or higher. Each child's development was monitored during the course of the study using selected items from Gesell's developmental scales (Gesell & Amatruda 1947); the gross motor maturation of all subjects remained within normal limits. Hearing acuity was not formally assessed, but all infants responded appropriately to auditory stimuli.

The study used a semilongitudinal approach. The age of subjects at the time of entry into the population ranged from 2 to 161 days; each infant was observed over a period of approximately four months at intervals averaging 28 days. From the 62 individual observation sessions a statistical consultant selected four consecutive observations of each of the ten infants, providing a statistically useful sample of respiratory behavior over the age range in question (2–255 days). For data analysis these observations were grouped into eight 32-day age intervals, roughly representing age in months. Observation of each of the infants used in the analysis of data are summarized in Figure A.

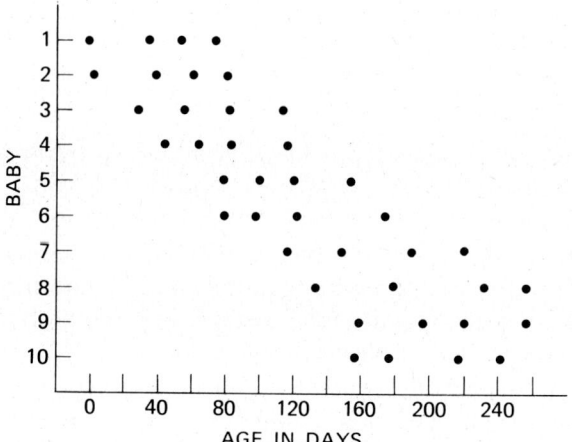

Figure A. Distribution of the 40 sample observations among the study population.

SOURCE: Wilder, C. N., & Baken, R. J. (Winter 1974–75). Respiratory patterns in infant cry. *Human Communication*, No. 3, pp. 18–34.

Correlational Research

Correlational research plays an important role in speech pathology and audiology. Correlational studies are found in research on test reliability and validity, in factor analyses of large groups of variables, in studies aimed at predicting behavior from knowledge of certain variables, and in studies of the interrelations of many clinical variables. There is a broad spectrum of correlational research to be found in the field and no single example can typify correlational research. Nevertheless, a specific example would be helpful to illustrate briefly the manner in which a researcher might go about assembling important variables for correlational analysis.

Excerpt 7.43 is taken from a study of the relationship between esophageal speech proficiency and various measures of auditory function. The basic goal of the research was to determine if the ability of laryngectomees to understand esophageal speech was related to ease of learning esophageal speech. The Method section of the study is presented in Excerpt 7.43 and details the measurement of the auditory variables to be correlated with ratings of esophageal speech proficiency of the subjects. The first section of the excerpt describes the subjects used and the other four sections describe the test materials and procedures used for making the auditory and speech measures. Minimization of threats to internal and external validity is difficult in such a correlational study because the researchers do not have the ability to manipulate the independent (predictor) variables. That is to say, these predictor variables are attribute variables, the values of which depend on subject selection and careful measurement procedures. The authors have described the subjects and measurements carefully and the attempts to reduce internal validity threats in the measurement of predictor variables can be seen in their description of the measurements.

EXCERPT 7.43

METHOD

Subjects

The subjects were 21 male laryngectomees enrolled in therapy in a large metropolitan treatment center. They were consecutive admissions to the center over a three-month period. No subject produced esophageal speech at the time he began participating in this study or exhibited disruption of oromotor function as determined by examination of the oral peripheral speech mechanism. Furthermore, all subjects were capable of silently reading the stimulus items used in testing. The subjects ranged in age from 44 to 73 years; the mean age was 60 years. Time since surgery ranged from three to 32 weeks; the mean was nine weeks.

An audiologic test battery that included special tests of ability to discriminate esophageal speech was administered to each subject two weeks after the beginning of the esophageal speech training. The 21 subjects were recalled four months after the beginning of therapy to have their speech recorded. Four months was the average duration of therapy in this clinic. During this period, subjects received six to 10 hours a week of individual and group therapy from the same instructor. Subjects recorded the first paragraph of the Rainbow Passage (Fairbanks, 1960), using high-quality recording equipment. The first two sentences from each full paragraph recording were extracted and used as the material for the speech-rating sessions.

Test Materials

The subjects could not be expected to respond to conventional audiometric procedures requiring a verbal response. Therefore, the test materials that were used to assess SRT and speech discrimination were selected to obviate the need for oral responses.

A modification of the Verbal-Auditory Screening Test for Children described by Griffing, Simonton, and Hedgecock (1962) was used to obtain SRTs. The discrimination ability of laryngectomees for normal speech was assessed with Form 1A of the multiple-choice discrimination test described by Schultz and Schubert (1969).

Multiple-choice discrimination tests for eosphageal speech, based on the Schultz and Schubert (1969) test, were developed by the investigator. These tests differ from the Schultz and Schubert test in that the stimulus words were recorded by esophageal speakers rather than by normal laryngeal speakers.

Three speech pathologists, experienced in esophageal speech instruction, selected 10 esophageal speakers, representing a range of speaker proficiency, from a file of former patients. Three speakers, judged to represent good, average, and poor esophageal speech proficiency, were screened from the original group of 10 by the judges. The good, average, and poor speakers then recorded multiple-choice discrimination test Equivalent Forms, 1B, 2B, and 4B, respectively, using high-quality recording equipment. The VU meter on the recorder was peaked at zero on each test word to provide a constant intensity level for the test stimuli. A normal speaker recorded a carrier phrase, which preceded each test word. A 10-second silent interval was included between test words. A 1000-Hz calibration tone was recorded at the beginning of each of the three tapes.

Auditory Tests

A series of audiologic tests was administered to each subject two weeks after the beginning of therapy. Hearing tests were administered in a sound-treated, two-room, IAC test suite. An Allison Model 2B two-channel audiometer, calibrated to ISO 1964 standards, was employed for both pure-tone and speech audiometry. TDH–39 earphones were used for air-conduction testing. Prerecorded cartridge tapes containing speech stimuli were introduced to the speech circuit of the Allison unit from an Elcomatic cartridge tape recorder and reproduced over a Regal Electro-Voice loudspeaker.

All subjects received a pure-tone, air-conduction threshold test in both ears at 250, 500, 1000, 2000, 4000, and 8000 Hz. They also received a pure-tone, bone-conduction threshold test in both ears at 250, 500, 1000, 2000, and 4000 Hz. The ascending technique of Hughson and Westlake (1944) was employed for threshold determination.

Free-field SRTs were obtained using the modified Verbal-Auditory Screening Test. The subject responded to this recorded material by pointing to a picture of the word he heard.

Discrimination ability for normal speech was assessed with Form 1A of the multiple-choice discrimination test materials (Schultz & Schubert, 1969). The subject was presented the appropriate multiple-choice response form and instructed to draw a line beside the word he believed to be the stimulus word. The 50-item word list was presented free field at 40 dB above SRT.

Discrimination ability for esophageal speech was evaluated by means of the multiple-choice discrimination test for esophageal speech. Each subject was informed before administration of the test that the stimulus words had been recorded by esophageal speakers. The order of presentation of the three forms was Form 1B (good), Form 2B (average), and Form 4B (poor esophageal speech). The subject was given the appropriate multiple-choice response form and asked to draw a line beside the word he believed to be the stimulus word. Each of the three word lists was presented in the field at 40 dB above SRT.

Judges

The listeners were 20 college-age students drawn from introductory public-speaking courses. All judges had normal hearing as determined by a screening test. They were considered to be inexperienced in that they had never listened to esophageal speech nor received any formal training in speech pathology.

Judgments

The judges were instructed to rate each speech sample on a seven-point global scale of esophageal speech proficiency. A rating of 7 represented most proficient and a rating of 1 represented least proficient, with the remaining ratings equally spaced between 1 and 7. The order of presentation of samples was rerandomized between presentations to minimize order effects in the judgment technique. Rating sessions were conducted in a sound-treated listening room using a high-quality reproduction system. The tapes were presented at a comfortable listening level of 70 dB SPL.

SOURCE: Martin, D. E., Hoops, H. R., & Shanks, J. C. (1974). The relationship between esophageal speech proficiency and selected measures of auditory function. *Journal of Speech and Hearing Research, 17,* 80–85.

Another example of a correlational study can be seen in Excerpt 7.21, which was presented earlier in this chapter as an example of the selection of appropriate measures. As the text in Excerpt 7.21 indicates, the study attempted to correlate certain pretreatment variables with the outcome of stuttering therapy. Pretreatment variables were used as predictors of the relative degree of success in stuttering therapy. The correlational research in Excerpt 7.21 was aimed at verifying the prognostic value of different measures of stuttering severity, personality, and attitude by examining their correlations with, and their ability to predict, success in stuttering therapy.

Retrospective Research

In Chapter 2, we cited some of the problems associated with retrospective research studies. Excerpt 7.44 presents two selections from the Method section of a study by Carhart and Porter on the relationship between pure-tone and spondee thresholds for subjects with various audiometric configurations. The first paragraph is important because it details subject selection criteria that are significant for both internal and external validity. Note, for example, that satisfactory reliability during testing was one important criterion, that very young and very old patients were eliminated (probably because of the difficulty they present in testing), and that normal hearing persons were excluded. The sample ultimately chosen was large and included subjects with a variety of audiometric configurations (described in other parts of the Method section) that were probably reasonably representative of hearing-impaired patients seen in many audiology clinics.

The second paragraph is even more important because it directly addresses the main problem in retrospective research, namely, under what conditions were the data collected. In this brief paragraph, Carhart and Porter indicate the following steps that were taken to overcome the problems associated with retrospective research: (1) that the data were collected in sound-treated test environments, (2) that testing was performed by trained and qualified clinicians, (3) that calibration was checked frequently, (4) that the Carhart-Jerger technique was used to measure pure-tone thresholds and that a 2-dB bracketing method was used for all speech threshold measurements, (5) that tape-recorded spondee words were employed and that the speaker was Tillman, and (6) that the calibration values conformed or were made to conform to current reference standards. Only the authors' assurance that all of the data were collected under the conditions as described makes it possible for the critical reader to give any weight to the subsequent Results section. The evaluator of retrospective research, whether it be comparative or correlational, must be painstaking, indeed, when reading the Method section for such research may stand or fall on this section alone.

EXCERPT 7.44

PROCEDURE

We explored the relationship between audiometric contour and threshold for spondees by performing a retrospective statistical analysis of records obtained in the Northwestern University Hearing Clinics between January 1966 and September 1968.Patients seen in these clinics were judged suitable for inclusion in the study provided they (1) were between 10 and 80 years old, inclusive; (2) had exhibited satisfactory reliability during both pure-tone and speech testing; (3) did not have two or more thresholds better than 10 dB ISO 1964 in either ear; (4) had recordable thresholds from 250 through 4000 Hz for the better ear; and (5) yielded a measurable threshold when tested with spondees. Two thousand one hundred thirty-five cases satisfied these criteria. Every seventh record was then removed so as to yield an audiometrically hetero-geneous pool for purposes of comparison with earlier studies. The audiograms for the better ears of the remaining 1823 persons were classified as to pattern into six groups.

. . . .

Before considering the findings that emerged, a word must be said about the conditions in which the data under consideration had previously been gathered. All tests were administered in adequately sound-proofed booths. Testers were either full-time audiological clinicians or well-trained student clinicians working under the immediate supervision of full-time clinicians. All audiometers were monitored frequently with Bruel and Kjaer equipment to assure proper calibration. Pure-tone thresholds were obtained by the Hughson-Westlake method (Carhart & Jerger, 1959) with audiometers adjusted to the ISO 1964 standard. Speech thresholds were obtained by a bracketing method em-ploying 2-dB steps. Test materials were spondee words spoken by Tillman and recorded on magnetic tape. The O-dB hearing level was set at 22 dB SPL as determined by a 1000-Hz calibration tone recorded to equal the frequent peaks for spondees as viewed with a VU meter. This setting conformed to the ASA 1953 standard for speech audiometers. However, for purposes of this paper, all spondee thresholds are reported re a reference level of 20 dB SPL because this value is specified for the TDH-39 earphone in the new ANSI standard for audiometers (1969). This change was made to bring the regression equations emerging from this study into conformity with current reference levels.

SOURCE: Carhart, R., & Porter, L. S. (1971). Audiometric configuration and prediction of threshold for spondees. *Journal of Speech and Hearing Research, 14*, 486–495.

Survey Research

We come next to the evaluation of survey research. Although there is an extensive body of literature on survey research methodology, questionnaire development, interview techniques, and the like (e.g., see Babbie, 1973; Davis, 1971; and Slonim, 1960), such research does not appear with much frequency in the speech and hearing research literature. Thus, we will focus here on only a few selected issues that need to be identified by the critical evaluator of survey research and hope that the interested reader who wishes to delve more deeply into the area will consult the sources noted above.

The choice of a survey research design should be consistent with, and appropriate to, the purpose of the study. The first question the critical reader must raise, then, is whether the research reported was best conducted by means of a survey design or whether there were alternative, and perhaps better, research designs that could have been used to answer the research questions. Assuming that the survey design was appropriate, the next ques-tion deals with the adequacy of the sample surveyed. As we pointed out in Chapter 2, it is difficult, if not impossible, to survey the entire population of interest (e.g., all speech pathologists in the United States, all speech and hearing facilities in the country). As a result, survey researchers often draw a sample of subjects that presumably is representative of the total population. On the surface, this may appear to be a relatively simple task. In reality, the task can be quite complex. Fortunately, there are a variety of sampling techniques that can be employed. These include random sampling, stratified sampling, cluster sampling, systematic sampling, and the like. We cannot address here the technical aspects of sampling or the advantages and disadvantages of various sampling techniques. Suffice it to say that the critical reader must address the issue of the adequacy of the sample used in survey research. It may not be readily apparent but the sampling issue in survey research is analogous to the differential-selection-of-subjects threat to internal validity as well as the subject-selection threat to external validity.

The mortality threat to internal validity is a common problem in survey research. Mortality in this context is represented by the number of people surveyed who failed to respond to the survey instrument. Babbie (1973) points out that a response rate of at least 50% can be considered adequate for analysis and reporting purposes, that a response rate of 60% is good, and that a response of 70% or greater is very good. If the nonresponse rate is high, the researcher may have a biased sample, a sample that may not be representative of the population of interest, and a sample of responders who are quite different, on important dimensions, from individuals who failed to respond. It is for these reasons that survey researchers spend considerable time, effort, and money on attempts to enlist the cooperation of individuals who failed to respond to the initial request to participate in the survey. The careful reader of survey research must identify the mortality rate and determine if the number of nonresponders poses a threat to both internal and external validity.

The instrumentation threat to internal validity is directly related to the adequacy of the survey instrument, be it a questionnaire or an interview. Good questionnaire development is a difficult and complex task, one not readily undertaken by the novice. Are the questions clear and unambiguous? Do the questions address the issues under study? Are the questions objective and nonthreatening? Do the questions lead to nonbiased responses? In an attempt to ensure the adequacy of a questionnaire, researchers often pretest the instrument. That is, a small sample of representative individuals is given a trial questionnaire for their reactions, their suggestions, and their comments. The pretest is an extremely important part of questionnaire development and the critical reader should be alert to the researcher's reference to the use of a pretest. It should be noted that the questionnaire itself is usually not available for the reader's inspection but should be made available to an interested reader if requested from the researcher. In longer articles or in books reporting the results of survey research, the questionnaire is usually included for the reader's inspection. Remember, a questionnaire survey is only as good as the questions asked.

The survey research interview has several advantages over the questionnaire format. Interviewing permits probing to obtain more or different data, allows for greater depth, and enables the interviewer to assess rapport and communication between interviewer and respondent and to determine if these factors are affecting the data-collection process. On the other hand, interviews are costly and time consuming, the interviewer needs to be trained, and the interaction between interviewer and respondent can have a strong influence on the data collected. In this context, of course, the interviewer and the interview format (e.g., structured vs. unstructured interviews) can pose an instrumentation threat to internal validity.

Excerpt 7.45 is from an article that reports Part I of a two-part survey of characteristics of hearing-impaired children in the public schools. The excerpt includes a two-paragraph introduction that explains the rationale for the survey and the specific purpose of Part I. The Method section outlines the areas covered in the survey questionnaire and how it was administered with the school audiologists. In addition, the Method section includes a description of the classification of the schoolchildren and how the random sampling was conducted within each classification. Also described is a procedure for follow-up on missing information and a statement regarding final missing data and the expected margin of error for all values reported for the random sample.

The random sampling within each classification is a procedure that ensures good external validity: consumers can be confident of generalizations made to subjects of the same kind in similar settings because of the random sampling within each classification that took place. Generalization to other kinds of settings or subjects, of course, would require replications. But the stratified random sampling used in this study is a strong procedure for improving external validity.

Also note that the entire questionnaire is available on request from one of the authors. This would enable interested consumers to review the questions and evaluate the instrument directly. The classification of subjects is quite detailed as indicated in the Method section and in the Appendix. Internal validity is improved by using the strict criteria for defining subject groups and the subjects to whom generalization is appropriate is well specified. Note, too, the attempt to preserve the anonymity of the children, yet ensure the ability to follow up on missing data. In summary, this survey has included a number of steps to bolster both internal and external validity, yet deal with the practical realities of surveying 13 Area Education Agencies spread over an entire state.

Excerpt 7.45

Attempts by state and local educational agencies to implement Public Law 94–142 have highlighted the paucity of information on which educational programming is based for certain groups of handicapped children. Of particular concern at present are unserved and underserved populations, including children with hearing impairment. Although the educational and demographic characteristics of severely-to-profoundly hearing-impaired children are well-documented (Gentile, 1972; Balow & Brill, 1975; Moores, 1970; Trybus & Karchmer, 1977), less severely hearing-impaired children have not been studied systematically. Ross (1977) estimates that there are at least 20 times as many moderately hearing-impaired children as severely-to-profoundly hearing-impaired and that they can be found in every school building in the country. Many of them are unidentified or misdiagnosed (Ross, 1977), others are identified but do not have access to special support services (Davis, 1977), while others receive extensive educational support (Peterson, 1972). Unfortunately, little is known about the status and needs of moderately hearing-impaired children in general or the relations among important factors such as degree of hearing loss, hearing-aid use, classroom placement, and, in particular, psychoeducational status. The few studies in existence reporting educational achievement data on small numbers of moderately hearing-impaired children indicate that they are underachievers, delayed in academic skills, and in jeopardy regarding social relationships (Kodman, 1963; Quigley & Thomure, 1968; Davis, 1974; Peterson, 1972). Although these studies provide helpful information, they are not designed to answer specific questions about the prevalence of patterns of hearing loss among school children, their use of amplification, educational placement, and special support services, or their psychoeducational status and needs. Without these types of demographic and educational data, it is unlikely that adequate educational programming will be developed and implemented for this population.

This study was designed to collect both demographic and psychoeducational data for a large number of randomly sampled hearing-impaired children enrolled in the public schools of Iowa. Only demographic data will be reported here. Psychoeducational data will be reviewed in a subsequent paper. The state's plan for providing services to hearing-impaired children has resulted in an unusually comprehensive identification and follow-up program, involving employment of about 70 audiologists, 500 speech-language pathologists, and 100 teachers of the hearing-impaired. The availability of so many special personnel makes it likely that moderately hearing-impaired children will be identified and evaluated, resulting in a pool of available data for a large number of children.

METHOD

A survey questionnaire was developed[1] that included inquiries about age, sex, onset of hearing loss, hearing status, educational placement and services, use and monitoring of amplification, and language and academic achievement. School audiologists were paid an hourly wage to perform the sampling and complete the questionnaires. All but two of the state's 15 Area Education Agencies (AEAs) participated in the study. The AEAs are multi-county agencies in Iowa charged with providing special support services to handicapped children within their geographic boundaries.

A total of 1250 hearing-impaired children were included in the sample. On

[1]The survey questionnaire is available on request from Julia M. Davis, Department of Speech Pathology and Audiology, University of Iowa, Iowa City, Iowa 52242.

the basis of their most recent audiograms, the children were stratified into three main groups:

Group A consisted of those children with a bilateral or unilateral conductive hearing loss as defined by the existence of normal hearing by bone conduction and air-bone gaps greater than 10 dB. After the sampling was completed, children in group A were assigned to three subgroups based on degree of hearing loss, as shown in the Appendix.

Group B_1 consisted of those children with a bilateral or unilateral high frequency hearing loss. For sampling purposes, children were required to have air and bone conduction thresholds greater than 25 dB HL (ANSI, 1969) at frequencies only of 4,000 and/or 6,000 Hz and above.

Group C consisted of children with sensorineural or mixed hearing loss at more than one of the standard audiometric test frequencies, and not included in groups A or B_1. Within group C, children were assigned to six subgroups on the basis of the degree and configuration of their hearing losses, as shown in the Appendix.

In addition to the above predetermined major groupings (A, B_1, and C) and post-hoc subgroups (A_1, A_2, A_3, C_1, C_2, C_3, C_4, and C_5) three post-hoc classifications were made to allow for a more detailed analysis of high frequency hearing. As described in the Appendix, subgroups B_2, B_3, and B_4 represent high-frequency hearing loss with decreasing cutoff frequencies. When these three groups are viewed with the major group B_1, the result is a continuum of high-frequency hearing loss. That is, group B_1–B_4 represent a reduction in hearing sensitivity at increasingly lower frequencies. The three major groups, A, B_1, and C, are mutually exclusive. In addition, all of the A and C subgroups are derived solely from the A and C groups, respectively. In contrast, the B_2, B_3, and B_4 subgroups are derived from the major group C.

Each of the main groups in each AEA was randomly sampled; groups A and B_1 were sampled at a 5% rate and group C was sampled at a rate of 20%. Different sampling rates were employed to insure approximately equal numbers of children in each of the main groups. The AEA audiologists were provided with randomly generated numbers (between 1 and 20 for groups A and B_1 and between 1 and 5 for group C) for entry into their lists of children who exhibited hearing loss.

A questionnaire was then completed on each of the children sampled. The survey information was obtained from all available records on the children. Answers to all questions were not available for all children, however. Each child was coded with a 12 digit alphanumeric code that only the AEA employees could decipher. This code was used by the authors to request further clarification on individual children and yet preserve anonymity. The most recent copy of each child's audiometric evaluation was included with each questionnaire. Questionnaire information was coded for computer analysis.

It was not unusual for data to be missing from a particular child's files, resulting in a variable n for many questions. Computation of an error prediction for a random sample indicated, however, that all demographic data are accurate to within ±6% for the total groups A, B_1, and C.

SOURCE: Shepard, N. T., Davis, J. M., Gorga, M. P., & Stelmachowicz, P. G. (1981). Characteristics of hearing-impaired children in the public schools: Part I demographic data. *Journal of Speech and Hearing Disorders, 46*, 123–129.

Case Study Research

Our last evaluation example concerns case study research, a type of descriptive research that is frequently found in the speech pathology and audiology research literature. As we have pointed out earlier, case study research has both advantages and disadvantages. Case studies lay the groundwork for future research that will use larger groups of subjects by identifying variables that can or should be experimentally manipulated and by generating hypotheses that need to be tested. A case study obviously allows for intensive exploration of the phenomenon of interest and may shed light on rare phenomena or raise questions about the adequacy of well-established theoretical formulations (Hersen & Barlow, 1976). On the other hand, without replication, case studies may have limited generalizability. Also, case studies are especially vulnerable to subjective biases. A case may be studied because it fits the researcher's preconceptions or because it is especially dramatic. Whatever the advantages and disadvantages of case study research, the task that remains is to identify the evaluative criteria that can be used by the consumer of this research. It should be noted that case study research is the only descriptive design that is not altogether amenable to an analysis that incorporates the Campbell and Stanley evaluation framework, a framework we have employed throughout. In actuality, the factors that threaten internal validity in experimental research and in other descriptive research may be the factors that are the substance of the case study approach. As one example, history may be a contaminating influence in a variety of research designs. In case study research, a "history" event may provide considerable insight about the phenomenon under study. For instance, one of the child's parents separates from the household, producing a marked decrease (or increase) in the behavior being observed. Maturational influences, another contaminating variable, may, in fact, be the primary variable under investigation in case study research. Biases introduced by subject selection are inherent in case study research because subjects are selected for their uniqueness.

The evaluation of case study research revolves around the following considerations: (1) Is the approach appropriate to the purpose of the study? (2) Have methods been employed to control for experimenter bias (videotaping the subject and allowing other clinicians or researchers to evaluate the behavior observed)? (3) Have careful measurements been made of the behavior or phenomenon under study? (4) Is sufficient detail provided about the procedures so that the procedures can be replicated by other interested parties? (5) Does the research lead to hypotheses that can be tested experimentally or to research questions that can be explored with other research designs? (6) Are the conclusions drawn by the researcher couched in appropriately cautious and conservative terms? and (7) Does, in fact, the case study reported contribute to our understanding of behavior, even if that behavior is restricted to a single subject? The evaluation of a case study must encompass the entire article from the introduction through the discussion.

Space limitations prevent us from including an entire case study here. Instead, we have reprinted abstracts from two recent case studies in Excerpts 7.46 and 7.47. These abstracts describe briefly one speech pathology and one audiology case study. Readers are referred to the entire articles from which the abstracts are excerpted for further details regarding the specific cases and the methods used to study these cases.

EXCERPT 7.46

Palilalia is an acquired speech disorder characterized by reiteration of utterances in a context of increasing rate and decreasing loudness. The condition has been associated with bilateral subcortical neuropathology. The relationship of palilalia to other adult disfluency syndromes, aphasia, and motor speech disorders requires a thorough understanding of the nature of palilalic speech. To date no detailed description of the nature and severity of palilalic reiteration has appeared in the literature. This case report systematically describes seven distinct types of reiteration, frequency (severity) of reiteration relative to seven types of speech tasks, and consistency and adaptation effects observed in a 29-year-old male.

SOURCE: LaPointe, L. L., & Horner, J. (1981). Palilalia: A descriptive study of pathological reiterative utterances. *Journal of Speech and Hearing Disorders, 46,* 34–38.

EXCERPT 7.47

A well-documented case report is presented in which the use of a high-output hearing aid over a 10-year period resulted in significant threshold shifts in the aided as compared to the unaided ear. At no time did the user experience loudness discomfort and she consistently wanted more gain from the hearing aid, indicating that there is no relationship between loudness discomfort levels and the sound pressure levels at which damage to the auditory system occurs. Difficulties in detecting the cause of the threshold shifts and recommendations for case management are discussed.

SOURCE: Hawkins, D. B. (1982). Overamplification: A well-documented case report. *Journal of Speech and Hearing Disorders, 47,* 382–384.

Summary

This chapter has illustrated the typical parts of the Method section of the research article. Examples from the literature have been presented to show how researchers have described the subjects, materials, and procedures used in empirical studies. The section on subjects showed several examples dealing with problems of sample size and subject selection criteria. The section on materials dealt with examples of hardware instrumentation and calibration, reliability and validity of behavioral instruments, and some miscellaneous measurement considerations such as experimenter bias. The section on procedures included examples that demonstrated the ways in which researchers had designed a variety of research studies, including many that had been outlined in Chapter 2. It is in the Method section that a critical reader is most likely to find the researcher's attempts to deal with the major threats to internal and external validity. Careful scrutiny of the Method section is necessary to determine the degree of internal and external validity of any research article.

EVALUATION CHECKLIST

Instructions: The four-category scale at the end of each part of the *Method* section checklist may be used to rate these parts of an article. The *Evaluation Items* help identify those topics that should be considered in arriving at the ratings. Comments on these topics, entered as *Evaluation Notes*, should serve as the basis for the ratings. An additional scale is provided to allow for an overall rating of the Method section.

Evaluation Items (Subjects)   *Evaluation Notes*

1. Sample size was adequate.
2. Subject selection and exclusion criteria were adequate and clearly defined.
3. Subjects were randomly selected and randomly assigned.
4. Overall or pair matching was employed.
5. Differential selection of subjects posed a threat to internal validity.
6. Subjects were selected on basis of extreme scores.
7. Interaction of subject selection and treatment posed a threat to external validity.
8. Miscellaneous.

Overall Rating (Subjects):   _____ _____ _____ _____
                                  Poor   Fair   Good   Excellent

Evaluation Items (Materials)   *Evaluation Notes*

1. Instrumentation (hardware and behavioral) was appropriate.
2. Calibration procedures were described and were adequate.
3. Evidence presented on reliability and validity of hardware and behavioral instrumentation.
4. Experimenter and human observer bias was controlled.
5. Test environment was described and was adequate.
6. Instructions were described and were adequate.
7. There were adequate selection and measurement of independent (classification, predictor) variables.
8. There were adequate selection and measurement of dependent (criterion, predicted) variables.
9. Miscellaneous.

Overall Rating (Materials):

____	____	____	____
Poor	Fair	Good	Excellent

Evaluation Items (Procedures)   *Evaluation Notes*

1. Research design was appropriate to purpose of study.
2. Procedures reduced threats to internal validity arising from:
   (a) history
   (b) maturation
   (c) pretesting
   (d) mortality
   (e) Hawthorne effect
   (f) interaction of above

3. Procedures reduced threats to external validity arising from:
   - (a) reactive arrangements
   - (b) reactive effects of pre-testing
   - (c) subject selection
   - (d) multiple treatments

4. Miscellaneous.

Overall Rating (Procedures):

Poor	Fair	Good	Excellent

Overall Rating (Method):

Poor	Fair	Good	Excellent

References

Arndt, W. B. (1977). A psychometric evaluation of the Northwestern Syntax Screening Test. *Journal of Speech and Hearing Disorders, 42,* 316–319.

Babbie, E. R. (1973). *Survey research methods.* Belmont, CA: Wadsworth.

Barber, T. X. (1976). *Pitfalls in human research.* New York: Pergamon.

Barber, T. X., & Silver, M. J. (1968). Fact, fiction, and the experimenter bias effect. *Psychological Bulletin Monograph Supplement, 70* (6, Pt. 2).

Barlow, S. M., Cole, K. J., & Abbs, J. H. (1983). A new head-mounted lip-jaw movement transduction system for the study of motor speech disorders. *Journal of Speech and Hearing Research, 26,* 283–288.

Buros, O. K. (1972). *The seventh mental measurements yearbook.* Highland Park, NJ: Gryphon Press.

Christensen, L. B. (1977). *Experimental methodology.* Boston: Allyn & Bacon.

Darley, F. (Ed.). (1979). *Evaluation of appraisal techniques in speech and language pathology.* New York: Wiley.

Davis, J. A. (1971). *Elementary survey analysis.* Englewood Cliffs, NJ: Prentice-Hall.

Guillemin, B. J., & Nguyen, D. T. (1984). Microprocessor-based speech processing system. *Journal of Speech and Hearing Research, 27,* 311–317.

Hersen, M., & Barlow, D. H. (1976). *Single case experimental designs: Strategies for studying behavior change.* New York: Pergamon.

Hipskind, N. M., & Rintelmann, W. F. (1969). Effects of experimenter bias upon pure-tone and speech audiometry. *Journal of Auditory Research, 9,* 298–305.

Hixon, T. J., Bless, D. M., & Netsell, R. (1976). A new technique for measuring velopharyngeal orifice area during sustained vowel production: An application of aerodynamic forced oscillation principles. *Journal of Speech and Hearing Research, 19,* 601–607.

Hixon, T. J., Hawley, J. L., & Wilson, K. J. (1982). An around-the-house device for the clinical determination of respiratory driving pressure: A note on making simple even simpler. *Journal of Speech and Hearing Disorders, 47,* 413–415.

Lee, L. L. (1977). Reply to Arndt and Byrne. *Journal of Speech and Hearing Disorders,* *42,* 323–327.

Levitt, H. (1983). Issue X: Advancing technology. *Proceedings of the 1983 National Conference on Undergraduate, Graduate, and Continuing Education. ASHA Reports, 13,* 87–89.

McCauley, R. J., & Swisher, L. (1984). Psychometric review of language and articulation tests for preschool children. *Journal of Speech and Hearing Disorders, 49,* 34–42.

Netsell, R., & Hixon, T. J. (1978). A noninvasive method for clinically estimating subglottal air pressure. *Journal of Speech and Hearing Disorders, 43,* 326–330.

Plutchik, R. (1974). *Foundations of experimental research* (2nd ed.). New York: Harper & Row.

Rosenthal, R. (1966). *Experimenter effects in behavioral research.* New York: Appleton-Century-Crofts.

Rosenthal, R., & Rosnow, R. L. (Eds.). (1969). *Artifact in behavioral research.* New York: Academic Press.

Rosenthal, R., & Rosnow, R. L. (1975). *The volunteer subject.* New York: Wiley.

Slonim, M. J. (1960). *Sampling.* New York: Simon & Schuster.

Smitheron, J. R., & Hixon, T. J. (1981). A clinical method for estimating laryngeal airway resistance during vowel production. *Journal of Speech and Hearing Disorders, 46,* 138–146.

Ventry, I. M., Woods, R. W., Rubin, M., & Hill, W. (1971). Most comfortable loudness for pure tones, noise, and speech. *Journal of the Acoustical Society of America, 49,* 1805–1813.

Wood, G. (1974). *Fundamentals of psychological research.* Boston: Little, Brown.

8
The Results Section

Introduction

Basic terms, concepts, and procedures employed in organizing and analyzing data derived from research in speech pathology and audiology were described in Chapter 5. This chapter will consider the evaluation of the Results section of a research article through the use of examples that illustrate many of those basic terms, concepts, and procedures.

An important consideration in the evaluation of the Results section is the manner in which the results are related to the research problem. It is imperative that the Results section be organized in a clear fashion with regard to the general research problem and the various subproblems delineated under it. Without clear articulation of the results to the problem, even relatively simple data may be confusing and frustrating to the reader, whereas tight organization of the results around the research problem may make complex data comprehensible to most readers. Just as the writer has a responsibility to maintain the problem as the focus of the Results section, the reader must constantly bear the problem in mind while reading and evaluating the Results section.

Organization of Results

Upon completion of data collection, the researcher's first task is to organize the raw data to present a coherent picture of the results to readers. This section will present examples from the speech pathology and audiology literature that illustrate some of the ways in which raw data have been organized for presentation. In reality, an author may have gone through several steps of organizing and reorganizing raw data on paper before arriving at a solution that enables him or her to present the results in as clear, complete, and efficient a manner as possible within the confines of a short journal article. What the reader eventually sees in print is usually a capsuled or boiled down version of the raw data that renders them more palatable, yet still gives a clear indication of the general behavior or characteristics of subjects in the various conditions of the research design. The results may be organized for the reader by tabular or graphic presentation of the frequency distribution of the data or through the use of summary statistics that may describe the distribution more succinctly.

Frequency Distributions: Tabular and Graphic Presentations

It was stated in Chapter 5 that whenever variables are measured in a research study, the obtained values of the measurements form a distribution. The distribution may be in the form of category frequencies (for nominal data), ranks (for ordinal data), or score values (for interval or ratio data). Both tabular and graphic presentation of the frequency distribution may be effective means of data organization in order to begin making comparisons of results within subjects or between groups of subjects. Although any frequency distribution may be presented in either tabular or graphic form, there are some advantages unique to each type of illustration. In general, frequency distributions presented in graphic form (i.e., frequency histograms or polygons) give a more immediate overall picture of the distribution and have a more dramatic effect on the reader in showing the characteristics of the distribution. On the other hand, frequency distributions presented in a table are generally more convenient for inspection of specific values of the data or for making exact within-subjects and between-subjects comparisons. In some articles, authors have taken advantage of both types of presentations and included both a tabular and a graphic presentation of a frequency distribution.

Excerpt 8.1 shows the use of a table that includes both a frequency distribution and a cumulative frequency distribution of the scores of stutterers and nonstutterers on a scale of communication attitudes. Attitude scores are shown in the left-hand column, with the lower scores on the top of the table and the higher scores on the bottom of the table. The next column to the right (*f*) shows the number of nonstutterers who obtained each score. The next column (*crf*) shows the cumulative relative frequency (expressed as a decimal fraction of the number of subjects) of the nonstutterers obtaining each score on the attitude scale. The next two columns on the right-hand side show the data for the stutterers displayed in the same format. In addition, summary statistics (means and standard deviations) are shown at the bottom

EXCERPT 8.1

TABLE 1. FREQUENCY (*f*) AND CUMULATIVE RELATIVE FREQUENCY (*crf*) DISTRIBUTIONS OF *S*-SCALE SCORES IN THE NONSTUTTERING AND STUTTERING GROUPS

Score	Nonstutters (n = 144)		Stutterers (n = 120)	
	f	crf	f	crf
1	0	0.00		
2	7	0.05		
3	5	0.08		
4	11	0.16		
5	9	0.22	0	0.00
6	6	0.26	1	0.01
7	5	0.30	0	0.01
8	9	0.36	1	0.02
9	6	0.40	1	0.02
10	7	0.45	1	0.03
11	7	0.50	2	0.05
12	4	0.53	0	0.05
13	5	0.56	1	0.06
14	6	0.60	4	0.09
15	3	0.62	2	0.11
16	6	0.67	2	0.12
17	6	0.71	4	0.16
18	5	0.74	4	0.19
19	2	0.76	5	0.23
20	4	0.78	3	0.26
21	5	0.82	4	0.29
22	3	0.84	2	0.31
23	2	0.85	2	0.32
24	3	0.88	6	0.38
25	5	0.91	8	0.44
26	1	0.92	6	0.49
27	3	0.94	4	0.52
28	0	0.94	6	0.58
29	3	0.96	3	0.60
30	1	0.97	12	0.70
31	2	0.98	8	0.77
32	2	0.99	3	0.79
33	1	1.00	7	0.85
34	—	—	11	0.94
35	—	—	3	0.97
36	—	—	2	0.98
37	—	—	2	1.00
Mean	13.24		26.65	
SD	8.20		7.24	

SOURCE: Erickson, R. L. (1969). Assessing communication attitudes among stutterers. *Journal of Speech and Hearing Research, 12,* 711–724.

of the table for both groups of subjects. Inspection of the table reveals both the degree of separation and overlapping of the two groups in their scores on this communication attitude scale.

The next excerpt (8.2) shows a frequency distribution presented in the form of a histogram. This illustration shows the scores of a group of stutterers and a group of nonstutterers on two tests of phonetic ability. The bar heights in the histograms indicate the number of subjects in each group who achieved each score on the tests. The top two histograms present the stutterers and nonstutterer's data on the phonetic anagrams test and the bottom two histograms show the data for the backward speech test. Inspection of the four histograms reveals that more nonstutterers achieved higher scores on the two tests than did stutterers.

The histograms in Excerpt 8.2 give a more immediate and dramatic picture of the overall results than does Table 1 shown in Excerpt 8.1. On the other hand, closer inspection of the exact frequency of subjects obtaining each specific score is easier when inspecting the frequency table.

Excerpts 8.1 and 8.2 illustrate how tabular or graphic frequency distributions would appear in a journal article when the dependent variable data are scores at the interval or ratio level of measurement. The next two excerpts (8.3 and 8.4) show frequency distributions for data at the nominal and ordinal levels of measurements. In other words, they show the distribution of frequencies of categories (nominal level) or frequencies of rankings (ordinal level).

Excerpt 8.3 is from a study on predicting hearing loss from acoustic reflex thresholds in which each subject was predicted to have "normal hearing," "mild-moderate hearing loss," or "severe hearing loss," on the basis of certain acoustic reflex results. Excerpt 8.3 illustrates the use of a frequency distribution table for displaying the number of subjects who fell into each of the three nominal categories. Eight different groups of subjects (each group had a different type of pure tone audiogram) are listed in the left column and the number of subjects in each of the eight audiogram-type groups listed is shown in the second column. The next six columns toward the right show the number and percent of subjects from each of the eight groups who were classified by the Jerger acoustic reflex procedure as having normal, mild-moderate, or severe hearing loss. Subject group number one actually consisted of 17 normal hearing subjects. Readers will note on inspection of the first row of the table, that ten of these subjects (i.e., 59%) were correctly classified by the acoustic reflex procedure as having normal hearing, whereas seven subjects (41%) were predicted to have a mild-moderate hearing loss. The other seven groups displayed various types of hearing loss in their audiograms, and none of these (i.e., 0%) were predicted to have normal hearing by the Jerger acoustic reflex procedure. Readers should now be able to inspect the other rows to determine how many subjects in each of these groups were classified as mild-moderate or severe.

EXCERPT 8.2

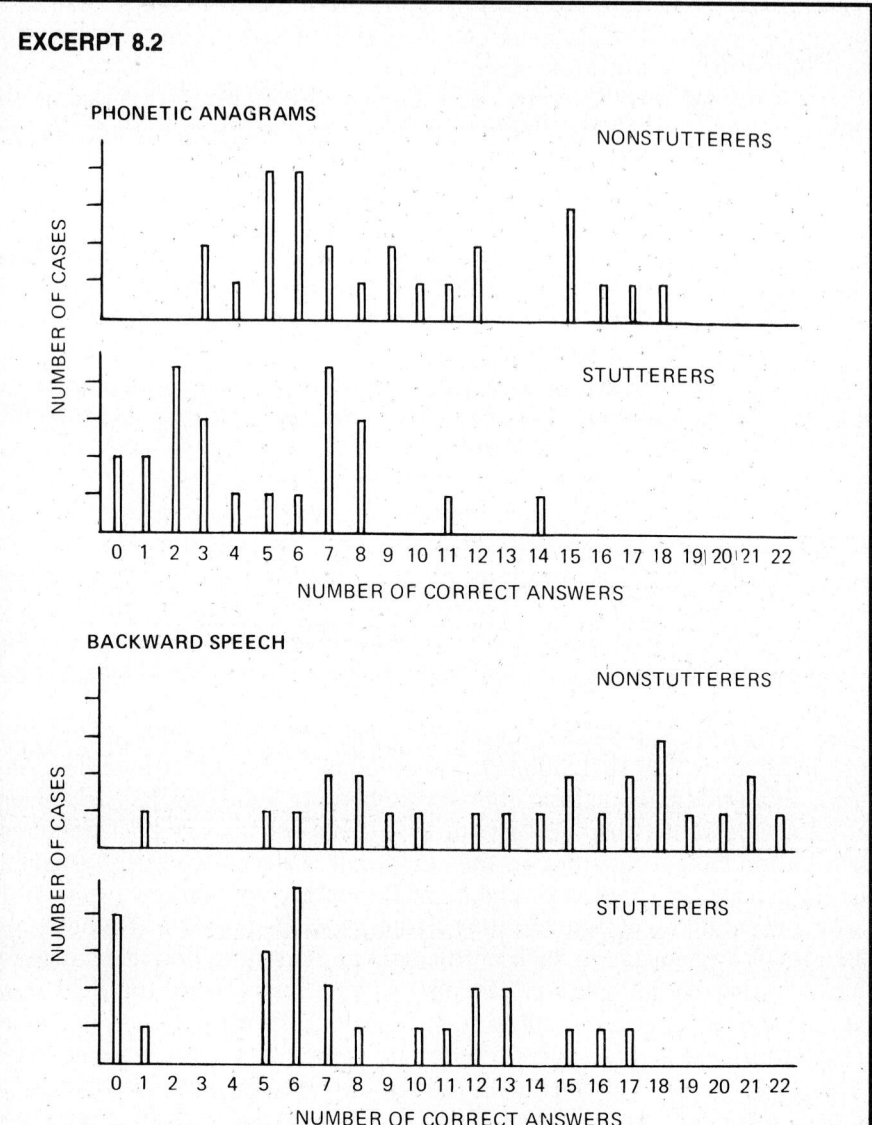

Figure 1. Distributions of individual success in solving items of the two

SOURCE: Wingate, M. E. (1971). Phonetic ability in stuttering. *Journal of Speech an Hearing Research, 14*, 189–194.

EXCERPT 8.3

TABLE 5. NUMBER OF SUBJECTS. CLASSIFIED BY JERGER ET AL. (1974) PROCEDURE AS NORMAL, MILD-MODERATE, OR SEVERE FOR EACH SUBJECT GROUP

		\multicolumn{6}{c}{Prediction}

Group	N	Normal N	Normal %	Mild-Moderate N	Mild-Moderate %	Severe N	Severe %
1	17	10	59	7	41	0	0
2	12	0	0	9	75	3	25
3	8	0	0	1	13	11*	87
4	2	0	0	1	50	1	50
5	12	0	0	3	25	9	75
6	13	0	0	7	54	6	46
7	9	0	0	5	56	4	44
8	4	0	0	1	25	3	75

*The correct number is 7.

SOURCE: Margolis, R. H., & Fox, C. M. (1977). A comparison of three methods for predicting hearing loss from acoustic reflex thresholds. *Journal of Speech and Hearing Research, 20*, 241–253.

Excerpt 8.4 illustrates the use of a frequency histogram to show the distribution of data for a dependent variable at the ordinal level of measurement. The example is from a study of quality judgments of speech transduced through hearing aids. The histogram shows the frequency of listeners response rankings from best to worst (1 to 5 on the abscissa) of each of five different hearing aids (labelled A through E). The height of each bar represents the number of times each hearing aid was ranked at each position from best to worst by the listeners. Inspection of Figure 2 in Excerpt 8.4 reveals that hearing aid E was most often ranked as the best aid and hearing aid D was most frequently ranked as the worst aid. Hearing aids C, B, and D received more frequent rankings in the intermediate stages between best and worst.

Although histograms probably are used more often for graphical presentation of frequency distributions, frequency polygons are sometimes used to present a frequency distribution as a line graph. Excerpt 8.5 illustrates the

EXCERPT 8.4

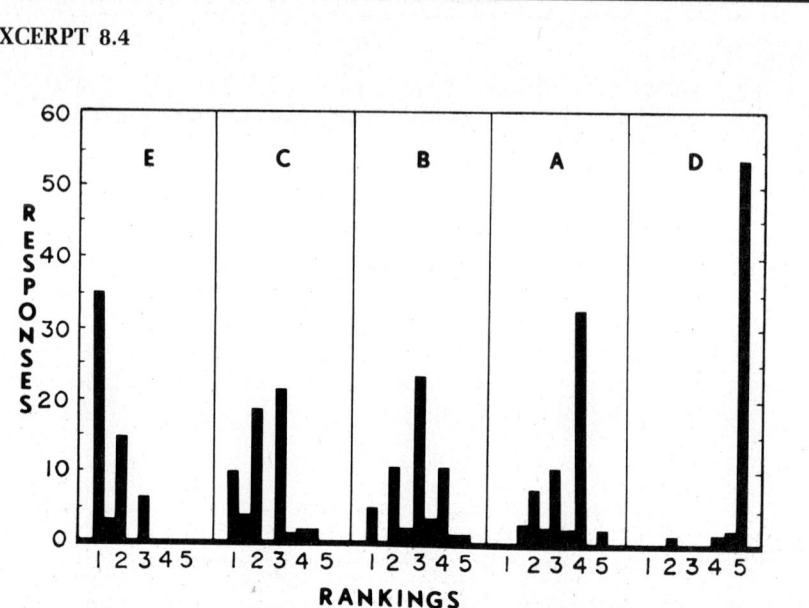

Figure 2. Histograms representing frequency distributions of listener's response rankings of the aids, A through E. Each bar on the graph shows the number of times an aid was ranked in a given position, based upon the ratings across all listeners. Thirty subjects judged the aids on two different listening sessions, making 60 the total number of possible responses per aid. This figure is the responses for the female voice.

SOURCE: Witter, H. L., & Goldstein, D. P. (1971). Quality judgments of hearing aid transduced speech. *Journal of Speech and Hearing Research, 14,* 312–322.

use of a frequency polygon in a study of audiometric evaluation of adult aphasics. Aphasic subjects who responded adequately to audiometric testing were compared with aphasics who responded inadequately by plotting the frequency of subjects in each group at each score (from low on the left to high on the right) on the Understanding score of the Functional Communication Profile. Inadequate responders can be seen to cluster on the lower end of this profile score in the frequency polygon, whereas adequate responders show a wider distribution of scores, many of which are higher than those of the inadequate responders.

The frequency histograms shown in Excerpts 8.2 and 8.4, the frequency polygon shown in Excerpt 8.5, and the frequency tables shown in Excerpts 8.1 and 8.3 all show the absolute frequencies at each score, ranking, or

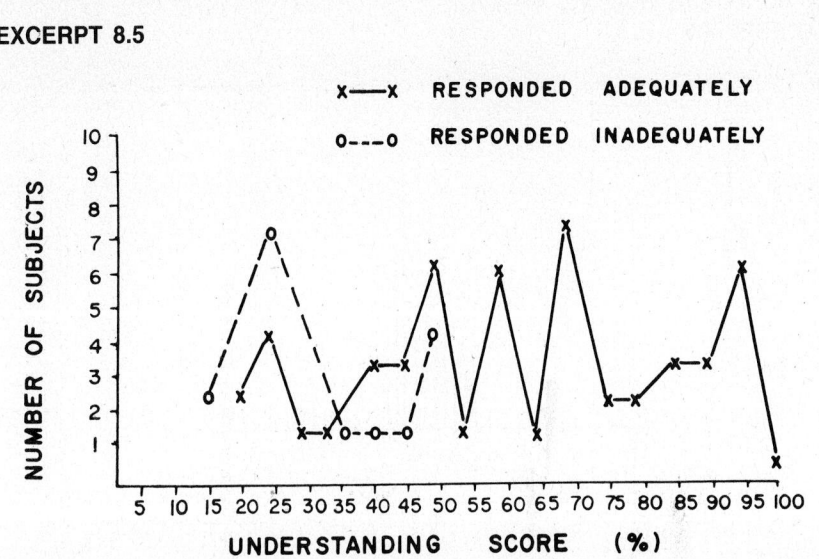

EXCERPT 8.5

x——x   RESPONDED   ADEQUATELY

o---o   RESPONDED   INADEQUATELY

NUMBER OF SUBJECTS

UNDERSTANDING   SCORE   (%)

Figure 1. Distribution of Functional Communication Profile Understanding scores for two groups of subjects. One group responded adequately to audiometric testing, the other did not.

SOURCE: Ludlow, C. L., & Swisher, L. P. (1971). The audiometric evaluation of adult aphasics. *Journal of Speech and Hearing Research, 14,* 535–543.

category. In addition, the table in Excerpt 8.3 shows the percentage of cases represented by each absolute frequency and the table in Excerpt 8.1 shows the cumulative relative frequency. Readers may also expect to encounter frequency distributions that present all data as relative frequencies, expressed as a percentage or proportion of total cases in the distribution. Excerpt 8.6 shows the use of a relative frequency histogram to display voice onset time (VOT) data for the voiced plosive /b/ for three groups of subjects of different ages. The ordinates for the three histograms are labelled as Relative Frequency (%) and the abscissa of each histogram indicates VOT in milliseconds from −5 on the left to +30 on the right. The height of each bar in the histogram, then, does not represent the number of subjects at each VOT value but rather the percentage of subjects in each group at each VOT value. These relative frequency distributions give a very clear picture of the distribution (central tendency and variability) of the data, but readers should be careful to note whether they are reading absolute number of subjects or relative number of subjects (e.g., percentage) at each score value.

EXCERPT 8.6

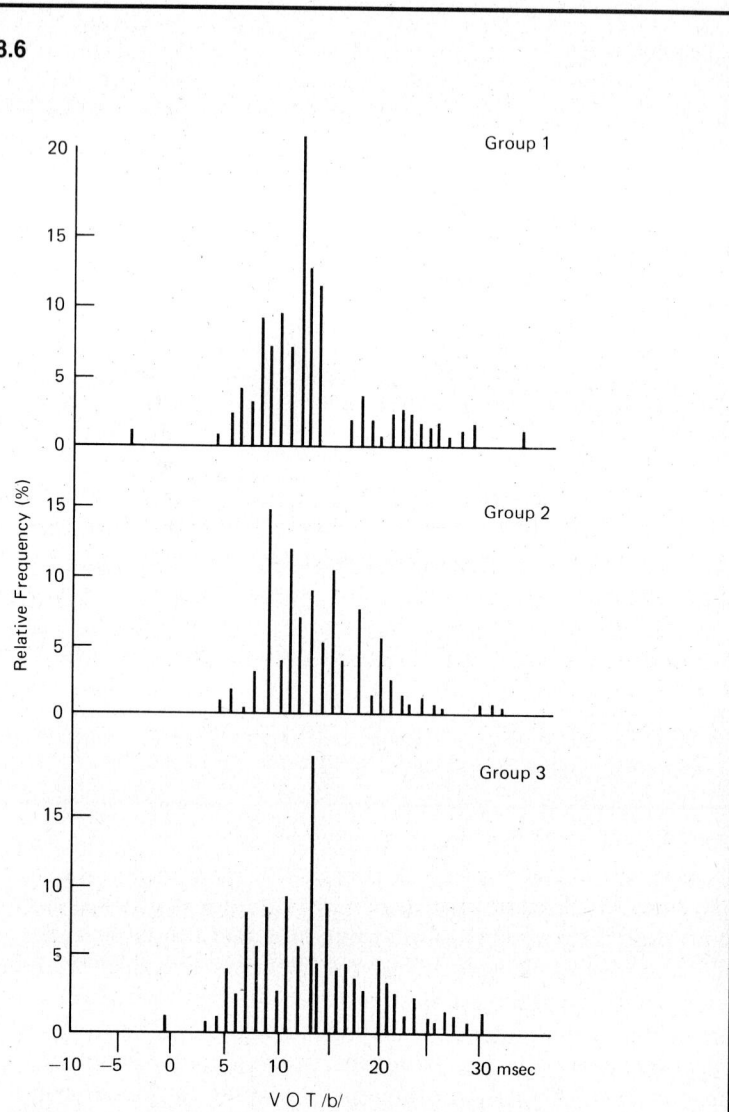

Figure 1. Relative frequency distribution for all productions of /b/ for three experimental groups. Group
1, aged 25 through 39; Group 2, aged 65 through 74;
Group 3, over 75.

SOURCE: Sweeting, P. M., & Baken, R. J. (1982). Voice onset time in a normal-aged population. *Journal of Speech and Hearing Research, 25,* 129–134.

As seen in the foregoing examples, frequency distributions can be a valuable addition to the Results section, in that they provide a description of the overall distribution of the data. We noted in Chapter 5 that the selection of a format for organizing the data may depend partly on the author's style and partly on the requirements of the data. Nevertheless, the format chosen should: (1) present the data accurately, (2) be clearly labelled for easy reading and interpretation, and (3) relate well to the textual description of the data.

One other point should also be mentioned: the problem of accounting for missing data. Occasionally some data may be lost or not available for analysis, perhaps owing to equipment failure or failure of some subjects to complete all tasks (i.e., mortality). Authors should make a point of explaining to readers what happened in the particular study to account for any missing data. They should also comment on the implications (if any) of missing data for the validity of the study. Whenever the number of data entries in tables or figures varies from the number stated in the text or varies from condition to condition, the author should explain the reason for the discrepancy in the text or, perhaps, in a footnote. Some authors may offer an explanation of missing data or fluctuations in number of scores in the Method section, whereas other authors may wait and explain discrepancies as they arise in the Results section. Again, this is usually a matter of individual style, but all authors have a responsibility to their readers to explain number discrepancies or missing data somewhere in the article.

Summary Statistics: Central Tendency and Variability

A second way of organizing data in addition to, or instead of, the use of frequency distributions, is the use of summary statistics. Summary statistics are parsimonious because they describe the overall distribution of a body of data in a simple numerical form that uses less space than does the presentation of the entire frequency distribution. Also, the summary statistics help to provide the foundation on which most analysis techniques are based, and, therefore, the selection of appropriate summary statistics is critical to appropriate analysis of the data. Most articles encountered in the speech pathology and audiology literature present data that are organized through the use of summary statistics.

Summary statistics are used to describe the central tendency and variability of a distribution of data with a few numbers. The central tendency statistics describe what is "typical" or "average" in a distribution and the variability statistics describe how the data spread out from the "typical" or "average" case in the distribution. In many articles, different conditions or groups of subjects are compared so that summary statistics are used to organize the data for each condition or subject group. Later, analysis of relationships or differences will refer to the summary statistics of each condition or group for the purpose of making comparisons.

Various summary statistics are available for describing distributions, and the selection of appropriate statistics depends on such factors as the level of measurement of the data, the number of observations, and normality or skewness of the distribution. Normal or nearly normal distributions of a fairly large number of interval or ratio measurements are usually summarized by reporting the mean and standard deviations of the measurements. Lack of one or more of these data characteristics (i.e., small N, skewed distribution, or nominal or ordinal level of measurement) usually means that data should be summarized with the median or the mode as a measure of central tendency and some form of the range (e.g., total range or interquartile range) as a measure of variability.

In some instances, summary statistics may be included only in the textual narrative, especially if only a few numbers are presented. Excerpt 8.7 is an example from an article on sentence familiarity and lipreading that includes a small number of summary statistics. The authors apparently felt that the data were simple enough to include in textual presentation and that the use of tabular or graphic presentation was not warranted in this situation. Readers should have little or no difficulty digesting the summary statistics included in the paragraph.

EXCERPT 8.7

RESULTS AND DISCUSSION

In analyzing the data obtained from the 102 hearing-impaired college students, familiarity values were computed for the 60 sentences. The sentence familiarity values covered nearly the total range offered the raters, 1.05 to 4.62, with a median of 2.67, a mean of 2.74, and a standard deviation of 0.88. These data indicate a relatively normal distribution of values. Although these data suggest a degree of construct (face) validity, it was decided that a follow-up study be conducted on a different class of students. One hundred thirty hearing-impaired college students enrolled in a freshman communication class served as raters. The testing procedure was identical to that used with the preparatory students. The familiarity values were computed for the 60 sentences. The sentence familiarity values ranged from 1.07 to 4.58 with a median of 2.91, a mean of 2.87, and a standard deviation of 0.82. These data for this freshman group are in general agreement with the preparatory group and indicate a normal distribution.

SOURCE: Lloyd, L. L., & Price, J. G. (1971). Sentence familiarity as a factor in visual speech perception (lipreading) of deaf college students. *Journal of Speech and Hearing Research, 14,* 291–294.

The more usual case, however, involves presentation of summary statistics in tabular or graphic form, or, sometimes, in both forms. Graphic presentation (i.e., histograms, polygons) of summary statistics has the advantage of providing an easily viewed overall summary of results for different conditions or groups of subjects. Differences between subject groups, changes in dependent variables as a function of changes in independent variables, or differences in performances on different measures can often be immediately impressed on the reader by a well-formulated graphic presentation of summary statistics. On the other hand, graphic figures may suffer from a disadvantage: the difficulty in locating exact values of the summary statistics for each condition or group, especially when the ordinate or the abscissa is labelled with gross intervals. Some figures are labelled only at every tenth- or fifth-score interval and interpolation of exact scores between such gross intervals may be difficult. Tabular presentation of summary statistics may be less dramatic or immediately impressive to the reader, but it does have the advantage of allowing easier retrieval of exact values of summary statistics for any group or condition.

The process of graphical and tabular presentation of summary statistics is illustrated in Excerpt 8.8, which includes both a table and a figure presenting the same summary statistics on the effects of noise on speech intelligibility.

Examination of the table and figure in Excerpt 8.8 reveals that the latter provides a more immediate overall picture of the general pattern of results. Normals show better performance than either group of hearing-impaired subjects and normals show only a small performance decrement from quiet listening to more difficult noise situations. Hearing-impaired subjects with flat audiograms perform better than do subjects with high-frequency hearing loss and they show less dramatic performance decrement as noise level increases in the background. These conclusions are easily drawn from a brief perusal of Figure 1 in Excerpt 8.8. On the other hand, readers may wish to examine more closely the exact values of means and standard deviations of the word recognition scores of the different subject groups in the different listening conditions in order to make specific within-subjects or between-subjects comparisons. Readers will find such information more readily available in the table that displays in digital form the means, standard deviations, and ranges of word recognition scores of the three subject groups in each of the three listening conditions. By making the data available in both tabular and graphic form, these authors have judiciously organized their data in a fashion that allows readers the opportunity to view the overall pattern of results and to inspect exact values for within-subjects and between-subjects comparisons.

Excerpt 8.9 includes a bar graph that was used to display summary statistics (means) in a study on vowel duration of normal and esophageal speakers. Duration is indicated on the ordinate and the four vowels studied are indicated on the abscissa. The bar heights indicate the mean duration of each

EXCERPT 8.8

TABLE 2. MEAN, STANDARD DEVIATION, AND RANGE OF SCORES OBTAINED IN EXPERIMENT 1

Group	Measure	Experimental Condition		
		Quiet	-4 S/N	-12 S/N
Normals	$\bar{X}$	99.2	94.8	92.4
	SD	2.5	3.0	4.4
	Range	92–100	90–100	82–96
High-frequency loss	$\bar{X}$	93.2	70.5	55.4
	SD	4.6	18.5	30.6
	Range	88–100	39–90	4–86
Flat loss	$\bar{X}$	94.6	85.4	80.5
	SD	6.4	6.9	12.3
	Range	80–100	74–96	54–94

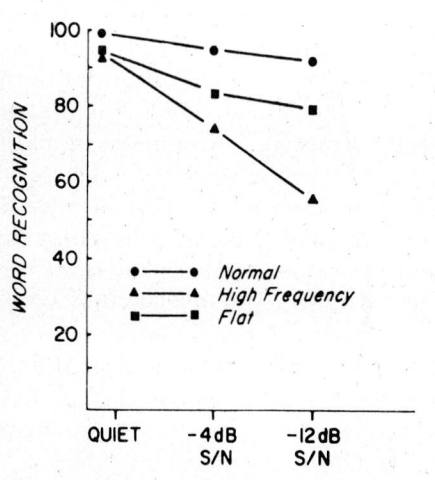

Figure 1. Test results of Experiment 1 in which word-recognition scores are plotted as a function of the three experimental test conditions.

SOURCE: Cohen, R. L., & Keith, R. W. (1976). Use of low-pass noise in word recognition testing. *Journal of Speech and Hearing Research, 19,* 48–54.

of the four vowels (averaged across several consonant environments) for the normal and esophageal speakers. This general presentation of results provides readers with a good overall comparison of normal and esophageal speakers. Christensen and Weinberg followed up this general presentation with specific comparisons of mean vowel durations in several consonant environments in additional tables and figures.

EXCERPT 8.9

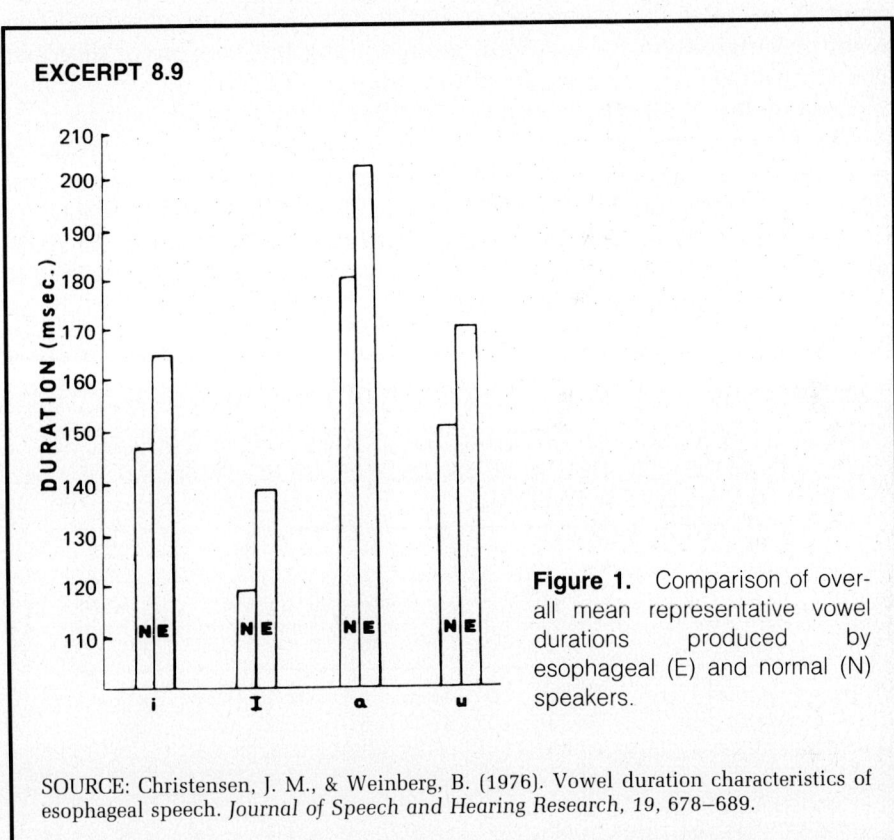

Figure 1. Comparison of overall mean representative vowel durations produced by esophageal (E) and normal (N) speakers.

SOURCE: Christensen, J. M., & Weinberg, B. (1976). Vowel duration characteristics of esophageal speech. *Journal of Speech and Hearing Research, 19,* 678–689.

Table 1 in Excerpt 8.10 illustrates a relatively large body of summary statistics that has been well organized in a compact table. Despite the relatively large number of entries in this table, readers will be able to appreciate the results quite easily once the organization of the table is understood. The 10 dependent variables are listed in the first column under the heading "Tests." Note that the table footnote gives the maximum value attainable on each test for reference. The independent variables are two subject classifications. First, the subjects were classified relative to their manual communication backgrounds as native ASL signers or as delayed sign language users. Then, within each of these two groups, subjects were further subdivided by sex as males or females. The mean (M) and standard deviation (SD) on each test is then tabulated for each of the sexes for each of the sign language groups. The first two columns of numbers give the means and standard deviations for the female native ASL subjects, the next two columns give the means and standard deviations for the male native ASL subjects, and so on. Despite the fact that there are 80 numbers (2 statistics × 2 sexes × 2 sign groups X 10 tests), the reader can easily locate any measure of central tendency or variability for any subject group on any test because of the clear tabular organization. Reading down the columns or across the rows allows easy intergroup comparison for any test. Once the tabular organization is grasped by the reader, it is a relatively simple matter to make the appropriate comparisons in reading the array of entries in the table. As mentioned earlier, even a large array of data can be made simple if the author takes the proper steps to organize the data with regard to the original problem statement.

EXCERPT 8.10

TABLE 1. MEAN SCORES OF FEMALES AND MALES IN THE TWO DEAF GROUPS ON TESTS OF COGNITIVE SKILLS, ENGLISH COMMUNICATION SKILLS, AND FIELD INDEPENDENCE

	ASL				Delayed Sign Language			
	Females		Males		Females		Males	
Tests[a]	M	SD	M	SD	M	SD	M	SD
Abstract reasoning	35.40	7.09	36.86	4.41	33.87	12.24	36.18	7.99
Spatial relations tests	36.40	9.91	47.25	8.01	33.75	13.77	38.65	11.71
Reading	7.96	1.41	7.90	1.97	8.62	1.37	7.79	.94
Writing	7.24	.83	6.94	1.18	7.04	1.14	6.97	.61
Speechreading with sound	21.40	10.71	12.75	9.62	36.25	14.16	33.65	28.15
Speech intelligibility	2.68	1.42	1.55	.65	2.80	.98	2.96	1.04
Speechreading without sound	28.00	17.22	20.87	10.75	47.25	14.77	31.29	17.07
Manual reception	84.40	16.33	81.50	11.35	92.00	4.00	78.12	13.08
Simultaneous reception	80.00	13.42	68.25	13.62	77.25	11.11	68.71	15.06
Group Embedded Figures Test	5.00	3.39	12.12	4.91	8.62	3.81	10.76	4.51

[a]The highest possible scores on the tests are as follows: abstract reasoning test = 50, spatial relations test = 60, reading test = 12, writing test = 10, Group Embedded Figures Test = 18, speech intelligibility = 5. All other tests = 100.

SOURCE: Parasnis, I. (1983). Effects of parental deafness and early exposure to manual communication on the cognitive skills, English language skill, and field independence of young deaf adults. *Journal of Speech and Hearing Research, 26,* 588–594.

Figure 1 in Excerpt 8.11 illustrates the use of a line graph to present *both* central tendency and variability data together in one graph. The independent variable on the abscissa is sensation level (in dB re: SRT) and the dependent variable shown on the ordinate is percentage correct score on the nonsense syllable test (NST) of speech sound discrimination. The authors investigated the ability of the NST to assess speech sound discrimination of three groups of listeners: English, Spanish, and bilingual native speakers. The three lines, E, S, and B, indicate the mean performance of each of the three subject-classification groups at each of the five sensation levels at which the test was presented. The vertical bars connected to each filled circle within each line indicate plus-and-minus one standard deviation above and below the mean for each subject group at each sensation level. Thus, the reader can compare the mean performance of each group at each sensation level and also determine if the groups differed in variability as

EXCERPT 8.11

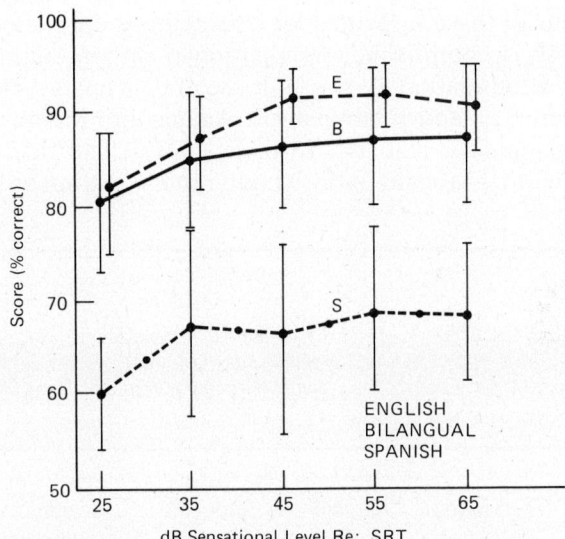

Figure 1. Phoneme-scored NST articulation functions plotted from the mean and standard deviation scores for the English (E), bilingual (B), and Spanish (S) groups.

SOURCE: Danhauer, J. L., Crawford, S., & Edgerton, B. J. (1984). English, Spanish, and bilingual speakers' performance on a nonsense syllable test (NST) of speech sound discrimination. *Journal of Speech and Hearing Disorders, 49,* 164–168.

well as central tendency. For example, it can be seen that the Spanish group means were lower than the means of the other two groups at all sensation levels and that the variability of the members of the Spanish group was generally greater than the variability of both of the other groups at all sensation levels except for the lowest one (i.e., 25 dB).

As mentioned earlier, not all articles will contain data that would be organized with means and standard deviations as the summary statistics. Often the summary statistics will be in the form of medians and ranges, perhaps because of small number of subjects, skewed distributions, or lack of interval or ratio-level measurements. Excerpt 8.12 presents Table 1 from the Results section of Adams and Moore's study on the effects of auditory masking on stuttering frequency, anxiety level, vocal intensity, and reading time of stutterers. Twelve stutterers served as subjects in the study, so the authors decided against the use of mean and standard deviation summary statistics and decided to employ the median and semi-interquartile range to show central tendency and the variability of the data. Inspection of the excerpt's Table 1 reveals that medians and semi-interquartile ranges are entered for each of the dependent variables listed across the top of the table and comparisons of these measures for a masking and a no-masking condition can be easily accomplished. As mentioned earlier, summary statistics help to provide a foundation for the later use of data analysis techniques for examining differences and relationships. Adams and Moore appropriately employed nonparametric statistics in their analysis and this particular example will be referred to again in this chapter in the section on data analysis.

EXCERPT 8.12

TABLE 1.   MEDIAN AND SEMI-INTERQUARTILE RANGE (Q) VALUES FOR SUBJECTS' FREQUENCY OF STUTTERING, VOCAL INTENSITY, READING TIME, AND PALMAR SWEAT ANXIETY IN THE MASKING AND NO-MASKING (CONTROL) CONDITIONS

Condition	Frequency of Stutter	Vocal Intensity (dB)	Reading Time (Secs)	Palmar Sweat Anxiety (Microamperes)	
Masking	4.0	83.50	91.08	5.0	*Median*
	7.5	4.50	91.13	5.0	*(Q)*
No-masking	19.0	74.50	85.83	4.5	*Median*
	17.5	3.50	132.83	5.5	*(Q)*

SOURCE: Adams, M. R., & Moore, W. H. (1972). The effects of auditory masking on the anxiety level, frequency of dysfluency, and selected vocal characteristics of stutterers. *Journal of Speech and Hearing Research, 15,* 572–578.

Some Characteristics of Good Data Organization

Results that are included in the text, table, and figures of an article should be organized in a manner that allows the reader to understand immediately the author's empirical statement regarding the problem posed in the introduction to the article. Readers should expect some of the following characteristics of good data organization when reading the Results section of an article.

First, table and figure captions should be brief but informative, and they should quickly convey the organization of the particular illustration. After reading the caption, the reader should know immediately where to find data entries for each subject group, experimental condition, or dependent variable that is included in the illustration. The caption should act as a clear road map to direct the reader through the illustration in the most efficient manner possible. Occasionally, a complex illustration may require a longer caption. There is nothing wrong with a lengthy caption per se as long as it is clearly written and the length is justifiable in helping the reader to understand the illustration. The Information for Authors section on the inside back cover of every issue of *JSHR* emphasizes the importance of captions by stating:

> Table titles and figure caption should be concise but explanatory. The reader should not have to refer to the text to decipher the information.

Readers should expect the table titles and figure captions that they read to be prepared according to this statement.

One further point should be made with regard to figure captions. There should be a key either in the caption or in the field of a figure that identifies the meaning of the symbols used in the figure. For example, Figure 1 in Excerpt 8.9 includes bars labeled N and E and the figure's caption indicates that N refers to normal speakers and E refers to esophageal speakers. In Excerpt 8.5, a key is set in the field of the graph that identifies solid lines as plotting the data for aphasics who responded adequately and dashed lines as plotting the data for the subjects who responded inadequately. Readers should expect to find such keys in either the caption or the field of a figure to provide ready understanding of the organization of the figure.

Second, each table or figure should be capable of standing alone as an illustration of the results. That is, the table should be sufficiently clear and complete so that the reader can spend some time studying it without having to refer constantly to the text to understand it. The text may summarize and analyze the results in the illustration, but the illustration should be well constructed so that it can act as an independent display of the results. If the reader has great difficulty understanding an illustration without constantly referring back to the text to make sense of the illustration, there is probably something wrong with its construction.

Third, a good illustration should dovetail quite nicely with the description of the data in the text. The textual narrative should contain references to the illustrations, usually in consecutive order of presentation. This narrative will often summarize overall patterns of results in the illustration and may mention specific values of data in the illustration. The text and illustrations should be parallel in the results presentation so that the reader does not have to jump back and forth in the Results section to understand the organization of the results in relation to the research problem. A good Results section contains a smoothly flowing narrative with tables and figures integrated into the text so that the flow of the narrative is not interrupted awkwardly by the references to illustrations.

A fourth point is that figures should be accurately proportioned so that the visual impression created for the reader actually reflects the data. Fortunately, the editorial boards of professional journals usually scrutinize figures to ensure accurate representation of results. Nonetheless, readers should be sure that values represented in tables or text are carefully presented in figures so that the overall effect is not a distortion of actual data values.

Finally, tables and figures should be as consistent and complete as possible. All available data or summary statistics should be displayed in similar manner for all groups or conditions to facilitate within-subjects and between-subjects comparisons. Consistency of tabular entries or graphic configurations are important for meaningful comparisons between such elements as experimental and control groups. Once a particular organization has been set up, readers should be able to follow it through different illustrations in an efficient manner. If it is necessary for an author to change the organization in presenting a large number of illustrations, the new organization should be clearly described so that readers are not confused by the change.

Many research articles present only descriptive statistics to organize the data with no further analysis included in the Results section. There may be a variety of reasons for an author's decision to exclude the analysis techniques. For example, the descriptive statistics employed to organize the data may show such striking differences or lack of differences that further data analysis might only belabor the obvious. Or the research questions might have been phrased in such a way that descriptive measures of central tendency and variability would suffice for answering them. In any case, consumers of research should be aware that they may encounter articles that present only a descriptive organization of the data and that this may be entirely appropriate in many cases.

Analysis of Data

Once the data of a study have been organized so that readers may peruse them to grasp the pattern of results in relation to the original research problem, certain statistical procedures may be employed to analyze the results. These statistical procedures may be generally classified as the analysis of relationships and the analysis of differences, although these two kinds of analysis may overlap somewhat, as pointed out in Chapter 5. This section will begin with examples of data analysis employing correlational statistics to examine relationships among variables and then proceed to examples of data analysis using inferential statistics (also called significance tests) to examine differences between subjects or conditions.

Correlational Analysis

Researchers often wish to examine (1) the strength and direction of relationships among two or more variables and (2) the manner in which performance on one variable may be predicted from performance on another variable. The first examination is accomplished through the calculation of correlation coefficients and the plotting of scattergrams (also called scatterplots), and the second examination is accomplished through the use of regression analysis. Correlation and regression are intimately related statistical procedures that are often completed together as one analysis package to examine relationships among variables. Some researchers, however, complete only one of the two analyses as they may be more interested in the strength and direction of the relationship than in predicting performance on one variable from another (or vice versa).

Correlation and regression analysis may be done in the relatively simple case of the relationship between two variables or it may be attempted for the more complicated case of the relationships among several variables. We will begin with examples of correlation and regression analysis of some simple bivariate examples to show how the results of such analysis could be presented in a journal article and then progress to some more complicated multivariate examples.

As mentioned in Chapter 5, the scattergram graphically depicts the relationship between two variables by showing the intersection point of the two measurements for each subject. If the two variables are positively correlated, subjects would tend to have high scores on both measures, medium scores on both measures, or low scores on both measures so that the pattern of dots on the scattergram slopes upward to the right of the graph. If the two variables are negatively related, subjects who score high on one variable tend to have low scores on the other variable so that the pattern of dots on the scattergram slopes downward to the right of the graph. Uncorrelated variables result in a scattergram that has dots spread around the graph in no particular order.

The strength of the relationship between the two variables can be roughly observed in the scattergram. A tight clustering of the dots around the center of an upward slopping pattern indicates a strong positive correlation, whereas a more diffuse pattern of dots spread around the center of an upward sloping pattern indicates a weaker positive correlation. By the same token, the clustering or dispersion of the dots around the center of a downward sloping pattern indicates the strength or weakness of a negative correlation.

Excerpt 8.13 includes a scattergram that depicts the relationship between onset of lingual movement (indicated on the abscissa) and onset of velar movement (indicated on the ordinate) for subjects saying the words "three" and "answer" embedded in different sentence contexts. Open circles indicate data for utterances spoken with unmarked boundaries between "three" and "answer" and filled circles indicate data for utterances spoken with marked boundaries between the two words. McClean found that the correlation coefficient for these two variables was $r = .94$ and concluded that the

EXCERPT 8.13

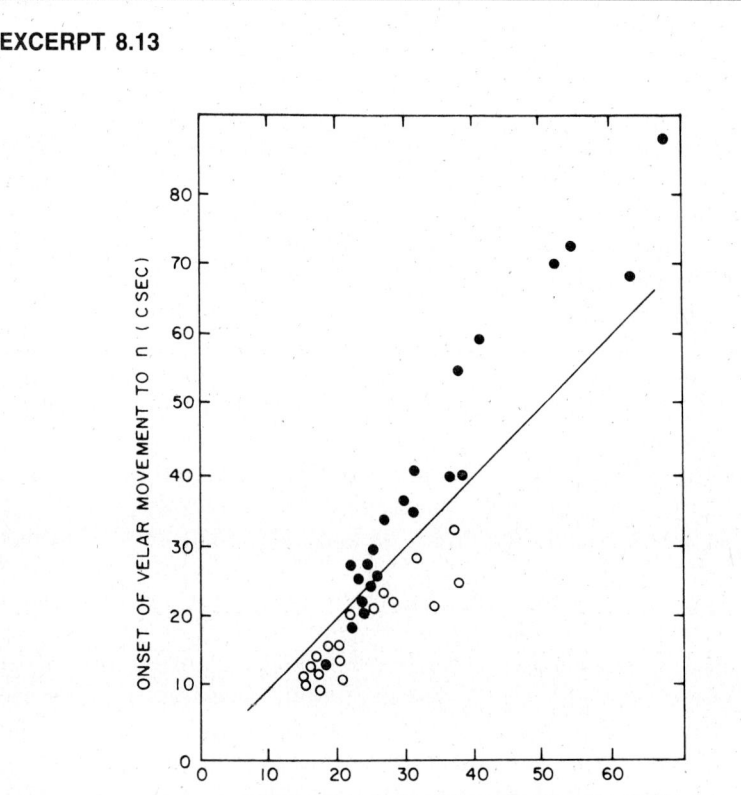

Figure 5. A plot of the temporal onset of velar movement to /n/ as a function of the temporal onset of lingual movement to æ. Time zero on the axes represents the last frame on which the tongue tip made contact with the central incisors for the consonant /θ/ in the word *three*. The open circles represent the unmarked boundary cases (Utterances 1–3) and the filled circles, the marked boundary cases (Utterances 4–7). The diagonal running through the plot represents the situation where onset of velar movement precisely coincides with the onset of lingual movement.

SOURCE: McClean, M. (1973). Forward coarticulation of velar movement at marked junctural boundaries. *Journal of Speech and Hearing Research, 16,* 286–296.

two variables were "very closely related." The tightness of the clustering of the dots around the center of the pattern as well as the upward slope to the right confirms the strong positive correlation between the two variables.

Tweney and Hoemann's study contains a scattergram showing the relationship between age (in months) and paradigmatic responses of deaf children to word association tasks (Excerpt 8.14). The correlation coefficient reported by the authors is + .40 which was found to be significant at p < 0.01. Although this correlation is moderately positive and significantly different from zero, it is obviously much lower than the correlation reported for the data shown in Excerpt 8.13. Comparison of the scattergrams in the two excerpts reveals a much tighter clustering of the data points in the former and a greater dispersion of the data points in the latter. Both scattergrams contain dot patterns that slope upward to the right, indicating positive correlations in both cases. The comparison of these two scattergrams indicates quite well the manner in which the correlation coefficient and the scattergram go hand-in-hand to convey to the reader a summary of the strength and direction of the relationship between two variables.

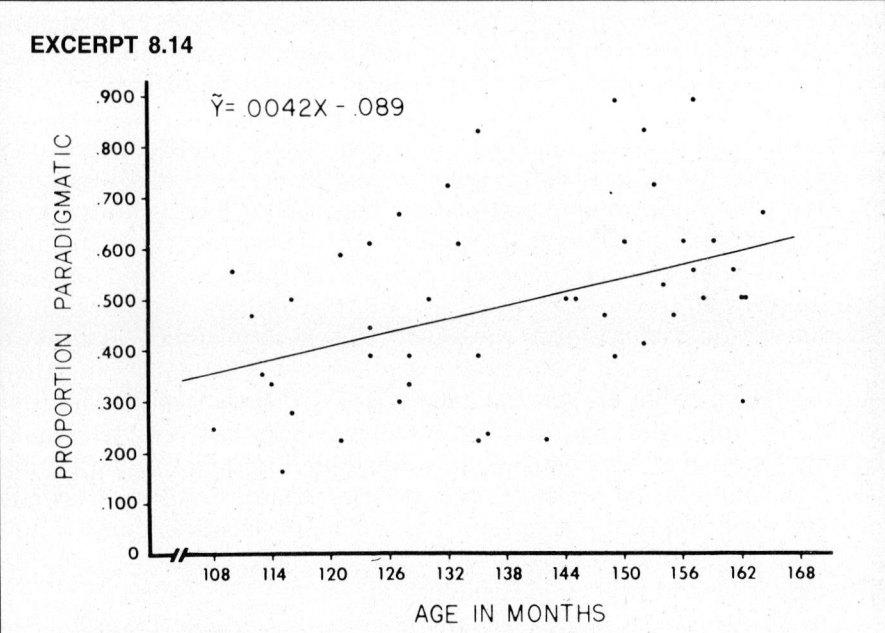

EXCERPT 8.14

$$\tilde{Y} = .0042X - .089$$

Figure 1. Proportion of paradigmatic responses as a function of age for 46 deaf children.

SOURCE: Tweney, R. D., & Hoemann, H. W. (1973). The development of semantic associations in profoundly deaf children. *Journal of Speech and Hearing Research, 16,* 309–318.

The reader should also notice that Figure 1 in Excerpt 8.14 contains the regression formula for predicting proportion of paradigmatic responses (Y in the formula) from age (X in the formula). The line through the dots is the best fit regression line drawn according to the predicted values of Y for each X-value according to the equation. The authors emphasized in the text of the article that this particular graphic method of displaying the data was selected because they wished to convey the fact that there was much variability in the relationship between these two variables. The spread of the dots around the regression line in the center of the dot pattern and the moderate value of the correlation coefficient are consistent in conveying the impression of the variability in the relationship.

Many studies involve an examination of the relationships among several variables and correlation coefficients must then be calculated for all possible combinations of two variables. In such a case, presentations of all possible scattergrams would be cumbersome and would use too much journal space, so a tabular matrix is presented that shows all of the correlation coefficients calculated. Usually, the variables are listed down the vertical axis of the table and across the horizontal axis of the table. The correlation coefficient for each pair of variables is then entered into the cell of the table that represents the intersection of the two variables. Excerpt 8.15 shows two such correlation matrices taken from a study on the equivalence of different lists of CID sentences (an original set of 10 sentence lists and a revised set of 10 sentence lists) used for measuring speech intelligibility. Table 1 in Excerpt 8.15 illustrates the correlation coefficients between the intelligibility scores on each pair of the 10 original CID sentence lists (lists A through J) and Table 2 in Excerpt 8.15 illustrates the correlations between the intelligibility scores on each pair of the 10 revised CID sentence lists. The authors noted that the correlations were generally low and that few of them reached statistical significance.

If, indeed, the lists had been equivalent, higher correlations would have been found between the intelligibility scores of each combination of two sentence lists for both the original and revised CID sentences. These lower correlations indicate, then, that most sentence lists did not yield intelligibility scores that were equivalent to intelligibility scores of most other lists. If the authors had wished to present scattergrams to further illustrate the interrelationships of the various lists, a total of 90 scattergrams would have been needed: 45 scattergrams for the original 10 CID lists; and 45 scattergrams for the 10 revised CID lists!

The intercorrelation matrix taken from Weiner's article (Excerpt 8.16) presents a similar type of analysis of data on intelligence test performance of children with delayed language development. Seven intelligence test scores were intercorrelated in this study: three different administrations of the Arthur Adaptation of the Leiter International Performance Scale (AALIPS); three different administrations of the Peabody Picture Vocabulary Test (PPVT); and the verbal, performance, and total IQ scores of the Wechsler

EXCERPT 8.15

TABLE 1. PEARSON PRODUCT-MOMENT CORRELATIONS BETWEEN CID SENTENCE LISTS

	A	B	C	D	E	F	G	H	I	J
A	—	0.21	0.51*	0.08	0.39	0.65*	0.12	0.43	0.53*	0.38
B	—	—	0.24	0.31	−0.01	0.26	0.45	−0.05	0.10	0.16
C	—	—	—	0.41	0.19	0.44	0.41	0.30	0.41	0.65*
D	—	—	—	—	−0.29	0.29	0.37	0.04	0.06	0.32
E	—	—	—	—	—	0.19	0.29	0.37	0.36	0.15
F	—	—	—	—	—	—	0.27	0.42	0.39	0.33
G	—	—	—	—	—	—	—	0.18	−0.07	0.81
H	—	—	—	—	—	—	—	—	0.46	0.30
I	—	—	—	—	—	—	—	—	—	0.19
J	—	—	—	—	—	—	—	—	—	—

*Significant at the 0.01 level or better.

TABLE 2. PEARSON PRODUCT-MOMENT CORRELATIONS BETWEEN REVISED CID SENTENCE LISTS

	A	B	C	D	E	F	G	H	I	J
A	—	0.09	0.44	0.05	0.64*	0.50	0.04	0.31	0.63*	0.05
B	—	—	0.20	0.45	0.36	0.43	0.42	0.48*	0.13	0.27
C	—	—	—	0.30	0.56*	0.34	0.21	0.11	0.30	0.19
D	—	—	—	—	0.09	0.58*	0.69*	0.30	−0.02	0.41
E	—	—	—	—	—	0.32	0.26	0.22	0.47*	0.14
F	—	—	—	—	—	—	0.54*	0.45	0.37	0.20
G	—	—	—	—	—	—	—	0.44	0.10	0.33
H	—	—	—	—	—	—	—	—	0.37	0.34
I	—	—	—	—	—	—	—	—	—	0.01
J	—	—	—	—	—	—	—	—	—	—

*Significant at the 0.01 level or better.

SOURCE: Giolas, T. G., & Duffy, J. R. (1973). Equivalency of CID and revised CID sentences lists. *Journal of Speech and Hearing Research, 16,* 549–555.

Intelligence Scale for Children (WISC). Each test is listed by abbreviation on the left side of the matrix and indicated by a number along the top of the matrix (e.g., AALIPS first administration = 1; WISC Total IQ = 7). The correlation coefficient for each possible pair of intelligence tests is entered in the table cell representing the intersection of the two tests. Note that the correlation coefficients in all of the diagonal cells are entered as 1.00 because the correlations in those cells are the correlations of each test with itself. This tabular entry option for organizing the correlations was not used in the matrices shown in the previous excerpt, and its use is usually a matter of the individual style of the author; some authors prefer to leave these cells blank, whereas others enter the value of 1.00 in each diagonal cell. Note also the empty cells in the top of the Table 2 in Excerpt 8.16 and in the bottom of Tables 1 and 2 in Excerpt 8.15. These empty cells would contain the same correlation coefficients that are in the filled cells in the other half of the table because there are two possible cells in a matrix for each combination of two variables. The other half of the matrix is usually left blank to make the table easier to read, although some authors believe that the redundant correlations should be entered throughout the table for a more complete presentation of the correlations. Because this is also a matter of individual style, readers may expect to find tables containing an intercorrelation matrix to be constructed in different manners by different authors.

Inspection of the matrix in Excerpt 8.16 reveals that eight of the correlations were not significantly different from zero, and the author simply entered "n.s." in each cell in which the correlation between the two variables was not significant. Thirteen of the correlations were significantly different from zero and their values are entered in the appropriate cell for each pair of variables. Asterisks refer to the footnote at the bottom of the table, which indicates whether the correlations were significant at the 0.05 or 0.01 level. Obviously, the higher correlations are significant at the 0.01 level and the more moderate correlations are significant at the 0.05 level. Note also that all of the correlations are positive.

The interpretation of these correlations is of particular interest because Weiner was concerned with the reliability and validity of the AALIPS and PPVT. Reliability was assessed by comparing the subjects' performances on the three test administrations of both the AALIPS and the PPVT (only the first and third administrations are shown in the table; the correlations between the first and second administrations are presented in the text). Criterion validity was assessed by comparing subjects' performances on the AALIPS and PPVT with their performances on the WISC. In other words, the WISC acted as an outside validating criterion against which the AALIPS and PPVT were compared. Comparison of the first administration of the AALIPS and PPVT with the WISC scores provided information about their predictive validity. The comparison of the later AALIPS and PPVT administration with the WISC provided information about the concurrent validity of the AALIPS and PPVT. Readers of the remainder of this article will find a well-organized discussion of the reliability and validity of these tests. The article not only illustrates the concepts of reliability and validity but also provides a good example of how the statistical analysis of the test data may demonstrate the degree of reliability and validity of the tests.

EXCERPT 8.16

TABLE 2. PRODUCT-MOMENT COEFFICIENTS OF CORRELATION AMONG RESULTS ON THREE INTELLIGENCE TESTS OF CHILDREN WITH DELAYED LANGUAGE DEVELOPMENT

Variable		1	2	3	4	5	6	7
AALIPS I†	(N = 22)	1.00	—	—	—	—	—	—
AALIPS III‡	(N = 22)	0.63**	1.00	—	—	—	—	—
PPVT I†	(N = 21)	n.s.	n.s.	1.00	—	—	—	—
PPVT III‡	(N = 21)	n.s.	n.s.	0.66**	1.00	—	—	—
WISC Verbal IQ	(N = 21)	0.50*	0.75**	n.s.	0.59**	1.00	—	—
WISC Perf. IQ	(N = 22)	0.51*	0.83**	n.s.	n.s.	0.67**	1.00	—
WISC Total IQ	(N = 21)	0.55*	0.86**	n.s.	0.48*	0.92**	0.91**	1.00

*$p < 0.05$
**$p < 0.01$
†First administration
‡Third administration

SOURCE: Weiner, P. S. (1971). Stability and validity of two measures of intelligence used with children whose language development is delayed. *Journal of Speech and Hearing Research, 14,* 254–261.

Excerpt 8.17 contains a table and three scattergrams that illustrate the use of the Spearman correlation with rank-order data in a study of vocal characteristics and male-female quality of the voice. Rank-order data were used in the analysis of the relationships among three variables: rating of male–female voice quality, fundamental frequency of the voice, and vocal tract resonance. Spearman rank-order correlations (rhos) are entered in the table for each of the three pairings of the variables: male–female voice quality with fundamental frequency, male–female voice quality with vocal tract resonance, and fundamental frequency with vocal tract resonance. These three relationships are indicated under the table heading "Comparison." The three columns of Spearman rhos include the correlations calculated for male speakers only, female speakers only, and male and female speakers combined. These same relationships are also depicted in the corresponding scattergrams. Male data are indicated by filled circles and female data are indicated by the open circles. The correlations for male and female data combined correspond to the entire scattergram for each variable pair.

The correlations of male–female voice quality with fundamental frequency are the highest ones and the scattergram in Figure 2 depicts these correlations and shows the tightest clustering of the pattern of dots. In fact, the dot pattern clusters more tightly for the females than for the males, and the correlation for the female speakers only is higher than the correlation for male speakers only. The correlation for male and female data combined is highest of all because this correlation is based on a larger number of observations with a greater range of scores on both variables. The correlations of male–female voice quality with vocal tract resonance and of vocal tract resonance with fundamental frequency are much lower, and a more widely dispersed pattern of dots can be seen in Figures 3 and 4 in Excerpt 8.17 that are the corresponding scattergrams for these correlations. Significance of all the correlations is indicated by the asterisks in Table 1 that identify those correlations that were significantly different from zero at the .01 level. Readers should find it a relatively simple matter to compare the correlations and scattergrams for each pair of variables for each subject group because of the effective manner in which the correlational analysis has been displayed.

The Pearson correlations shown earlier were computed from interval- or ratio-level data and the Spearman correlations (Excerpt 8.17) were computed from ordinal-level data. It was mentioned in Chapter 5 that correlational analysis may be performed with nominal-level data through the use of the χ^2 statistic to evaluate the significance of the association between nominal level variables. Excerpt 8.18 illustrates this use of χ^2. In this example, Conture, McCall, and Brewer investigated the association between the occurrence of various laryngeal behaviors (adduction, abduction, and a combination of the two) and three different types of stuttering (part-word repetition, sound prolongation, and broken words). Table 1 in Excerpt 8.17 shows the frequency and percent of occurrence of each laryngeal behavior during the occurrence of each of the three types of stuttering. In the text, the authors reported a χ^2 value of 22.4 that was calculated from the frequencies of these nominal data and indicated that a significant ($p < .001$) association between type of stuttering and laryngeal behavior was evident. The authors used the remainder of the Results section to analyze the specific laryngeal behaviors observed for each type of stuttering.

EXCERPT 8.17

TABLE 1. SPEARMAN RANK-ORDER CORRELATION COEFFICIENTS (RHOs) BETWEEN DEGREE OF MALE-FEMALE VOICE QUALITY (M-F VOICE QUALITY), FUNDAMENTAL FREQUENCY (F_0), AND VOCAL TRACT RESONANCES (VTR)

	Rhos		
Comparison	Males and Females	Males Only	Females Only
M-F voice quality with F_0	0.94*	0.65*	0.88*
M-F voice quality with VTR	0.59*	0.00	0.27
VTR with F_0	0.56*	0.14	0.17

*$p < 0.01$.

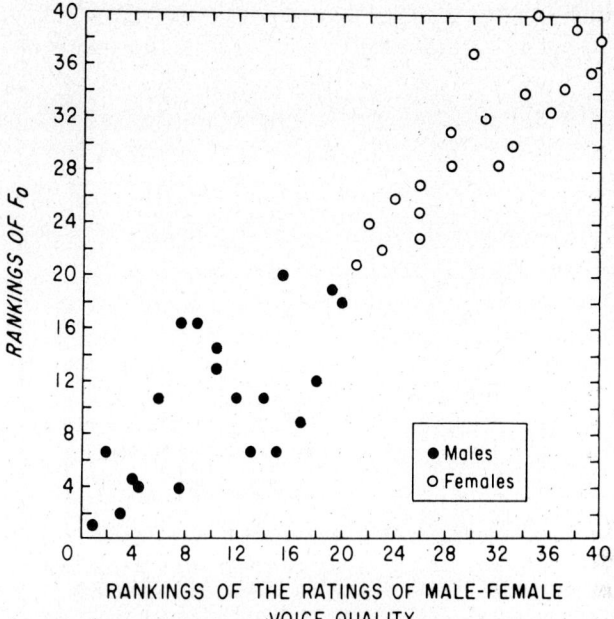

Figure 2. Rankings of listener ratings of degree of male–female voice quality compared with rankings of fundamental frequency.

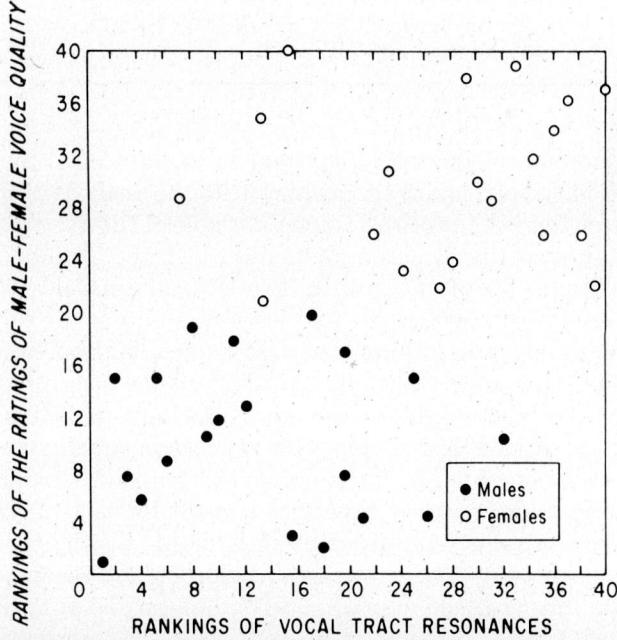

Figure 3. Rankings of individual vocal tract resonances compared with rankings of listener ratings of degree of male–female voice quality.

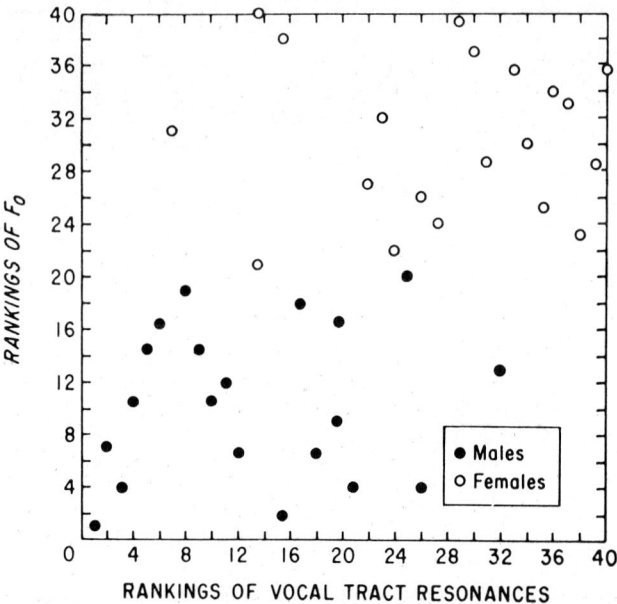

Figure 4. Rankings of individual vocal tract resonances compared with rankings of fundamental frequency.

SOURCE: Coleman, R. O. (1976). A comparison of the contributions of two voice quality characteristics to the perception of maleness and femaleness in the voice. *Journal of Speech and Hearing Research, 19,* 168–180.

With the exception of the data displayed in Excerpt 8.14, the examples shown thus far have been mainly concerned with the analysis of the strength and direction of the relationships among variables. The prediction of one variable from another that is accomplished through the development of regression equations is also important in correlational analysis. Excerpt 8.19 displays a table taken from Carhart and Porter's study of the relationships among thresholds at various pure-tone frequencies and speech reception threshold (SRT). This table shows the correlations between predicted SRT and actual SRT (i.e., the multiple correlations) for each combination of predictor variables. The table also displays the regression equations for predicting SRT from each combination of pure-tone thresholds. A separate listing of these correlations and regression equations is made for each of six groups of hearing-impaired subjects with different audiometric configurations. Three sets of equations are included: zero-order, first-order, and second-order. The zero-order equations are used to predict SRT from the one pure-tone threshold that is most highly correlated with SRT. The first-order equations are

EXCERPT 8.18

RESULTS

Table 1 shows the laryngeal behavior associated with each of the three types of stuttering. The association between the type of stuttering and laryngeal behavior was statistically significant ($X^2 = 22.4$; df = 4; $p < 0.001$). The nature of this association is considered from each of the three types of stuttering.

TABLE 1. JUDGMENTS OF SEPARATION OF THE POSTERIOR ASPECTS OF THE VOCAL FOLDS ASSOCIATED WITH EACH OF THREE TYPES OF STUTTERING*

| | Type of Stuttering | | | | | |
| | Part-Word Repetition (N = 55) | | Sound Prolongation (N = 39) | | Broken Word (N = 7) | |
Laryngeal Behavior	Number	%	Number	%	Number	%
Abduction	33	60	11	28	7	100
Adduction	15	27	28	72	0	0
Combination	7	3	0	0	0	0

*Number and percentage of the total instances of stuttering associated with a particular category of laryngeal behavior is given for each of the three types of stuttering. Nine of the ten subjects produced the 55 part-word repetitions, eight of the ten subjects produced the 39 sound prolongations, and three of the ten subjects produced the seven broken words.

SOURCE: Conture, E. G., McCall, G. N., & Brewer, D. W. (1977). Laryngeal behavior during stuttering. *Journal of Speech and Hearing Research, 20*, 661–668.

used to predict SRT from the two pure-tone thresholds that are most highly correlated with SRT and the second-order equations are used to predict SRT from the three pure-tone thresholds that are most highly correlated with SRT. The prediction may become more accurate as more predictor variables are added to the regression equation, so several orders of equations are often run through in this fashion to find the most accurate prediction equation. Once the most accurate equation is found, it can be used to predict SRT from the pure-tone data of new patients who fall into the various categories of

EXCERPT 8.19

TABLE 7. COEFFICIENTS OF CORRELATION AND REGRESSION EQUATIONS FOR PREDICTION OF SPEECH RECEPTION THRESHOLD (SRT) FROM PURE-TONE THRESHOLDS (T's) FOR SIX GROUPS CLASSIFIED ACCORDING TO AUDIOMETRIC PATTERN*

Classification	Coefficient	SRT = Regression Equation
Zero-order	*r*	
Flat	0.975	$0.4 \text{ dB} + 0.94 \, T_{1000}$
Gradual	0.931	$3.4 \text{ dB} + 0.84 \, T_{1000}$
Marked	0.873	$12.0 \text{ dB} + 0.87 \, T_{500}$
Rising	0.929	$0.0 \text{ dB} + 0.92 \, T_{1000}$
Trough	0.951	$-10.6 \text{ dB} + 1.03 \, T_{1000}$
Atypical	0.882	$4.8 \text{ dB} + 0.76 \, T_{1000}$
First-order	*R*	
Flat	0.978	$-0.3 \text{ dB} + 0.77 \, T_{1000} + 0.19 \, T_{2000}$
Gradual	0.952	$2.6 \text{ dB} + 0.39 \, T_{500} + 0.53 \, T_{1000}$
Marked	0.891	$7.3 \text{ dB} + 0.63 \, T_{500} + 0.26 \, T_{1000}$
Rising	0.955	$1.6 \text{ dB} + 0.60 \, T_{1000} + 0.43 \, T_{4000}$
Trough	0.962	$-12.5 \text{ dB} + 0.68 \, T_{1000} + 0.41 \, T_{2000}$
Atypical	0.927	$2.0 \text{ dB} + 0.37 \, T_{500} + 0.51 \, T_{1000}$
Second-order	*R*	
Flat	0.979	$-1.1 \text{ dB} + 0.18 \, T_{500} + 0.62 \, T_{1000} + 0.18 \, T_{2000}$
Gradual	0.956	$-0.1 \text{ dB} + 0.38 \, T_{500} + 0.41 \, T_{1000} + 0.16 \, T_{2000}$
Marked	0.894	$3.0 \text{ dB} + 0.62 \, T_{500} + 0.21 \, T_{1000} + 0.11 \, T_{2000}$
Rising	0.958	$1.7 \text{ dB} + 0.48 \, T_{1000} + 0.21 \, T_{2000} + 0.38 \, T_{4000}$
Trough	0.966	$-10.9 \text{ dB} + 0.21 \, T_{500} + 0.44 \, T_{1000} + 0.45 \, T_{2000}$
Atypical	0.937	$-0.5 \text{ dB} + 0.40 \, T_{500} + 0.41 \, T_{1000} + 0.11 \, T_{2000}$

*The threshold for each frequency is designated by the appropriate subscript (for example T_{1000}= threshold for 1000 Hz). The right-hand section of each equation consists of a correction constant (first term) followed by one or more terms consisting of a beta coefficient multiplied by a threshold value.

SOURCE: Carhart, R., & Porter, L. S. (1971). Audiometric configuration and prediction of threshold for spondees. *Journal of Speech and Hearing Research, 14,* 486–495.

audiometric configuration. In the text of this article, the authors have suggested the best equations for making these predictions with patients having different types of audiometric configurations when various pure-tone data are available.

The focus in this last example is more on prediction of one variable from the others than on the analysis of strength and direction of the relationship among the variables. Both of these concepts are important and intimately related aspects of correlational analysis, but different authors may emphasize one of them over the other, depending on the purposes of a particular study. Traditionally, the analysis of the strength and direction of the relationship through presentation of correlation coefficients and scattergrams has been more prevalent in the research literature, but there has been more interest developing in the regression aspect of correlational analysis in recent years.

Analysis of Differences

Now that we have illustrated some of the typical formats in which correlational analysis may be presented in the Results section of a research article, we will present some examples of the use of inferential statistics to examine differences between subjects or to examine within-subjects differences between conditions. We will begin with cases of simple two-sample comparisons and progress to cases with more complicated comparisons of several samples.

The format for the presentation of inferential statistics to test the significance of differences may vary somewhat from article to article. Some authors prefer to include inferential statistics in a table that combines frequency distributions and summary statistics. The table may include values of central tendency and variability for the different groups or conditions that were compared and the values of the inferential statistics that were used to test the significance of the differences. The significance levels of the inferential statistics may be included in the table or may be placed in a footnote to the table. In other articles, the inferential analysis may be described in the narrative of the Results section, perhaps with the values of the inferential statistics and significance levels presented in parentheses. Such a narrative analysis may often make references to the summary statistics presented in a table of data organization. Some authors simply mention in the text that inferential tests were used and that differences were significant without specifically stating the values of the statistics or the significance levels that were reached. This latter alternative certainly provides less information than would be desirable for a complete evaluation of the article, but it has apparently come into vogue as a space-saving device because journal space is at such a premium.

The examples that follow will illustrate some of the diverse manners in which authors have presented inferential analysis in research articles in speech pathology and audiology. Although these examples do not provide an exhaustive treatment of the possible formats that readers may encounter in the literature, they should enable consumers of research to appreciate the general manner in which statistical inference may be presented in journal articles and enable them to locate and examine inferential analysis in the articles they will read in the future.

As mentioned in Chapter 5, bivalent, or two sample differences may often be evaluated statistically. These might involve between-subjects comparison of two different groups or within-subjects comparison of the same group under two different conditions. The two samples, then, represent two different levels of an *independent* or *classification* variable. These two samples may be compared to each other on one or, in some cases, on more than one *dependent* variable. When the data used in such comparisons meet the requirements of the parametric statistical tests, the *t*-test (sometimes called the "Student's test" after the pseudonym of its inventor, W. S. Gosset) is used to make the bivalent comparison. When the data do not meet the requirements of the parametric model, nonparametric tests for the bivalent comparisons are used instead.

Whenever two *different* groups of subjects are compared, the particular *t*-test used is called an independent *t*-test or a *t*-test for unrelated measures or uncorrelated groups. In addition to this independent *t*-test, there is another *t*-test called the dependent *t*-test or the *t*-test for related measures or correlated groups. This dependent *t*-test is used for making within-subjects comparisons on the *same* group, such as comparison of scores on a test before and after therapy. As mentioned in Chapter 5, larger values of the resultant *t*-statistic indicate a more significant difference between groups or conditions (i.e., a larger value of *t* would have a lower probability of occurrence if the two samples were indeed the same under the null hypothesis). Conversely, small values of *t*-scores indicate less significant differences.

Table 2 in Excerpt 8.20 illustrates the presentation of a *t*-test in the comparison of the means of two different groups of subjects (i.e., a between-subjects comparison). The subjects were two different groups of listeners:

EXCERPT 8.20

TABLE 2. COMPARISON OF THE INSTRUCTIONAL GROUPS FOR MEAN DISCREPANCY BETWEEN ACCURACY SCORES FOR ESTIMATING STUTTERING AND ACCURACY SCORES ON INFORMATION

	Number of Subjects	Mean Discrepancy Score	Standard Deviation	*t*-Value	*p*
Manner group	35	59.7	20.6	2.04	5%
Content group	32	46.4	25.3		

SOURCE: Bar, A. (1967). Effects of listening instructions on attention to manner and content of stutterers' speech. *Journal of Speech and Hearing Research, 10,* 87–92.

one group was instructed to listen to the content of a stutterer's speech and the other was instructed to listen to the manner of a stutterer's speech. Each group of listeners was given two tests: one for accuracy in estimating amount of stuttering and one for accuracy of retention of the content of the stutterers' speech. A discrepancy score was computed for these two tests for each group of listeners. The entries in Table 2 of Excerpt 8.20 indicate (from left to right) the number of subjects in each group, the mean discrepancy score of each group, the standard deviation of the discrepancy scores of each group, the value of the t-statistic computed for the comparison of discrepancy scores, and the level of significance (p) of the resultant t-statistic. Because the t-score of 2.04 reached significance at the .05 level as indicated by the 5% entry under p in the table, the author concluded that the two groups listening to the speech under different instructions performed differently from each other on this particular measure.

The textual example shown next (Excerpt 8.21) illustrates how a bivalent between-subjects comparison with a t-test was simply integrated into the Results section without using a separate table. Note how the authors have included summary statistics (mean and SD) in the short paragraph along with the resultant t-statistic and its significance level in this comparison of deaf and hearing subjects.

EXCERPT 8.21

RESULTS

The mean number of graphemically similar responses for the deaf and hearing groups was 2.74 (SD = 4.98) and 0.65 (SD = 1.25) respectively. These means were significantly different as determined by a t-test ($t = 3.72$, $p < 0.01$). That there was more between-subjects variation in the deaf is indicated by their larger standard deviation.

SOURCE: Blanton, R. L., Nunnally, J. C., & Odom, P. B. (1967). Graphemic, phonetic, and associative factors in the verbal behavior of deaf and hearing subjects. *Journal of Speech and Hearing Research, 10*, 225–231.

The example in Excerpt 8.22 illustrates a within-subjects comparison made with a t-test. In this example, Fristoe and Goldman compared listeners' scoring of a traditional articulation test with their scoring of a condensed version of the test used for examining the same number of sounds. Table 2 in Excerpt 8.22 shows the mean and the SD of the number of articulation errors noted by the listeners under traditional and condensed articulation test conditions. Also included is the t-statistic and level of significance (p). The resultant t-score was quite small and not significant (i.e., its probability was greater than .70, a level much higher than the usual .05 or .01 levels required by most investigators for statistical significance). The authors concluded that the number of articulation errors detected with the traditional and condensed form of the test were equivalent. This example is an illustration of the use of the *t*-test for making a within-subject comparison because the same listeners performed under the two conditions. It is interesting to note that the number of listeners used in this study was relatively small (12), so, a nonparametric alternative to the *t*-test could have been used for this within-subjects comparison. However, the *t*-test is used with small samples by some investigators because the degrees of freedom (as discussed in Chapter 5) associated with the number of observations made is taken into account in determining the significance of the resultant *t*-statistic. Although conservative statisticians generally recommend the use of nonparametric statistics with a small number of subjects (e.g., fewer than 20), the decision to use parametric statistics seems to be a matter of the individual preference of different investigators, as evidenced by the prevalence of articles in the literature that report *t*-tests with small samples. Note, also, that the degrees of freedom were not identified in Excerpts 8.20 to 8.22, but they can be calculated by the reader through examination of the Method section to determine the number of subjects in each group.

EXCERPT 8.22

TABLE 2. A COMPARISON OF THE MEAN NUMBER OF ARTICULATION ERRORS RECORDED BY THE 12 JUDGES UNDER THE TRADITIONAL AND CONDENSED TEST LISTENING CONDITIONS

	Mean	SD	*t*	*p*
Traditional	31.97	13.07	03796	>0.70
Condensed	31.81	12.29		

SOURCE: Fristoe, M., & Goldman, R. (1968). Comparison of traditional and condensed articulation tests examining the same number of sounds. *Journal of Speech and Hearing Research, 11,* 583–589.

The illustration in Excerpt 8.23 shows the use of the Mann-Whitney *U* test (a nonparametric test) to make a between-subjects comparison. The Mann-Whitney *U* test, as mentioned in Chapter 5, is often referred to as a nonparametric alternative to the *t*-test because it is used to make a two-sample comparison between subjects when the requirements for the t-test cannot be met by the data. In the example shown, Excerpt 8.23, two groups of subjects with cleft palates (one group with greater than 1 mm palatopharyngeal gap and one group with less than 1 mm palatopharyngeal gap) were compared on four different dependent (criterion) variables: syllable nasal manometer readings; vowel nasal manometer readings; oral breath pressure ratios; and articulation scores. The mean and range of each of the dependent variables for each of the two groups of subjects are shown in the table columns in the center. The Mann-Whitney U statistics are entered in the right columns and footnotes indicate the significance levels obtained. Vowel nasal manometer readings and articulation scores showed significant differences between the two groups, but syllable nasal manometer readings and oral breath pressure ratios did not show significant differences.

As mentioned above, the Mann-Whitney U test is often referred to as a nonparametric alternative to the independent t-test because it is used to make a bivalent between-subjects comparison. It should be noted, however, that the Mann-Whitney U statistic is calculated in a manner different from the manner in which the t-statistic is calculated. Smaller values of the Mann-Whitney U statistic indicate a more significant difference between groups and, conversely, larger values of Mann-Whitney U are nonsignificant.

When a nonparametric alternative to the t-test is used, the author may decide to include a central tendency measure other than the mean or a variability measure other than the standard deviation in the summary statistics table. This is because the mean and standard deviation are usually associated with parametric statistics. In the example in Excerpt 8.23 the authors did include the mean as the measure of central tendency, but used the range instead of the standard deviation as a measure of variability.

The Mann-Whitney U test operates on the ranks of the subjects in the two groups rather than on their actual test scores. Thus, the level of measurement used for the dependent variable is ordinal. The Mann-Whitney U test would be an appropriate alternative to the t-test when the original dependent variable data are at the ordinal level of measurement or when interval- or ratio-level original data are transformed to the ordinal level of measurement for use with a nonparametric test because one of the other assumptions of a parametric test (e.g., normal distribution) cannot be met. The Wilcoxon Matched-Pairs Signed-Ranks Test (to be illustrated in the next excerpt) also makes use of ranks rather than actual scores, so that it is also appropriate for analyzing data at the ordinal level of measurement.

Excerpt 8.24 contains an illustration of the use of the Wilcoxon Matched-Pairs Signed-Ranks Test to make a bivalent within-subjects comparison. Wilcoxon's Matched-Pairs Signed-Ranks Test is often referred to as a nonparametric alternative to the dependent t-test because it is used to make a comparison of the performance of one group of subjects in two different conditions when the data are not appropriate for the use of parametric statis-

EXCERPT 8.23

TABLE 2. COMPARISON OF CLEFT-PALATE SUBJECTS WITH MEAN PALATOPHARYNGEAL GAPS OF 1 MM OR GREATER WITH A GROUP OF CLEFT-PALATE SUBJECTS WITH MEAN GAPS OF LESS THAN 1 MM FOR DIFFERENCE IN U-TUBE MANOMETER READINGS, ORAL BREATH PRESSURE RATIOS, AND ARTICULATION TEST SCORES

	<1 mm Gap		>1 mm Gap		Mann-Whitney *U*
	Mean	Range	Mean	Range	
U-tube syllable readings[1]	2.06	0 to 6.2	2.71	.9 to 6.8	68
U-tube vowel readings[1]	.05	0 to .33	.18	0 to .58	55*
Oral breath pressure ratios[2]	.93	.80 to 1.0	.89	.50 to 1.0	89.5
Articulation scores[3]	86.20	65.67 to 100.00	72.50	46.26 to 94.02	40**

*Significant at the .025 level.
**Significant at the .01 level.
1. In cm of water.
2. Pressure in ounces nares open/pressure in ounces nares closed.
3. Percent of responses correct.

SOURCE: Shelton, R. L., Brooks, A. R., & Youngstrom, K. A. (1965). Clinical assessment of palatopharyngeal closure. *Journal of Speech and Hearing Disorders, 30*, 37–43.

tics. In the study by Adams and Moore, 12 stutterers were compared in two different conditions (with vs. without listening to masking noise) on four dependent variables: frequency of stuttering, vocal intensity, reading time, and palmar sweat anxiety. The Wilcoxon Matched-Pairs Signed-Ranks statistic (*T*) reported in the text showed significant differences only for frequency of stuttering and vocal intensity. Similar to the Mann-Whitney *U* test, a smaller value of the Wilcoxon statistic indicates a significant difference. Readers should observe that Adams and Moore (Excerpt 8.24) included the median and semi-interquartile range in their summary statistics as measures of central tendency and variability. The use of these descriptive statistics with a nonparametric inferential analysis is more consistent with the general practice of dealing with data for which parametric statistics are inappropriate.

EXCERPT 8.24

Statistical Analyses

Each of the four dependent variables (frequency of stuttering, palmar sweat anxiety, vocal intensity, and reading time) were compared across the two conditions. In every case, comparisons were conducted by using the nonparametric Wilcoxon Matched-Pairs Signed-Ranks Test (Siegel 1956).

RESULTS

Table 1 presents the median and semi-interquartile range values for the subjects' frequency of stuttering, vocal intensity, reading time, and palmar sweat anxiety in the two conditions.

TABLE 1. MEDIAN AND SEMI-INTERQUARTILE RANGE (Q) VALUES FOR SUBJECTS' FREQUENCY OF STUTTERING, VOCAL INTENSITY, READING TIME, AND PALMAR SWEAT ANXIETY IN THE MASKING AND NO-MASKING (CONTROL) CONDITIONS

Condition	Frequency of Stutter	Vocal Intensity (dB)	Reading Time (secs)	Palmar Sweat Anxiety (microamperes)	
Masking	4.0	83.50	91.08	5.0	Median
	7.5	4.50	91.13	5.0	(Q)
No-masking	19.0	74.50	85.83	4.5	Median
	17.5	3.50	132.83	5.5	(Q)

First, the reduction in stuttering in the presence of noise was highly significant ($T = 0$, $N = 12$, $p < 0.005$). All 12 subjects had fewer dysfluencies in the presence of noise than in quiet. The increase in vocal intensity in the presence of noise was also significant ($T = 0$, $N = 12$, $p < 0.005$). Each of the 12 stutterers used greater vocal intensity while reading in noise than in quiet. Reading time did not differ appreciably across conditions. Six subjects took less time to read the passage in the masking condition, four took less reading time in quiet, and two exhibited no difference in reading time between conditions. The median palmar sweat measures for subjects in the two conditions are almost identical. Five of the stutterers had no difference in their palmar sweat anxiety between conditions, four subjects had higher palmar sweat readings in the masking condition, and three individuals had lower palmar sweat readings with masking present. None of these previous four comparisons were influenced in any way by the order in which the subjects encountered the two conditions.

SOURCE: Adams, M. R., & Moore, W. H. (1972). The effects of auditory masking on the anxiety level, frequency of dysfluency, and selected vocal characteristics of stutterers. *Journal of Speech and Hearing Research, 15*, 572–578.

In the example in Excerpt 8.25, deaf students who had been exposed to manual communication from infancy were compared to deaf students who had been exposed to oral communication. The χ^2 test was used to test the significance of the difference between oral and manual students in their performance on Gallaudet College Entrance Examinations. Scores on this examination were dichotomized into "pass" and "fail" categories and the frequencies of oral and manual students falling into the pass and fail categories are shown in the 2 by 2 contingency table in the excerpt. The χ^2 for this comparison was 5.23, which, as the authors indicated, was significant at the .05 level. The χ^2 statistic is similar to the t-statistic in the determination of its significance; that is, higher values of χ^2 are needed to indicate significant differences.

EXCERPT 8.25

TABLE 5.   STUDENTS OF IQ 110 OR BETTER WHO PASSED GALLAUDET COLLEGE ENTRANCE EXAMINATIONS

	Oral	Manual
Passed Gallaudet Exams	17	18
Did not pass Gallaudet Exams	16	4

$\chi^2 = 5.23$ df $= 1$ $p < .05$

SOURCE: Vernon, M., & Koh, S. D. (1970). Early manual communication and deaf children's achievement. *American Annals of the Deaf, 115*, 527–536.

The example in Excerpt 8.25 shows the use of the chi square (χ^2) as a test of the significance of the difference between two groups of subjects. As mentioned in Chapter 5, χ^2 has a variety of uses. We have already seen its use as a measure of association in the example in Excerpt 8.18 in the correlational section of this chapter. It can also be used to show the significance of the difference between the performance of two groups of subjects on nominal level variables.

The χ^2 test may also be encountered when more than two groups are compared or when groups are compared on a nominal variable that can be categorized in more than two ways.

These comparisons can become somewhat cumbersome and difficult to interpret if there are many categories, but χ^2 can be useful with several categories. An example is shown in Excerpt 8.26 of the comparison of two groups on a nominal-level variable that is categorized in three ways.

In this example, χ^2 is used to test the significance of the difference between stutterers and nonstutterers in their identification of an unseen speaker while viewing listener reactions to the speaker. On viewing the listener, the subjects were given the choice to identify the unseen speaker as: a "Stutterer," a "Nonstutterer," or "Can't Tell." Wingate and Hamre considered these three judgments to be three levels of a nominal variable and, therefore, used the χ^2 statistic to test the difference between stutterers' and nonstutterers' identifications. Inspection of the table entries in Excerpt 8.26 reveals that the frequencies of each of the three judgments made by the stutterers are similar to the frequencies of each of the three judgments made by the nonstutterers. The χ^2 value computed from these data was lower than the χ^2 value needed to reach significance at the .05 level for this comparison (2 by 3 contingency table), so, the authors concluded that there was no difference between the two groups in their identifications of the speaker.

EXCERPT 8.26

TABLE 1. STUTTERERS' AND NONSTUTTERERS' IDENTIFICATIONS OF THE UNSEEN SPEAKER

	Identifications			
Subjects	"Stutterer"	"Nonstutterer"	"Can't Tell"	χ^2
Stutterer	117	52	31	
Nonstutterer	108	64	28	1.68*
Total	225	116	59	

*With 2 degrees of freedom, a χ^2 value of 5.991 is required for significance at the 0.05 level.

SOURCE: Wingate, M. E., & Hamre, C. E. (1967). Stutterers' projection of listener reaction. *Journal of Speech and Hearing Research, 10,* 339–343.

The bivalent inference tests discussed above were used for making comparisons between two groups of subjects or for comparing the same subjects' performances in two different conditions on one or more dependent variables. However, when more than two samples are compared simultaneously (as in multivalent or parametric studies), these two sample comparison statistics are inappropriate and multivariate statistics such as the analysis of variance (ANOVA) should be used. ANOVA would be appropriate, for example, if three or more groups of subjects were compared on a dependent or criterion variable or if one group of subjects were tested in three or more different conditions. ANOVA would also be appropriate if two groups of subjects were compared under two different conditions because this would involve two simultaneous bivalent comparisons, one between-subjects comparison and one within-subjects comparison. The ANOVA allows the researcher to test the main effect of each independent or classification variable and also allows for the analysis of any interaction effects among the independent variables. As indicated in Chapter 5, analysis of variance techniques are available for making between-subjects comparisons, within-subjects comparisons (sometimes called "repeated measures" comparisons), and simultaneous between-subjects and within-subjects comparisons (sometimes called "mixed model" ANOVAs).

Excerpt 8.27 illustrates the use of an analysis of variance for the comparison of two groups of subjects (children with normal articulation vs. children with impaired articulation) performing under three different conditions (responding to digits, random words, and words in sentences). A mixed model ANOVA was used to compare the performances of the two groups of children (between-subjects comparison) as the first main effect. The second main effect examined was the difference between the three stimulus presentation conditions (within-subjects comparison). Finally, the interaction effect between subject groups and stimulus conditions was evaluated. The results of these three parts of the analysis of variance are shown in the figure, table, and text that are included in the excerpt.

Figure 1 in Excerpt 8.27 is a bar graph depicting the mean number of stimuli correctly recalled by the two groups of children in each of the stimulus conditions. The table is a complete ANOVA summary table similar to the one described in Chapter 5. The between-subjects and within-subjects main effects and the interaction effect are listed in the left column and the degrees of freedom, mean squares, F-ratios, and significance levels are listed in the other columns for each main effect and interaction. In such an ANOVA, significant differences are indicated by large F-ratios and nonsignificant differences are indicted by smaller F-ratios, although the absolute value of a significant F depends on the number of degrees of freedom associated with each comparison.

The F was significant for the main effect of the between-subjects comparison, indicating that the normal and articulation-impaired children performed differently on the recall task. The within-subjects F for the comparison of the effects of the different stimulus materials was also significant, indicating that recall performance was not the same for the different stimuli. The stimulus material by groups interaction was also significant, indicating that the two groups of children performed differently on the different types of material. This interaction effect is further explored in the text with references to the figure. Saxman and Miller indicated in the text that follow-up comparisons with contrast tests of specific pairs of means (e.g., normal vs. articulation-impaired children on recall of words in sentences) revealed that the two groups of children did not perform differently on recall of digits or random words but that they did perform differently on recall of words in sentences. This finding is the essence of the interaction effect and the most important result of this analysis of variance.

EXCERPT 8.27

RESULTS

Number of Items Recalled

Figure 1 is a graph of the mean number of items recalled correctly by the two groups of children for the three types of stimulus material. A groups-by-stimulus-material-type analysis of variance (ANOVA), with repeated measures on material type (Winer, 1962), was performed on the number of items recalled to determine which of the recall performance differences were statistically significant. Results of the ANOVA (summarized in Table 1) were that the groups-by-stimulus-material interaction was significant ($p < 0.01$), as were each of the main effects. Because of the significant interaction, group means for each of the stimulus-material-type conditions were analyzed. The group with good articulation recalled significantly more items than did the group with poor articulation when the word items were cast as sentences ($F = 29.61$; df 1,108; $p < 0.01$). The two groups did not perform differently on the digit or random-word tasks. Both groups were found to recall significantly ($p < 0.01$) more items on the sentence task than on the digit or random-word tasks. (See Figure 1.)

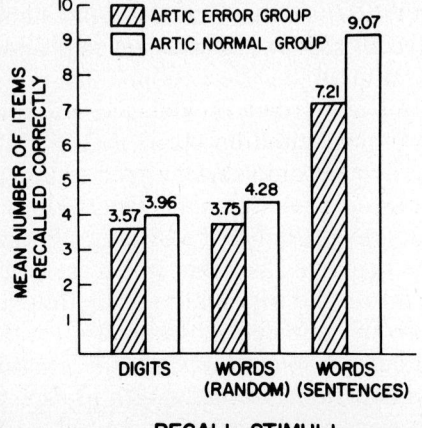

Figure 1. The mean number of items (string length) recalled correctly by the articulation-error ($N = 28$) and articulation-normal ($N = 28$) groups for each of the three types of stimulus material.

TABLE 1. SUMMARY OF ANOVA TO TEST FOR DIFFERENCES IN MEAN NUMBER OF ITEMS RECALLED FOR 28 CHILDREN WITH POOR ARTICULATION AND 28 CHILDREN WITH GOOD ARTICULATION FOR THREE STIMULUS MATERIAL TYPES

Source	df	MS	F	p
Between subjects	55	2.22	—	—
Groups (B)	1	36.21	22.77	<0.01
Error (S within B)	54	1.59	—	—
Within subjects	112	10.11	—	—
Stimulus material (A)	2	338.04	206.11	<0.01
Stimulus material × groups (A × B)	2	9.13	5.57	<0.01
Error (A × S within B)	108	1.64	—	—

SOURCE: Saxman, J. H., & Miller, J. F. (1973). Short-term memory and language skills in articulation-deficient children. *Journal of Speech and Hearing Research, 16*, 721–730.

Inspection of Figure 1 in Excerpt 8.27 confirms the notion that the two groups of children were different in their recall of words in sentences but not in their recall of either digits or random words. A greater separation of the means of the two groups can be seen for the words in sentences than for the digits or random words when the figure is inspected closely.

In this example, a rather thorough recounting of the analysis of variance was provided that included the ANOVA summary table, the figure, and a narrative description of the comparisons. Not all presentations of ANOVA are this complete, as the basic findings may be sometimes capsuled into a textual description. The next excerpt (8.28) illustrates a more abbreviated presentation of an analysis of variance, with the values of inferential statistics, df, and significance levels included in the text rather than in a table.

In this example, Webster and Dorman studied the effects of practice vs. no practice (first independent variable) and of normal vs. delayed auditory feedback (second independent variable) on articulation errors and reading time (two dependent variables). Subjects were randomly assigned to one of four conditions in this between-subjects design: (1) normal feedback without practice, (2) normal feedback with practice, (3) delayed feedback without practice, and (4) delayed feedback with practice. The table in Excerpt 8.28 shows the mean number of articulation errors and the mean reading time for each of the four conditions represented by the parametric combination of the two independent variables. The textual description of the ANOVA contains a neat summary of the independent and dependent variables as a preface to the analysis. All main effects and interactions are described in the text, with the values of F, *df* and significance levels indicated in parentheses.

EXCERPT 8.28

RESULTS

A two-way analysis of variance, was performed using articulation errors as the dependent variable; another two-way analysis of variance was performed on reading durations. The independent variables were levels of practice and type of auditory feedback. For the articulation errors measure, feedback, practice, and the practice by feedback interaction were significant (the respective values being: $F = 29.89$, df $= 1/56$, $p < 0.01$; $F = 11.11$, df $= 1/56$, $p < 0.01$; $F = 11.79$, df $= 1/56$, $p < 0.01$). Table 1 shows the mean number of articulation errors for all groups. The difference in mean number of articulation errors made by the OP and NP subjects under NAF was not significant. However, under DAF the OP subjects made significantly fewer articulation errors than the NP subjects ($t = 3.40$, df $= 28$, $p < 0.01$). The same findings hold for the means of the reading duration scores (Table 1). The analysis of variance showed that feedback, practice, and the practice-by-feedback interaction were significant (the respective values being: $F = 61.90$, df $= 1/56$, $p < 0.01$; $F = 5.23$, df $= 1/56$, $p = 0.05$; $F = 6.50$, df $= 1/56$, $p < 0.05$). The difference between the means of the OP and the NP subjects under NAF was not significant. The mean reading duration under DAF for OP subjects was significantly lower than this same measure for NP subjects ($t = 2.60$, df $= 28$, $p < 0.05$).

TABLE 1. MEAN NUMBER OF ARTICULATION ERRORS AND MEAN READING TIMES FOR ALL TREATMENT CONDITIONS

	Normal Feedback		Delayed Feedback	
	Errors	Time	Errors	Time
No practice	2.0	101.6	19.7	131.5
Oral practice	2.3	101.0	6.1	118.4

SOURCE: Webster, R. L., & Dorman, M. F. (1971). Changes in reliance on auditory feedback cues as a function of oral practice. *Journal of Speech and Hearing Research, 14,* 307–311.

Specific bivalent comparisons were also carried out with contrast tests after each of the two ANOVAs. The contrasts were accomplished with follow-up t-tests to explore the specific differences underlying the significant interaction effects. Readers should recall that ANOVA indicates only the significance of overall main and interaction effects and that specific bivalent comparisons need to be made with contrast tests to find which pairs of significantly different means account for the significant main and interaction effects. In the example in Excerpt 8.27, supplementary F-tests were used for contrasts and in the example in Excerpt 8.28 supplementary t-tests were used for contrasts. As mentioned in Chapter 5, other methods for specific contrasts to follow up the ANOVA include the Sheffé test, the Newman-Keuls test, and the Bonferroni t- test. A comparison of the relative merits of the different contrast tests is beyond the scope of this book, but suffice it to say that the selection of a particular contrast test to follow up an ANOVA depends partly on the type of comparison to be made and partly on the individual preferences of the particular author. The important point for consumers of research is to recognize that contrast tests are used for making specific bivalent comparisons after the completion of the analysis of variance in order to find which pairs of means are significantly different from each other.

This last point exemplifies an important dilemma facing the consumers of research for whom this book is intended. Most consumers have not had sufficient course work in statistics to enable them to judge the relative merits of various statistical procedures for the analysis of relationships and differences. In this book we have tried to help consumers to recognize the general kinds of statistics that may be used to describe or analyze certain kinds of data in certain situations. This should help these readers to understand many of the Results sections that they will read and to recognize, in general, the appropriate or inappropriate use of statistical description and analysis. The finer points and nuances of statistical analysis must be left to course work and textbooks in advanced statistics. Our purpose will be fulfilled if the consumer can read a Results section and appreciate how the author has used the empirical data to answer the research question.

Some Characteristics of Good Data Analysis

The analysis of data in a Results section should present a clear picture of the strength and direction of relationships or of the significant differences that were found. Readers should expect some of the following characteristics of good analysis of data.

Illustrations that are used in the analysis of relationships or differences should conform to the same standards that were discussed earlier in the section on organization of data. Table and figure captions should be brief, but informative. Tables and figures should be capable of standing alone in presenting the analysis and the narrative should dovetail easily with the illustrations in the discussion of the data analysis.

The analysis of relationships should employ statistical techniques that are appropriate to such factors as the level of measurement of the data and the number of observations. Readers should be aware of the general appropriateness of indices such as the Pearson and Spearman correlation coefficients, the χ^2, and the contingency coefficient that are employed in the analysis of relationships. The significance levels of the correlations that are reported should be included when necessary, and consumers may also expect authors to comment on the practical meaning of correlations as well as their statistical significance. This may often be accompanied by reference to the index of determination (R^2) in discussing the overlap of variance among variables.

The evaluation of intercorrelation matrices or of multiple regression analyses may be particularly difficult for novice consumers. Authors may aid consumers in this task through careful presentation and discussion of these analyses, especially in the integration of the narrative with the illustrations. Despite this, evaluation of multiple correlation and regression analyses will usually require more time and effort from consumers. Frequent exposure to multiple correlation studies should serve to sharpen the reader's evaluative skills in this area.

The analysis of differences should employ statistical techniques that are appropriate to the level of measurement used, the number of observations, the number of comparisons, and so forth. Readers should be aware of the appropriateness of parametric and nonparametric inference tests. Readers should also be cognizant of the appropriate uses of two-sample comparison statistics and of the need for analysis of variance techniques for simultaneous comparisons. These analyses should present a clear and consistent summary of significant and nonsignificant differences and of main and interaction effects when necessary. Such analyses often include reference to both a table and a figure to clarify the narrative explanation of the differences found. Multiple comparisons with complex interactions may present some difficulty to novice consumers; once again, authors may aid these readers through careful integration of tables, figures, and text.

Summary

The examples presented in this chapter have been used to illustrate some of the basic terms, concepts, and procedures used in organizing and analyzing data derived from research in speech pathology and audiology. Some of the basic formats for data organization in text, tables, and figures were exemplified and some characteristics of good organization of data were discussed. Examples were presented of many of the ways in which the analysis of relationships among variables may be displayed in the Results section. Some of the more common inferential statistics that are used to analyze differences between-subjects or within-subjects were illustrated.

The next chapter will illustrate some of the important aspects of the discussion section of the research article in which the author draws conclusions concerning the data shown in the Results section.

EVALUATION CHECKLIST

Instructions: The four-category scale at the end of this checklist may be used to rate the *Results* section of an article. The *Evaluation Items* help identify those topics that should be considered in arriving at the rating. Comments on these topics, entered as *Evaluation Notes*, should serve as the basis for the overall rating.

Evaluation Items   *Evaluation Notes*

1. Results were clearly related to research problem.

2. Tables and figures were integrated with text.

3. Summary statistics were used appropriately.

4. Organization of data was clear.

5. Statistical analysis was appropriate to:
   (a) level of measurement
   (b) number of observations
   (c) type of sample
   (d) shape of distribution

6. There was appropriate use of correlational and inferential analysis.

7. There was clear presentation of significant and nonsignificant correlations.

8. There was clear presentation of significant and nonsignificant differences.

9. Miscellaneous.

Overall Rating (Results): _____ _____ _____ _____

                             Poor   Fair   Good   Excellent

9

The Discussion and Conclusions Section

Introduction

The last section of an article, usually titled "Discussion" or "Conclusions" or both, is written with somewhat more license than are the other sections, and readers may often notice more variation among authors in the organization of this section. In fact, consumers of research may encounter shorter articles that combine the results and conclusions into one section. Nevertheless, there are some general topics that are usually addressed at the end of an article and consumers of research should be aware of the importance of these in the culmination of a research article. Five general topics will be included in our evaluation checklist for the "Discussion and Conclusions" section:

Relationship of Conclusions to Preceding Parts of the Article

Relationship of Results to Previous Research

Theoretical Implications of the Research

Practical Implications of the Research

Implications for Future Research

Each of these general topics will be discussed separately in the next five sections.

Relationship of Conclusions to Preceding Parts of the Article

The discussion section should contain some material that relates the conclusions directly to the *Problem, Method,* and *Results* of the investigation and that unites the preceding sections into a coherent whole.

The Research Problem

The conclusions of a research article should be directed clearly toward the *research problem* that was presented in the first section of the article. Complete restatement of the problem and rationale would be cumbersome at this point in an article, but in many of the better articles in the literature, the discussion commences with a brief reminder of the problem and a general statement of the conclusion of the investigation regarding the problem or research questions.

Excerpts 9.1 and 9.2 present introductory paragraphs from two Discussion sections that neatly remind readers of the research problem and quickly summarize the results in relation to the problem. The conclusions of both studies reflect clearly and directly on the research problems and set the stage for further discussion of the limitations and implications of the research.

EXCERPT 9.1

DISCUSSION

The purpose of the present study was to develop a picture identification test for the measurement of speech discrimination ability in hearing-impaired children. The results of the study indicate that we have been successful in developing a reliable test of four equivalent lists. The words used were within the recognition vocabulary of the subjects, and the pictures appear to be adequate representations of the words.

SOURCE: Ross, M., & Lerman, J. (1970). A picture identification test for hearing-impaired children. *Journal of Speech and Hearing Research, 13,* 44–53.

EXCERPT 9.2

DISCUSSION

It will be recalled that this study was conducted to see if the reduction in stuttering during singing is related to altered vocalization as suggested by Wingate (1969) or to the familiarity of the lyrics of the song being sung, or both. The results of the present investigation clearly indicated that during singing altered vocalization in the form of extended utterance duration and the familiarity of the lyrics being sung are both associated with significant decrements in stuttering frequency.

SOURCE: Healey, E. C., Mallard, A. R., & Adams, M. R. (1976). Factors contributing to the reduction of stuttering during singing. *Journal of Speech and Hearing Research, 19,* 475–480.

Some of the longer research articles that include several specific research questions or subproblems may devote a section of the Discussion to a more complete review of the research questions and results as an overall summary. This is particularly appropriate when the results are lengthly, complex, or concern several related issues. Excerpt 9.3 shows how Folkins summarized four research questions and the manner in which his data addressed each of them in a separate conclusion section at the end of a lengthly article on muscle activity involved in jaw closing during speech.

EXCERPT 9.3

CONCLUSIONS

The following is a review of the above data in relation to the four issues raised in the introduction:

1. How is elevation of the mandible during speech divided between the muscles? Based on the data presented here medial pterygoid seems to be involved in all jaw-closing movements, but masseter and temporalis often play a role, especially for larger movements. Recordings from lateral pteryoid differed substantially between subjects and tasks. In future studies it will be important to develop techniques to specify whether recordings are from the inferior or superior heads of lateral pterygoid.

2. Do timing parameters vary between different muscles? As illustrated in Figure 3, no consistent differences in the timing of peak EMG activity were found between muscles. The duration of medial pterygoid activity tended to be longer than temporalis or masseter, as shown in Figure 4.

3. Are there relations between the timing of muscle activity and jaw-closing movements? In some instances peak EMG activity tended to occur later when displacement was increased, but this usually was not so.

4. Are the relative levels of involvement between muscles kept in the same ratio relations or are the relative levels of activity variable? When jaw-closing movements were repeated for a train of syllables, the muscles were sometimes maintained at similar levels from syllable to syllable, but in many instances the relative amounts of EMG activity changed dramatically for similar jaw movements.

SOURCE: Folkins, J. W. (1981). Muscle activity for jaw closing during speech. *Journal of Speech and Hearing Research, 24,* 601–615.

The Method of Investigation

The Discussion section should also present some remarks concerning the *method* of the investigation and how it relates to the conclusion of the study. Any limitations of the research imposed by the particular method should be considered. Qualifying remarks may be found concerning the subjects, materials, or procedures employed and how they may have limited the conclusions that may be drawn from the data.

Of particular concern is the manner in which the author discusses the potential threats to internal and external validity in the investigation and how these threats may have been reduced in the design of the study. As readers will have surmised from reading Chapters 3 and 4, every empirical investigation may be subject to some threats to internal and external validity, and the better studies are those that minimize these threats. Minimization implies, however, that there is usually some residue of jeopardy to internal and external validity. This residue should be addressed in the Discussion section in order to qualify the conclusions and, perhaps, to suggest future research possibilities to improve or extend the findings of the investigation. The better studies in the literature, then, are those that not only reduce the threats to internal and external validity but also discuss the residue of jeopardy with some candor in qualifying the results. Of course, if an inordinately large number of research design limitations are discussed, readers may question the wisdom of the journal editor for publishing the study in the first place. In other words, as the limitations become more extensive and significant, the value of the research is reduced accordingly.

The next four excerpts from Discussion sections illustrate the ways in which authors have considered various limitations of the method of investigation and discussed appropriate qualifications of their conclusions based on these limitations. Excerpt 9.4 is taken from a Discussion subsection, entitled "Some Qualifications," and considers some problems of internal validity associated with maturation (mood) and instrumentation and the problem of sample size related to external validity.

EXCERPT 9.4

DISCUSSION

Some Qualifications

The sampling procedure employed in this study was utilized as a means of insuring that the subjects' utterances would be directly comparable. Since this study examined semantic relations reflected in language usage, it was critical that utterances in response to the same stimuli be obtained from each subject. On the other hand, it is recognized that a complete set of proposition rules could not be written with a 50-utterance corpus. The proposition rules written merely represented some of the child's semantic relation system. The small sample size no doubt made the acquired data more likely to be altered by moods or other transitory factors affecting a child's linguistic performance. The questions asked of the child were quite open ended, however, and judging from the Morehead and Ingram (1973) finding that children's spontaneous and "response" utterances did not differ, we believed that the use of such questions would have benefits over comparisons of language samples in a setting with no controls. It appears that unless one can acquire utterances numbering in the several hundreds as seen in normative studies (Bloom, 1970; Brown, 1973) such "purely" naturalistic samples might be risky for comparative purposes. Nevertheless, the use of specific questions does leave the possibility that the child's language usage was influenced by his ability to comprehend the questions. It would also be difficult to dismiss the possibility that the experimenter's questions affected to some extent the form and content of the child's sampled language.

Though the language-disordered children in this study represented a random sample of children requiring language intervention, the number of disordered children employed (20) was not sufficiently extensive to rule out the exclusion of disordered children demonstrating language usage quite dissimilar to the usage described in this investigation. Caution should therefore be taken in interpreting the present data as representative of all language-disordered children's usage.

SOURCE: Leonard, L. B., Bolders, J. G., & Miller, J. A. (1976). An examination of the semantic relations reflected in the language usage of normal and language-disordered children. *Journal of Speech and Hearing Research, 19,* 371–392.

Excerpt 9.5 is from a study of physical and perceptual measures of hypernasality and discusses two limitations in method. The first limitation concerns the problem of using a perceptual measure of hypernasality as an outside criterion for validating physical measures of hypernasality and the second problem concerns the use of simulated hypernasality instead of samples of speakers who were actually hypernasal. Despite these admitted limitations, reasonable correlations were found between physical and perceptual measures of hypernasality and the author makes some valuable suggestions for collection of normative data with the physical measure.

EXCERPT 9.5

An inherent problem in establishing the validity of a method of measuring physical correlates of hypernasality stems in part from the fact that perceptual measures themselves are not highly reliable. The less-than-desirable reliability of hypernasal ratings, in turn, appears to result from the fact that the percept of hypernasality in speech is multidimensional in nature, being influenced by such factors as nasal emission noise, misarticulation, compensatory substitutions, loudness, and pitch, in addition to acoustic consequences of velopharyngeal incompetence. Observer bias and the amount of experience with the hypernasal speech of cleft palate, deaf, dysarthric speakers, and so forth, are also known to influence listener reliability of nasality ratings.

In view of the problem, it was encouraging to find a reasonably high correlation between the N/V ratio and the perceived hypernasality scores derived from

naive listeners. The paired-comparison paradigm undoubtedly helped to reduce the difficulty of the listeners' task in rating hypernasality in the speech
samples. Admittedly, the use of simulated hypernasality weakens the conclusion of this study, although all the speech samples were judged by three
speech-language pathologists experienced in voice evaluation as representative
of hypernasal speech of various degrees. Further investigation is needed to
examine how the N/V ratio would correlate with mechano physiological measures such as velar height, velopharyngeal wall distance, velopharyngeal ori-
face size, and so forth. Compilation of normative data on the N/V ratio for
children and adults also needs to be made for the method to be used as an aid to
diagnostic and therapeutic procedures.

SOURCE: Horii, Y. (1983). An accelerometric measure as a physical correlate of perceived hypernasality in speech. *Journal of Speech and Hearing Research, 26,* 476–480.

Excerpt 9.6 presents a caveat regarding a possible carry-over sequencing
effect that could not be controlled by counterbalancing or randomizing conditions or using a between-subjects design. Notice how the author tries to
entertain three possible explanations for the results in light of this problem
and suggests that future research is needed to examine these possible
explanations.

EXCERPT 9.6

Before offering possible explanations for these results, a caveat is in order. This
experiment required that the subject perform the speech task first to increase
the possibility that stuttering samples would be obtained in addition to the
fluent tokens. It is possible that the state of excitability for the speech task
carried over into the finger counting task. Thus, we must view our conclusions
with caution. We are left with at least three possibilities: (a) a *radiation effect:*
discoordination of fine motor control in severe stutterers that includes not only
speech muscles but hand muscles, (b) a *generalized arousal effect:* carry over
effects of performing the speech task before the finger task, and/or (c) a *speech
mediation effect:* greater execution time for the finger task not due to difficulties in hand coordination but possibly because subjects were "speaking to
themselves" as they counted on their fingers. Further research is needed to test
these possibilities.

SOURCE: Borden, G. (1983). Initiation versus execution time during manual and oral
counting by stutterers. *Journal of Speech and Hearing Research, 26,* 389–396.

Excerpt 9.7 is from a study of visual evoked-response correlates of speechreading and concerns the subject-selection threat to external validity. This
excerpt shows how it may be difficult to generalize to more experienced
speechreaders, but that inexperienced speechreaders with normal hearing
had to be selected for this original study to minimize confounding effects of

variation in speechreading experience and linguistic abilities. In other words, the authors have followed the pattern of paying attention to internal validity first and being concerned with external validity in replications later, as was discussed in Chapter 4. Note that the authors have indicated in the excerpt that a follow-up study with hearing-impaired subjects was already underway.

EXCERPT 9.7

It should be pointed out that results obtained from unpracticed, normal-hearing subjects do not necessarily generalize to the hearing-impaired population. Many hearing-impaired individuals are experienced, competent speech-readers, unlike the subjects in this study. However, by choosing to study initially a normal-hearing population, we minimize the confounding effects of both experience with speechreading and large variations in linguistic abilities characteristic of the hearing-impaired population. This allows us to detect additional dimensions of individual differences relevant to speechreading ability which might otherwise be masked by experience and general language factors and provides baseline information for designing future studies of speechreading ability in the hearing-impaired population. For example, to the extent that VF16 reflects a generalizable aspect of information processing, the ability to control the variance in speechreading skills due to this factor will help determine the contributions of other factors such as language exposure, etiology of deafness, and the like. Experimental studies designed to determine the nature of VF16 and its relevance to speechreading skills in the hearing-impaired population are currently underway in our laboratory.

SOURCE: Samar, V. J., & Sims, D. G. (1983). Visual evoked-response correlates of speechreading performance in normal-hearing adults: A replication and factor analytic extension. *Journal of Speech and Hearing Research, 26,* 2–9.

The Results of the Investigation

The conclusions in the Discussion section should be drawn directly and fairly from the results. Although the Discussion section should not be merely a rehashing of the results, authors often refer to the data to support their conclusions. Occasionally, authors may even include a table or figure in the Discussion section to summarize their own results and, perhaps, the results of other studies to aid in the presentation of the conclusions. The important point is that the conclusions should be tied directly and fairly to empirical results, and comments that are not empirically based should be labeled as speculations, not as conclusions. Speculations are often important in the generation of new research and contribute to the creativity that is important in designing new research, but authors and readers alike must be aware of the difference between solid conclusions drawn directly from empirical data and intuitive speculations about the nature of phenomena.

Excerpt 9.8 is from a study that compared different methods of brief-tone audiometry for the measurement of auditory threshold and shows a rather straightforward conclusion regarding which method would be most adaptable for clinical measurement.

EXCERPT 9.8

The 1-dB/sec tracking task presented problems not encountered using the 2-dB/sec method. Under the former method, the subjects tended to lose track of signals during its slow attenuation. Frequently, an error of expectation occurred before the tone became audible again, causing the subject to further attenuate the signal. When this occurred, the tracings become erratic. The test-retest reliability coefficients (Table 2) and the standard errors of measurement (Table 3) for the 1-dB/sec tracking task results appear to reflect the greater difficulty associated with the reduced attenuation rate. The 2-dB/sec attenuation rate is rapid enough to overcome this problem. Certainly the foregoing does not support Martin and Wofford's (1970) contention that a 1-dB/sec tracking rate would increase the precision of the obtained thresholds. In summary, practical considerations are such that of the three tasks examined here, the 2-dB/sec tracking procedure represents the method which appears most easily adaptable to the clinical measurement of brief-tone audiometric thresholds.

SOURCE: Richards, A. M., & Dunn, J. (1974). Threshold measurement procedures in brief-tone audiometry. *Journal of Speech and Hearing Research, 17,* 446–454.

Excerpt 9.9 is from the study of factors contributing to reduction of stuttering during singing that Excerpt 9.2 came from. Again, the conclusions are drawn directly from the results, which were reasonably straightforward.

EXCERPT 9.9

Taken alone, our finding that subjects significantly extended utterance durations during song provides a measure of support for Wingate's "modified vocalization" hypothesis. At the same time, certain of our results indicate that extended utterance duration, and by implication, modified vocalization, can only account for part of the reduction in stuttering during singing. It appears as though the familiarity of the melody and lyrics of the song being sung also has an important effect on stuttering frequency. More specifically, our subjects experienced the greatest decrement in stuttering when they sang the melody and lyrics of a song with which they were familiar. Consequently, the construct of "familiarity" should be added to Wingate's formulation so that we can more completely specify the variables that are associated with the diminution of stuttering during singing.

In this experiment, familiarity was defined by the stutterer's ability to reproduce from memory the melody and lyrics of one of three songs well known to him. Such familiarity is most likely to develop with repeated practice or exposure to the songs. The fact that all of our subjects were able to correctly produce from memory the melody and lyrics of at least one test song is important. This observation strongly suggests that each of these individuals was indeed familiar with both the vocal patterns and articulatory gestures associated with the conventional lyrics of the material he sang in Condition 2. Evidently, the stutterers had repeatedly practiced, prior to the experiment, the requisite physiologic maneuvers essential for the production of the melody or words, or both, of one of the test songs. That this type of repeated motor practice could promote a decrease in stuttering should not be surprising in view of the results obtained in three earlier studies by Wingate (1966), Besozzi and Adams (1969), and Bruce (1974).

SOURCE: Healey, E. C., Mallard, A. R., & Adams, M. R. (1976). Factors contributing to the reduction of stuttering during singing. *Journal of Speech and Hearing Research, 19,* 475–480.

Results are not always clear-cut, however. Occasionally the researcher may run into puzzling results that are difficult to interpret or that may not reflect a valid measure of what the researcher sought in the original problem statement. In that case, the researcher is faced with the dilemma of trying to explain a difficult result and may need to speculate on the problem of interpretation of results and suggest future research for solving the dilemma. Excerpt 9.10, from a study of auditory speech perception of hearing-impaired children shows how the author tried to grapple with a puzzling result that accompanied a number of other, more interpretable results. Note how he has suggested several possible explanations for the result and suggested future research to clear up the issue.

EXCERPT 9.10

Experiment 2 was also designed to provide information on the perception of pitch and intonation. Subjects in the 75–89 dB HL and 90–104 dB HL groups had little difficulty identifying talker sex, but the mean score of the 105–114 dB HL group failed to reach the 1% level of significance. All subject groups performed at chance levels on the intonation subtest. There are, however, several reasons for believing that this subtest did not provide a valid measure of perceptual ability. Many of the subjects, for example, exhibited natural intonation patterns in their own speech, strongly suggesting that they had auditory access to intonation. Moreover, the ease of access shown by many subjects to the 0.6 octave difference of average fundamental frequency between the male and female talkers is inconsistent with their failure to perceive the 1.26 octave range of fundamental frequencies in the natural intonation contours. It seems probable that the poor performance of all subjects on the intonation subtest was due to their lack of experience in making conscious judgments about intonation patterns and in interpreting those patterns in terms of emotional state. It may also have been that the monotone was confusing because it is not a normal intonation pattern. The issue of the perception of intonation contours by subjects with sensorineural hearing loss clearly requires further research.

SOURCE: Boothroyd, A. (1984). Auditory perception of speech contrasts by subjects with sensorineural hearing loss. *Journal of Speech and Hearing Research, 27*, 134–144.

Relationship of Results to Previous Research

The Discussion section should relate the results of the investigation to the findings of previous research. Scientific research is a cumulative endeavor that relies on the results of many studies for a broad understanding and explanation of phenomena. One research study cannot cover sufficient territory to answer completely all of the relevant questions regarding a given topic. Therefore, it is important for a researcher to inform consumers of research about the relationship of his or her findings to other research findings in the literature.

The Discussion section should provide both completeness and accuracy of references to previous research. Completeness demands that the author be aware of the literature in the area of his or her investigation and that he or she relate the findings to as many relevant studies as possible within the space limitations of the journal article format. In some cases, reference to certain previous research may have to be omitted if the manuscript is too long, and only the most directly related articles can be covered. References to previous research findings should also be accurate. Occasionally, an author may seriously misinterpret the findings of a previous study and go awry in discussing the relationship of his or her findings to that study. If such errors go undetected, the development of knowledge on a given topic may become confusing and misleading to consumers of research.

It is important also for authors to provide an objective and balanced account of both the agreements and disagreements of their results with those of previous research. Sometimes the findings of a particular article dovetail quite nicely with previous results in the research literature. For example, the results of a study with children may show evidence of an orderly developmental trend in some behavior or characteristic when compared with the results of studies with children of other ages. On the other hand, an article may present results that are at odds with previous research. For example, a replication study may find a pattern of results different from those that have been previously reported. Or a study employing a new procedure to study a well-researched phenomenon may reveal that previous data can be obtained only with a certain procedure and that procedural changes may yield conflicting answers to the same question.

Those points on which there is agreement may provide material for the discussion of theoretical and practical implications of the research as we will see in the next section of this chapter. When there is disagreement, however, the author has a special responsibility to the readers to try to explain *why* there were disagreements between his or her results and those of previous research. For example, there might have been methodological, subject, or statistical differences between two investigations that could explain the discrepant results and such differences should be explored in the Discussion section. Often, the author may suggest avenues for future research that may help to explain why two studies show discrepant results.

Occasionally, the discussion of the relationship of results to previous research must cover some difficult and tricky territory. Subtle differences between studies must be analyzed to determine if the differences found are really meaningful or if they represent small fluctuations in human performance due to sampling or measurement errors. Also, very obvious differences between studies may involve controversial topics that promote acrimonious debates that are subject to theoretical or institutional bias. Sometimes such biases may subjectively color the discussion to the detriment of intradisciplinary or interdisciplinary communication and the advancement of scientific knowledge.

The important point is for consumers to look for an objective attitude on the part of an author who is discussing discrepancies between the results of various studies. The writer of a research article has a responsibility to readers to present a balanced and objective analysis of the discrepancies and agreements between his or her findings and the body of research in existence on a particular topic. The writer should also be certain to identify the theoretical or institutional biases in the field on *both* sides of the issue at hand to indicate the merits and demerits of *each* side in the interpretation of a cumulative body of research data. Too often in the past, a name or a school of thought has been associated with a particular theoretical inclination on a particular topic and a personal stake has been involved in the controversy over the relationship of the findings of different studies. There is no room in scientific research endeavors for a personality clash between researchers. These conflicts usually retard rather than advance the development of knowledge.

How can the reader determine if previous research has been completely and accurately referred to and if the discussion of agreements and disagreements has been fairly and objectively treated? First, consumers need to be aware of the important research that already exists on the topic covered in an article they are reading. Students and clinicians new to the field will develop this awareness over time as they read and assimilate more and more research. Second, for consumers who have questions about previous research, the best course of action is to find the references cited in the article's bibliography or reference list (that is one reason for appending a bibliography to an article) and read the original references (and the articles listed in those bibliographies) to check an author's interpretation of previous research.

The next three excerpts are taken from Discussion sections that illustrate balanced and objective approaches to the consideration of agreements and disagreements of the results with previous research results. In Excerpt 9.11 Manning and Riensche discuss the results of research on auditory assembly abilities of stuttering and nonstuttering children. The first two paragraphs indicate how their results agree with certain previous research and the next two paragraphs point out how their results disagree with previous research. Note their attempt to explain the discrepancy on the basis of subject-selection differences.

EXCERPT 9.11

The results of this investigation are in general agreement with the results of earlier studies employing these stimuli. Shriner and Daniloff (1970), Beasley and Beasley (1973), and Beasley et al. (1974) all found a significant effect for IPI similar to the one found in the present investigation. The consistency of this result provides added support for the contention that a breakdown in a child's ability to perceptually process such stimuli is likely to occur if the duration of the interphonemic interval exceeds approximately 200 msec. In the present investigation, this effect was found for both the stuttering and nonstuttering children.

Another finding consistent with the results of previous investigations was that the meaningful CVC stimuli were significantly easier to assemble than the meaningless stimuli. This result is in agreement with the previously reported performances of normal first- and third-grade children (Shriner & Daniloff, 1970), normal-speaking black and white children (Beasley & Beasley, 1973), and both normal and misarticulating children (Beasley et al., 1974). Apparently the children were able to apply stored semantic rules to aid in the perceptual processing of the meaningful stimuli while such rules were of minimal assistance when applied to the nonmeaningful stimuli. Again, both the stuttering and nonstuttering children performed in a similar manner on this factor.

The findings of this investigation indicate that the auditory processing skills of stutterers are similar to those of nonstutterers when there is appropriate control for relevant stimulus and subject variables. The present results, therefore, do not lend support to previous research which indicates that stutterers exhibit difficulties with certain auditory processing tasks. Shriner and Daniloff (1970) have suggested that the auditory task used in the present investigation involves short-term memory as well as competence and performance aspects of a child's language. To the degree that this task reflects these functions, stutterers appear to be similar to nonstutterers in their auditory abilities.

The finding of Williams and Marks (1972) that stutterers perform less well than normal-speaking children on auditory-vocal tasks was not supported by the stutterers' performance in the present investigation. A possible explanation for the relatively poor performance by Williams and Marks' subjects may lie in the selection process used to choose stuttering subjects for their study (nonstuttering subjects were not used in the investigation). While Williams and Marks stated that their subjects had "adequate articulation," their use of the Templin-Darley Screening Test of Articulation (1969) to screen their subjects may have resulted in some misarticulating children being included in their study. That is, since the age of the subjects in their study ranged from five years, three months to nine years, six months and the age norms of the Templin-Darley Screening Test permit specified misarticulations through age eight, it appears likely that several of the stuttering subjects used by Williams and Marks may have been children with one or more misarticulations. Beasley et al. (1974) found that misarticulating children performed significantly poorer than their normal-speaking counterparts in their ability to assemble meaningful CVC stimuli. Thus, the performance of any of Williams and Marks' subjects who also had misarticulations would possibly account for the poor performance of their stuttering subjects on auditory-vocal subtests of the ITPA.

SOURCE: Manning, W. H., & Riensche, L. (1976). Auditory assembly abilities of stuttering and nonstuttering children. *Journal of Speech and Hearing Research, 19,* 777–783.

Excerpt 9.12 is from the same study of visual evoked-response correlates of speechreading that was used in Excerpt 9.7. Both agreements and disagreements with previous research are discussed in a balanced and objective fashion and the authors speculated that the disagreements might have been at least partially due to subject or method differences. The authors also pointed out that the discrepancies between their results and previous findings indicate the need for more research before clinical applications should be considered.

Excerpt 9.13 illustrates an extended effort to compare the results of a study of tympanometric estimates of ear canal volume to previously published

---

EXCERPT 9.12

DISCUSSION

The relationship between VN130 latency and speechreading scores reported by Shepherd et al. (1977) appears to be a fundamentally replicable effect. This is supported both by the significant negative correlations we obtained and by the existence of two latency sensitive, objectively derived principal components which contributed to the prediction of speechreading scores. However, the correlations we obtained were significantly weaker than those of Shepherd et al. It is unclear whether this discrepancy is due to subject differences or to minor methodological differences, such as the size of the monitor used to present the speechreading test. Nevertheless, the failure of the latency-speechreading relationship to achieve the strength of prediction reported by Shepherd et al. should serve as a caveat to clinicians and researchers interested in the immediate clinical application of VN130 measurement. Further research is necessary to evaluate the generality of this relationship.

SOURCE: Samar, V. J., & Sims, D. G. (1983). Visual evoked-response correlates of speechreading performance in normal-hearing adults: A replication and factor analytic extension. *Journal of Speech and Hearing Research, 26,* 2–9.

EXCERPT 9.13

In summary, the data in Figure 3 show that different tympanometric estimates of ear canal volume produced admittance values at 0 daPa ranging from .804 acoustic mmhos (1312 acoustic ohms) to .484 acoustic mmhos (2187 acoustic ohms) for the 220-Hz probe tone and from 2.473 acoustic mmhos (461 acoustic ohms) to 1.750 acoustic mmhos (691 acoustic ohms) for the 660-Hz probe tone. For identical conditions encountered in the plane of the tympanic membrane, a difference in the assumptions made regarding the immittance characteristics of the ear canal volume produced a difference in the calculated admittance of 40% (impedance of 67%) at 220 Hz and of 29% (impedance of 50%) at 660 Hz.

As the data in Figure 3 demonstrate, static immittance values corrected to the plane of the tympanic membrane will vary substantially depending on whether the values are calculated at 0 daPa or at MAX and on the assumptions made regarding the immittance characteristics of the ear canal volume. These procedural and computational differences across studies make a direct comparison of admittance values with previous data difficult. In addition, most clinically available instruments measure only the magnitude of immittance and express this value in terms of an equivalent volume of air, which is dependent on altitude and barometric pressure (Lilly, 1973; Van Camp et al., 1976; Wiley & Block, 1979). The present admittance data, however, were directly comparable with data presented by Porter and Winston (1973) and by Margolis and Smith (1977). These investigators clearly specified the measurement and computational procedures used in their respective studies. Table 4 shows the mean and standard deviations (in parentheses) for conductance and susceptance (in acoustic mmhos) at 220 Hz and at 660 Hz obtained in these two studies compared with the results obtained in the present study. In all studies, ear canal volume was estimated from the tympanograms at high negative ear canal pressures (−200 to −400 daPa); ear canal conductance was assumed to be greater than 0 acoustic mmhos. The data from the three studies are in agreement,

TABLE 4. THE MEANS (STANDARD DEVIATIONS) FOR THE MAXIMUM CONDUCTANCE (*Cond*) AND SUSCEPTANCE (*Susc*) VALUES (IN ACOUSTIC MMHOS) AT 220 Hz AND AT 660 Hz REPORTED IN THREE INVESTIGATIONS. THE NUMBER OF SUBJECTS AND THE EAR CANAL PRESSURE USED FOR THE TYMPANOMETRIC ESTIMATE OF EAR CANAL VOLUME IN EACH INVESTIGATION ARE SHOWN IN PARENTHESES

Investigation	220-Hz Probe		660-Hz Probe	
	Cond	Susc	Cond	Susc
Porter & Winston (1973) (n = 16; −200 daPa)	.40 (.19)	.78 (.31)	2.41 (1.59)	1.62 (.51)
Margolis & Smith (1977) (n = 17; −300 daPa)	.30 (.12)	.73 (.27)	2.11 (1.33)	1.58 (.54)
Present investigation (n = 8; −400 daPa)	.31 (.16)	.80 (.35)	2.13 (1.46)	1.67 (.38)

although the susceptance values corrected to the plane of the tympanic membrane in this study are slightly larger than those reported in the other two studies. This difference is understandable when one considers the ear canal pressure used to estimate the ear canal volume. The ear canal pressure used in the current study was −400 daPa, which produces a slightly smaller ear canal volume estimate than would be obtained at −200 daPa (Porter & Winston, 1973) or at −300 daPa (Margolis & Smith, 1977).

Static admittance then was recalculated both at 0 daPa and at MAX using the recommended procedure to correct for the immittance characteristics of the ear canal volume. Table 5 shows the results of these calculations expressed in admittance and in impedance in both rectangular and polar notations. Ear canal volume was estimated from the 660-Hz susceptance tympanograms at an ear canal pressure of −400 daPa. This susceptance value divided by 3 was used to correct the 220-Hz data to the plane of the tympanic membrane. For both probe frequencies, ear canal conductance was assumed to equal 0 acoustic mmhos. Comparing these data with those in Table 4 again shows the importance of specifying the procedure used to correct for ear canal volume. Failure to do so undoubtedly has contributed to the variability in static immittance values reported in the literature.

TABLE 5. STATIC IMMITTANCE FOR 220-Hz AND 660-Hz PROBE TONES CALCULATED AT 0 daPa AND AT MAX USING THE RECOMMENDED PROCEDURE (−400 daPa at 660 Hz) TO CORRECT FOR THE IMMITTANCE CHARACTERISTICS OF THE EAR CANAL VOLUME. STATIC VALUES ARE EXPRESSED IN ADMITTANCE AND IMPEDANCE BOTH IN RECTANGULAR AND POLAR NOTATION.

	220-Hz Probe		660-Hz Probe	
Static Values	MAX	0 daPa	MAX	0 daPa
Admittance (acoustic mmhos)				
G_a	.36 (.15)	.27 (.06)	2.53 (1.59)	1.88 (.71)
jB_a	.93 (.37)	.75 (.18)	1.67 (.38)	1.54 (.37)
Y_a	.99 (.40)	.80 (.18)	3.09 (1.51)	2.45 (.74)
e	68.70 (3.12)	69.82 (3.87)	37.88 (11.31)	41.17 (8.54)
Impedance (acoustic ohms)				
R_a	407 (142)	456 (149)	289 (99)	326 (92)
$-jX_a$	1042 (329)	1235 (354)	260 (172)	313 (198)
Z_a	1121 (353)	1320 (374)	394 (186)	458 (205)
−e	69 (3)	70 (4)	38 (11)	41 (9)

SOURCE: Shanks, J. E., & Lilly, D. J. (1981). An evaluation of tympanometric estimates of ear canal volume. *Journal of Speech and Hearing Research, 24,* 557–566.

data. The first paragraph summarizes the influence of different measurement procedures and calculations on resulting admittance values. In the next paragraph, the authors point out the difficulties that procedural and computational differences cause in trying to compare the results of different studies and indicate that their data will only be compared with the data of two previous studies that were directly comparable regarding measurement and computational procedures. The data of the three studies are compared in the excerpt's Table 4; in addition, the recalculated data in the excerpt's Table 5 are compared to the Table 4 data. Note the last two sentences in the excerpt caution readers regarding specification of procedures when comparing values among studies in the literature.

Theoretical Implications of the Research

It is important for the author of a research article to articulate clearly the theoretical implications of the findings that are reported. Otherwise, the research article becomes nothing more than the sterile reporting of isolated facts without regard to past and current thinking in the field. In our last section, we discussed the relationship of the results to previous research. The theoretical implications of the results are closely tied to this relationship because the results of a single article are often juxtaposed with those of previous research to form the nomothetic network developed for any particular topic.

Implications may be drawn regarding the validity of a previously stated theory. Research results of a particular article may be supportive of an existing theory and further support may be gleaned from the agreement of that research article with previous research. Through the accumulation of more data in agreement with the predictions made by a particular theory, the theory gradually develops more plausibility as a valid explanation of the phenomenon under study. On the other hand, results of a particular study (and, possibly, other previous research) may be in disagreement with a particular theory. In such a case, the theory may need revision to account for discrepancies between the predictions made by the theory and the empirical evidence. In fact, so many data in disagreement with the theory may accumulate over the years that a theory may eventually be discarded because of its failure to find empirical support.

Theoretical implications are not limited to the discussion of previous theories in light of the data of a research article. The author may take the public opportunity to generate a new theory or to modify an old one so radically that it would no longer be recognizable in its revised form as a relative of the old theory. The data of a new article may be so provocative as to require new and original thinking for the explanation of the phenomenon under study. Readers will recall that two types of theory were mentioned in Chapter 1: those that are advanced before research is executed and await empirical confirmation and those that synthesize the existent empirical data.

Both types of theory may be entertained in the Discussion and Conclusions section when the theoretical implications of the research are discussed.

Where can the reader expect to find the discussion of the theoretical implications in the research article? This depends on the style of the particular author. Some authors prefer to combine the discussion of the relationship of results to previous research with the discussion of theoretical implications at the beginning of the Conclusions section. This makes particular sense if the results of a particular investigation are to be combined with those of previous research in commenting on a theory. Others prefer to separate the discussion of theoretical implications from the discussion of relationship of results to previous research. Some authors even give considerable attention to theoretical issues in the introduction, literature review, or rationale before reporting data and refer back to this material in the theoretical implications portion of the conclusion. The important point is that the author needs to lend theoretical perspective to the empirical data and to articulate the theoretical implications of his or her findings so that readers understand where the research fits in the nomothetic network regarding the particular topic.

Excerpts 9.14 and 9.15 present examples from two Discussion sections that illustrate two of the many ways in which theoretical implications of the results of a study may be discussed. The first excerpt is taken from an article on divergent semantic behavior in aphasia. The authors point out that their results support a theoretical model that had been previously neglected in aphasia research and therapy. They also mention the relationship of the neglected model to other theoretical models. The next illustration, excerpted from a discussion of the results of research on lipreading, presents a different kind of theoretical discussion. Here Erber and McMahan attempted to identify factors that might explain the pattern of their results. Perhaps further research may identify a combination of factors sufficient to explain and predict lipreading performance under a number of conditions so that a comprehensive theoretical model of lipreading may evolve.

EXCERPT 9.14

Traditional test of aphasia have typically involved one type of thought process, a convergent semantic thought process. Similarly, therapeutic models, defined on the basis of these traditional diagnostic models, have focused on the facilitation of highly organized, systematically stored, and knowledge-oriented responses, that is, convergent semantic responses.

The findings of the present study, however, support the existence of the divergent mental operation proposed by Guilford and indicate that persons with aphasia are impaired in their ability to generate semantic responses under this operation. This suggests that traditional definitions of aphasia and the diagnostic and therapeutic models which have been formulated on the basis of these definitions may have been too narrow. The definition of the aphasic impairment should be broadened to include a divergent as well as a convergent component. Specifically, aphasia should be redefined as an inability to generate a number and a variety of logical semantic alternatives to given information as well as an inability to converge upon semantic (lexical and syntactic) final products.

The results of the present study also lend strong support to the "propositional model" by Hughlings Jackson (1915), the "Abstract-Concrete Model" by Kurt Goldstein (1948), and the "Thought Process Model" by Joseph Wepman (1972). These models are concerned with the inability of aphasics to use propositional language, to express a number and a variety of different relationships, and to embellish ideas within a topic. Such models, interpreted in light of Guilford's research, show that there is a divergent component to the language impairment in aphasia.

SOURCE: Chapey, R., Rigrodsky, S., & Morrison, E. B. (1976). Divergent semantic behavior in aphasia. *Journal of Speech and Hearing Research, 19,* 664–677.

EXCERPT 9.15

Several factors may account for the difficulty demonstrated by deaf children in visual recognition of words when they occur in sentences. First, it is likely that the placement of a word within a list of other words creates "segmentation" problems for the lipreader. That is, coarticulation effects may make it difficult for the lipreader to specify word boundaries. In addition, coarticulation with segments of adjoining words, may modify the appearance of the key word and interfere with its recognition (Alich, 1967; Berger, 1972). It would seem that ordering this list according to a set of rules (as in a sentence) would aid the observer in the identification of constituent words. That is, the syntactic and semantic redundancy of language should help the observer to resolve ambiguities and to fill gaps in the perceived signal (Jeffers & Barley, 1971). In fact, this effect has been demonstrated clearly for normal-hearing adults in the classic auditory study of Miller et al. (1951). But many of the important word-segmentation cues that are available to the listener in an auditory task are carried by the prosody of the stimulus sentences (for example, syllable stress, intonation contour, and so on), and this sort of information is not normally apparent to the lipreader unless he is able to receive it through a hearing aid. Instead, in order to segment words, the lipreader must rely on vision for perception of articulatory rhythm and word prominence as well as refer to his knowledge of probable word sequences. These strategies appear to suffice for many experienced lipreaders.

Unfortunately, the linguistic organization of a sentence cannot help a lipreader to identify constituent words unless he has sufficient knowledge of typical language patterns to make use of this information. For example, to a deaf child with an adequate vocabulary but with an incomplete knowledge of language structure, a sentence may be perceived as a series of (stressed) words separated by nonspecific articulatory movements. To a younger child who does not yet understand what words are, the sentence may be perceived as a sequence of articulatory movements only.

For the children in this study, words were visually more intelligible in isolation than were the same words presented in sentence context. Except when animate nouns appeared in initial (subject) position, these children apparently were unable to fully use the syntactic and semantic redundancy of the stimulus sentences as an aid to recognition of words in a series. That is, the potentially negative effect of placing a word in a list may have offset the potentially positive effect of placing that word in a sentence (a list ordered by rules). The subjects did identify animate and inanimate nouns differently in sentences. Evidently, these children have sufficient knowledge of word probabilities to know that it is more likely for animate rather than inanimate nouns to be used as subjects in sentences with transitive verbs. That is, they apparently anticipate the occurrence of animate nouns in initial positions. Informal observations suggest that this type of sentence construction is commonly used by teachers and is one of the earliest forms introduced in the classroom.

SOURCE: Erber, N. P., & McMahan, D. A. (1976). Effects of sentence context on recognition of words through lipreading by deaf children. *Journal of Speech and Hearing Research, 19,* 112–119.

Excerpt 9.16 is an extended example of a thorough discussion of the theoretical implications of a cineflourographic study of kinematic aspects of speech during stuttering adaptation. The rather lengthly excerpt is included because it illustrates so well the schemapiric interplay of theory and data. The first part of the discussion concerns the negative impact of these data on previous theory and offers reasons why the previous theory may have been incorrect. An alternative explanation is then offered which may account for the data of the article and predictions are made from the alternative explanation that can be tested with future research. It is interesting to note that the original speculations that were not supported by the data of this article were put forth by one of the authors, yet he was able to criticize his own previous hypothesis in light of his new data and embark on a different path of reasoning. Good science demands this kind of candor in examining the relation between theory and data for the advancement of knowledge in any field and this example is a paragon of scientific excellence.

EXCERPT 9.16

DISCUSSION

These results show that practice may have certain effects on the kinematic parameters of the articulators as practice with a manual task has on limb kinematics. Specifically, practice, at least initially, seems to be associated with an increased velocity of the articulators. For both nonstutterers and stutterers the most consistent change was the increase in the peak velocities of the tongue tip between Trials 1 and 2—four of the five subjects showed increased velocities for this gesture.

The results, however, indicate clearly that the speculations of Zimmermann (1980c) and Zimmermann et al., 1981) are not supported. That is, the hypothesis that decreased velocities and displacements and increased movement duration are necessary conditions for fluency enhancement does not hold. The results show that the adaptation effect does not directly depend on a particular pattern, though an increased velocity of the tongue tip between Trials 1 and 2 seems to be a relatively consistent finding.

The hypothesis that the specific changes in the kinematics (velocity, displacement, and transition time) are necessary conditions for fluency in stutterers may have been, from the onset, naive. As mentioned, the speculations arose from the kinematic descriptions reported by Zimmermann (1980a, 1980c) and the premise that kinematic differences between stutterers and nonstutterers may be related to a compensatory sensory-motor strategy for aberrantly tuned pathways. The underlying premise was that movements of lower velocities, decreased displacements, and longer durations would have fewer and less disruptive afferent effects on the speech output process. Though our results do not disprove this position, they make the speculations less feasible.

The speculations of Zimmermann (1980a, 1980c) may have suffered from the implicit assignment of causal status to the surface (kinematic) descriptors of a system. Rather than viewing these descriptors as controlled variables (somehow represented and controlled in the brain), it may be more appropriate to view these parameters as "emergent qualities" of the speech production system, or the result of underlying control processes. This distinction arises from a dynamic perspective on movement systems rather than a model in which each parameter for each movement is programmed (Kelso, in press; Kelso, Holt, Kugler, & Turvey, 1980; Kugler, Kelso, & Turvey, 1980).[3] Hence, to afford causal status to these descriptors may have been a critical error. What level of analysis, then, can be used to understand better the principles of motor systems which must be related to the adaptation effect?

A Dynamic Perspective

A dynamic perspective on movement control has been developed that does not assume that the products of motor function are isomorphic with the underlying processes from which those products derived. Thus, as Kelso et al. (1980) pointed out, the surface (kinematic) descriptors do not attain ontological status. It is not necessary to assign causal status to kinematic descriptors; instead, the surface descriptors can be viewed as an a posteriori fact of the system and not as an a priori reference signal coded and stored in the brain and imposed on the system. In other words, the spatial-temporal organization is the result of the physical processes involved in movement control. A discussion of these principles is found in Werner (1977) and is reiterated in relation to movement control systems by Kugler et al. (1980).

The critical point to be made regarding the data presented is that a different approach toward stuttering and the control of movement may change the initial hypothesis. More heuristically valuable hypotheses may be developed by viewing stuttering—and speech in general—in terms of a physical analogue. This

---

[3]Much of the following discussion arose from discussions with J. A. Scott Kelso.

account of movement suggests that the final position of a limb, or other structure, is determined by the dynamic parameters of the system. While we observe the kinematic consequence of movement, the kinematic details are merely consequences of the system's dynamics and are determined by those dynamics (Fitch & Turvey, 1978; Kelso, 1981; Kugler et al., 1980).

Mass spring analogues of limb movements have been helpful in conceptualizing movement processes (Fel'dman, 1980; Kelso, Holt, & Flatt, 1980; Polit & Bizzi, 1978). If the articulators are viewed as a mass-spring system, certain predictions about the effect of fluency-enhancing conditions on movement arise. Zimmermann et al. (1981) suggested that stuttering behavior may be related to a variable background activity, tonic muscle action in the muscles involved in speech. Variable background activity in the muscles involved in speech may be depicted as continuous variation of the stiffness of a spring in a mass-spring system. Instantaneous velocities may be affected directly by variations in spring (muscle) stiffness.[4] If it is suspected that the adaptation effect is associated with a decrease in the magnitude and variability of tonic muscular activity, then one would predict that the variability of instantaneous velocities would decrease from Reading 1 to Reading 2. All three stutterers reduced the variability of the instantaneous velocities between Trials 1 and 2, whereas one of the nonstutterers remained the same while the other increased variability.

This directional change is consistent with the hypothesis that fluency enhancement in an adaptation procedure may be associated with the stabilization of background activity in the speech musculature. Furthermore, the data suggest that the oscillatory model approach may have at least heuristic value in the investigation of speech and its pathologies.

The data and the inferences from this post hoc analysis are consistent with hypotheses about the processes underlying the adaptation effect. The stabilization of background activity in the muscles of the articulators may be associated with a decrease in arousal. Thus, the kinematic variable that may be most appropriate for indexing psychophysiological factors (Wingate, 1966) may be that which indexes variations in tonic background activity of the muscles. The association between muscle activity and arousal makes this perspective compelling for accounting for the fluency enhancement in stutterers. That the reduction in the variability in instantaneous velocities is most consistent between Trials 1 and 2 agrees with the long-held belief that the greatest reduction in arousal occurs between Trials 1 and 2 in the adaptation procedure.

Practice also may play a role in the changes in motor organization that take place in the adaptation procedure. The increase in the velocity of the tongue tip for four of the five subjects between Trials 1 and 2 is consistent with the finding of Landa (in press), who studied the effects of practice on kinematic parameters in learning a simple manual task. Landa also found that the velocity of movement consistently increased with practice on this task.

That only the stutterers show a consistent reduction in the variability of instantaneous velocities may suggest differences in the processes underlying

---

[4]*Instantaneous velocity* refers to the velocity of movement between two points on the displacement-by-time graphs. These points are 10 msec apart at the filming speed of 100 fps. The mean is calculated by summing the instantaneous velocities between each pair of points and dividing by the number of pairs in the utterance /cæt/.

the adaptation effect in stutterers and nonstutterers. The adaptation effect in stutterers may be associated with (a) the stabilization of tonic muscle activity, which may be associated with a decrease in arousal, and (b) the effects of practice. For the nonstutterers, however, the most important variables may be the kinematic reorganizations associated with practice rather than the stabilization of tonic activity, that is, a reduction in arousal.

It may be misleading to suggest an "either/or" situation. Instead, the appropriate question can be phrased in terms of how much each of these variables accounts for the adaptation effect in any given subject. The most valuable perspective may be to view practice and arousal reduction as interacting or overlapping processes considered in terms of their relative weightings in a formula that may predict the outcome of an adaptation procedure. Stutterers and nonstutterers may simply fall on opposite ends of the continuum of values for the arousal coefficient.

The issue of relevant factors (e.g., psychomotor vs. motor-linguistic) in the adaptation process may be reduced to two questions suggested by Zimmermann et al. (1981): (a) How are inputs to motoneuron pools changed? and (b) What are the direct and indirect events leading to these changes? While each process must manifest its influence on the motoneuron pools associated with the muscles involved in speech, changes associated with practice and with arousal may be differentiable in terms of their effects on the pattern of muscle activity (at the motor unit level) and in terms of the variables affecting the different patterns.

It may be predicted then that stutterers and nonstutterers will show differences in the patterns of change in the motor unit behavior of speech muscles between Trials 1 and 2. The patterns for the nonstutterers would be associated with changes more connected with practice (i.e., changes in the patterning of phasic units) than with changes in arousal (fewer changes in the behaviors of small tonic motor units). The motor unit patterns of stutterers, on the other hand, would be associated with changes in both. Such speculations are open to empirical test.

SOURCE: Zimmermann, G. N., & Hanley, J. M. (1983). A cineflourographic investigation of repeated fluent productions of stutterers in an adaptation procedure. *Journal of Speech and Hearing Research, 26,* 35–42.

Practical Implications of the Research

In addition to the consideration of theoretical implications, the discussion and conclusions often address the question of practical implications of the results. As we mentioned earlier, it is often difficult to draw a true dichotomy between purely basic and applied research. Rather, there is usually a continuum along which research may fall with regard to its basic or applied orientation and with regard to whether practical implications are immediate or further off in the future. What some may consider to be pure research today may, surprisingly, turn out to have a practical implication tomorrow. The transistor, for example, was developed by scientists engaged in basic research in physics rather than by an inventor whose primary goal was to patent an invention for immediate sale.

In some cases an author may have no immediate practical application in mind as the research may have been more basic in its orientation or because applied considerations may have been reserved by the author until the accumulation of sufficient research to make judicious practical decisions. In such a case, the author may eschew the opportunity to discuss practical application if it is believed that such premature speculation would be unjustified or would be misconstrued by readers. On the other hand, the author might speculate about practical implications if he or she believed that appropriately cautioned speculation could be justified. For instance, the author might hope that this speculation would provoke readers with more practical inclinations to read his or her research or, perhaps, to begin applied research of their own. Readers should be careful to discern that such speculation is accomplished in a prudent and reasonable fashion. Some authors have become enmeshed in what is sometimes referred to as a "boilerplate problem," that is, the attachment of an uninteresting research problem to a "hot" topic in order to generate excitement when, in fact, the research is not relevant to the "hot" topic. Government and philanthropic agencies originated the term "boilerplate problem" to characterize research proposals that were obviously designed to secure grant money for research that was actually irrelevant to a granting agency's goals by attaching the irrelevant research to a "hot" topic on the agency's list. Consumers of research should also be wary of inflated practical implications that are no more than stretches of an overzealous author's imagination and to discriminate these from more genuine possibilities for future practical application. Consumers should also be cognizant of the need for patience in the anticipation of future practical applications when more research is necessary before a particular concept can be applied clinically in an ethical and professional manner.

Some research is undertaken with more immediate practical goals in mind and the author then has a special responsibility to delineate for the audience the implications of the research for assessment and management of communication disorders. General suggestions for clinical practice may be offered in a few sentences or the author may feel that a more thorough didactic presentation is necessary. Sometimes the author may even write a separate article on the clinical implications of the research, especially at the culmination of a series of related research articles on a particular topic.

Direct practical application of the results of research should be advocated only when the accumulated research has demonstrated the reliability and validity of techniques for assessment and management of communication disorders. In addition, the limitations of these techniques should be delineated in appropriate caveats to the readers. Unfortunately, some techniques have fallen into disfavor and been abandoned because practical applications were proffered before sufficient research was completed to ensure clinical success. In such cases, researchers may have suggested clinical application before they had collected sufficient data to warrant immediate use, or clinicians may have attempted to apply techniques that research had not yet confirmed as suitable for clinical use. In some cases *both* researchers and clinicians may have been guilty of overzealous and premature application of inchoate techniques that were destined to fail without extensive research into their proper development. Therefore, it is imperative for both producers and consumers of research to be aware of the limitations inherent in any technique and of the need for cautious clinical application during the development of new techniques.

The next four excerpts, taken from Discussion sections, illustrate the reasonable and cautious discussion of practical implications of research. Excerpt 9.17 contains the paragraphs that immediately follow the material shown in Excerpt 9.15 from the study by Erber and McMahan on contextual factors in lipreading. Note how logically the practical implications discussed in Excerpt 9.17 follow from the theoretical discussion shown in Excerpt 9.15. This is a good example of the unity that should be found in the various parts of a Discussion section and of the interplay between basic and applied considerations in research.

EXCERPT 9.17

A frequent activity of teachers of deaf children is the introduction of new vocabulary. It would be valuable for teachers to know the best linguistic context in which to place a new word for optimal comprehension through auditory or visual modalities. The results of this study indicate that words in isolation may be visually more intelligible to deaf children than are words in sentences. Thus, to increase a child's visual identification of an important word, a teacher should isolate the word while pairing it with the associated object or activity. For example, the teacher might say, "Ball!" (points to ball) "Throw the ball to me!" or alternately, "Throw the *ball* to me!," emphasizing the word *ball* to effectively isolate it from the other words in the sentence. Teachers have been observed to use techniques of this sort in their oral communication with deaf children (Erber & Greer, 1973). Yet, to increase a child's knowledge of the way in which words are joined to form sentences, and to familiarize him with the patterns of language, a teacher also should try to use connected discourse during oral communication with her pupils (Simmons 1964, 1966). Perhaps the best strategy is a compromise approach directed to both vocabulary growth and language development. This sort of orientation would include both the use of single words to label objects and events and also the use of sentences to describe the relation between language and the child's experience.

Sentence-recognition tests commonly are used to evaluate lipreading performance (see Jeffers & Barley, 1971). These tests are valid in the sense that the stimuli are similar to those which normally are received in conversation, and they are useful for obtaining a general impression of a child's lipreading ability. In our experience with this testing format, however, the sentence errors of some deaf children have varied in unusual ways, and neither main idea, correct syntax, nor number of words correct have been found to be completely appropriate criteria for scoring the written responses. In some cases, the scorers have found it difficult to specify the perceptual or linguistic nature of the error, and interjudge agreement occasionally has been poor.

A test of key-word recognition, such as the one used in this study, samples a deaf child's ability to extract information from sentences while avoiding most of the difficulties in scoring whole-sentence responses. Figure 2a, b indicates that teachers' ratings of a child's general lipreading performance are related much more closely to the child's recognition of words in sentences than to his recognition of isolated words, although the recognition scores generally are higher for isolated words. Therefore, it appears that a test which requires recognition of important (key) words in sentence context would be suitable for the assessment of lipreading performance of deaf children.

The key-word approach to lipreading evaluation is clinically feasible and has diagnostic potential. This testing format could be used to examine the relation between lipreading proficiency and certain characteristics of stimulus sentences. For example, a child may demonstrate an inability to identify key nouns in sentences longer than 10 syllables. A clinician could use this sort of information to diagnose a child's lipreading problems and to construct practice materials to help the child overcome his communication difficulties.

SOURCE: Erber, N. P., & McMahan, D. A. (1976). Effects of sentence context on recognition of words through lipreading by deaf children. *Journal of Speech and Hearing Research, 19,* 112–119.

Excerpt 9.18 is from the Discussion section of an article by Dever on morphological testing with retarded children. The results of that study had cast some doubt on the criterion validity of various measures of retarded children's use of morphemes. This excerpt includes judicious cautions regarding the use of such measures and suggests some possible practical improvements in testing to be examined in future research.

EXCERPT 9.18

It thus appears that whether nonsense syllables or real words are used as stimuli, the prediction of correct or incorrect free speech forms was not accomplished for educable mentally retarded children using the revised version of Berko's test of morphology. Therefore, the use of the test paradigm itself is questionable as a diagnostic indicator of the ability of EMR children to use the tested forms. This has important implications for the use of Berko's test as well as both the AVA subtest of the ITPA and the PTEI among retarded children as diagnostic tests of language development.

An additional word of caution concerning the possible uses to which the paradigm can be put is in order. Extreme care should be taken in making statements about what children "know" of English morphology (cf. Berko, 1958), "use of grammar" (cf. Bateman, 1967), and similar statements when they are based on the results of this test or any test using the paradigm. There are two reasons for this: (1) since the paradigm has been found, in the present experiment, not to reflect the use of the tested morphological forms in the free speech of retarded children, the same could well be true of normal children; and (2) inflectional morphology is such a minor aspect of a grammar of English, that, even had the test proven to be a good indicator of the items tested in the present experiment, the statements about the use of grammar would be overstepping the limits of generalization possibilities.

There is one remaining question: is it possible to devise an adequate way of testing for development of inflectional forms? Subjectively, it appears to the present author that one way may have been demonstrated in the present experiment. That is, in the process of obtaining the samples of free speech, an experimenter noticed that certain forms did not seem to be occurring in the first round of data-gathering. On the second round, an attempt was made to elicit these forms. The situation, although a free speech situation, closely paralleled the test paradigm in some respects. The major differences were the following: (1) the children probably perceived the situation differently from the test situation, (2) no pictures or objects were used during elicitation, (3) if one stimulus word did not appear to be working for a subject, a different one was tried, for example, the experimenter used a list of words rather than just one word, and flexibility was the keynote. The words used were quite common, such as *horse, lumpy*, etc., and (4) an attempt was made to get the subject to respond with the desired form by making conversation about the words, not by using a hard and fast paradigm. The conversation often came close to the test paradigm, for example, if a plural was the desired response, the experimenter tried to get the subject to talk about "more than one of them." This method appeared to be quite successful; in all cases in which it was used, the method produced scores which were higher than the test scores. Unfortunately, it is possible that not everybody could use such a method, because the tester's role needs to be such a flexible one, and flexibility does not make for standardization of procedure. In addition, we are still left with the problem of what happens if the form is not elicited because a nonresponse is still uninterpretable. Perhaps a way could be found to standardize such a procedure; only further experimentation could provide the answers which are needed.

SOURCE: Dever, R. B. (1972). A comparison of the results of a revised version of Berko's test of morphology with the free speech of mentally retarded children. *Journal of Speech and Hearing Research, 15*, 169–178.

Excerpt 9.19 is from a study of frequency variation within ANSI tolerance values on clinical auditory threshold measures. The author first briefly summarizes the results, then refers to previous research on calibration, presents examples of potential clinical problems in threshold measurement in light of the results, and refers to literature on threshold differences for different signals. Finally, he outlines both long-term and short-term solutions to improvement of measurement procedures. The long-term, and more far-reaching solution would be the reconsideration of frequency calibration tolerance by ANSI. The short-term solution of monitoring frequency and reporting actual outputs is discussed in the last paragraph. This article is a good example of the direct practical application of research results with an interim suggestion for clinicians to implement immediately and a more long-range suggestion for a standards group to reconsider the use of our current standard.

EXCERPT 9.19

DISCUSSION

Results of this study indicate that obtained estimates of auditory threshold for persons with some loss of hearing will vary depending upon actual frequency output within ANSI (1969) tolerance limits. This threshold variability may be as great as 20 dB, and both the probability and magnitude of these differences generally increase with frequency. This source of threshold variability can be expected to add to variability resulting from differences in earphone placement, manner of stimulus presentation, instructions to the client, and psychological factors. It will also interact with variability in sound pressure level output among audiometers within ANSI (1969) intensity tolerances, at times increasing variability resulting in threshold differences of up to 30 dB being obtained between audiometers, and at times counterbalancing the variability of intensity. This interaction effect will depend upon actual frequency and intensity output relationships of audiometers and the nature of an individual's hearing loss.

The above is based upon the assumption that the audiometers used are in fact calibrated within ANSI (1969) tolerances. It has been well substantiated that this is not always the case. In a survey of audiometers used in an industrial hearing conservation program, Pfieffer (1980) found 29.6% of his 128 audiometers were out of calibration in intensity output, and 8.4% exceeded frequency tolerances. Eagles and Doerfler (1961b) performed monthly calibration checks on six audiometers used to assess auditory threshold for school children. Their data indicate a 35.7% incidence of intensity output exceeding tolerances and a 6.3% incidence of frequency variations beyond tolerance values. The tolerance values used in this study were ± 5% for frequency and ± 4 dB at frequencies of 2 k Hz and below, and ± 5 dB at frequencies above 2 k Hz for intensity as per ASA (1951) recommendations. In a comprehensive study of the working condition of 100 audiometers from a variety of audiometric settings, Thomas et al. (1969) found 89% to exceed the ASA (1951) tolerance values for intensity and 31% to exceed the ± 5% tolerance values for frequency variability. The assumption that audiometers in use are in fact within calibration tolerance values is indeed optimistic.

The potential variability in clinically determined threshold attributable to frequency variations is larger than that due to intensity output variations. Also, unlike intensity output variations, it cannot be predicted from calibration data alone and subsequently eliminated via a correction factor, since it is extremely variable from person to person. When a large difference in results obtained on different audiometers is found, we may determine the probability of frequency output differences as a contributing factor if the actual frequency outputs of the audiometers are known. As indicated in Table 4, the direction of differences is quite predictable and therefore threshold differences between audiometers which are attributable to frequency variability should fit the frequency configuration of an individual's audiogram.

As an example, if we were to find that thresholds obtained at an actual frequency of 4100 Hz on one audiometer were 15 dB worse than those obtained earlier on another audiometer at an actual frequency output of 3900 Hz we must determine whether this threshold difference is due to deteriorating hearing or to artifact. If the individual in question were to present with an audiometric configuration sloping steeply between 3 k Hz and 6 k Hz we may be confident that the output frequency differences between the two audiometers has contributed to the threshold difference. If, on the other hand, the person's audiometric configuration is not consistent with the direction or degree of the threshold difference, we may suspect that loss of hearing has progressed, or that artifact of a different type has had an effect in one of the testing situations. As large scale analysis of audiograms becomes more common as in industrial audiometry and centralized processing of compensation claims, identification of comparison audiograms in which respective frequency outputs of audiometers used may well be a factor could be programmed into computer analysis. The requisite for such a procedure is that actual frequency output at each frequency setting for each audiometer be known and reported.

The magnitude of differences within the frequency triads tested and the tendency of differences to increase in magnitude with frequency in these subjects agree quite well with differences in threshold between pure tone, warble tone, and noise stimuli reported in the literature (Orchik & Mosher, 1975; Stephens & Rintelman, 1978; Orchik & Rintelman, 1978). Orchik and Mosher (1975), for instance, found average differences in obtained audiometric threshold of 31 dB when 2 k Hz pure tones and a narrow band of noise centered a 2k Hz with a 10 dB/octave rejection rate were used as stimuli. The noise stimulus yielded the better threshold values for the nine children with sharply sloping audiometric configuration used as subjects.

Stephens and Rintelman (1978) found average differences of from .6 to 1.9 dB across frequencies tested in thresholds obtained with pure tones and 3% frequency modulated warble tones in an adult population with sharply sloping audiometric configurations. As expected with this population, the warble tones yielded the better thresholds. Mean differences of from .1 to 3.9 dB were found for 10% warble tones, and from 0 to 22.2 dB for narrow band noise when these were compared to pure-tone results with the multi-frequency stimuli again yielding the better thresholds. No measures of variability were reported in this study.

These reports taken with the data presented here point out the importance of frequency variations as a factor in threshold determination, particularly with hearing-impaired persons. This is true whether the variation is controlled as is the case when warble tone or noise stimuli are used, or whether it is artifactual as in the case of output variations within calibration tolerances.

In light of the variable and potentially large differences in assessed threshold due to small frequency variations it may be appropriate for the American National Standards Committee to consider more stringent frequency calibration tolerances. At present it would certainly be prudent to carefully monitor frequency output and to indicate this in audiologic reports. Monitoring would be particularly important in cases where even small changes due to frequency variance could result in major differences in interpretation of findings, such as in brief tone audiometry. Reporting of frequency output increases in importance with the impact that findings will have on recommendations. Among situations in which reporting of actual frequency output is very important are evaluations for compensation purposes and audiograms obtained as a part of the hearing aid evaluation.

SOURCE: Woodford, C. M. (1984). The effect of small changes in frequency on clinically determined estimates of auditory threshold. *Asha, 26,* 25–30.

Excerpt 9.20 is from a study of acoustical characteristics of syllablic stress in esophageal speakers and includes two paragraphs from the Introduction and two paragraphs from the Discussion sections to illustrate how well part of the rationale and the problem statement integrated with the practical implications drawn at the end of the study. The first two paragraphs show part of the authors' rationale for studying prosodic variables in esophageal speech and the general purpose and specific research questions of the study. The next two paragraphs of the excerpt briefly summarize some of the results, suggest some possible physiological mechanisms, and indicate the direct clinical implications of the results regarding speech therapy with esophageal speakers.

EXCERPT 9.20

Because it appears that esophageal speakers exhibit reduced ability to manipulate fundamental frequency, sound pressure, and duration, clinical expectations for perfecting esophageal speech may be limited. Speech clinicians sometimes assume that esophageal speakers will be unable to approximate normal prosodic patterning associated with syllable stress and intonation.

   The present study was designed to explore the production of intended syllabic stress by excellent esophageal speakers. More specifically, do excellent esophageal speakers and normal speakers characterize primary syllabic stress with similar patterns of fundamental frequency, sound pressure, and duration? Further, are excellent esophageal speakers able to produce normal patterns of stress-associated acoustical characteristics irrespective of stress position within syllables and within sentences?

. . . .

   In general, the results of this study suggest that some laryngectomees are able to manipulate f_0, SPL, and duration in a manner reasonably comparable to normal speakers. The physiological factors contributing to these abilities are unknown at this time, but the amount of remaining musculature and the integrity of its neural innervation as well as the nature of the surgical reconstruction may be relevant (Simpson, Smith, & Gordon, 1972). Precise tension control of the neoglottic folds combined with optimal tissue viscoelasticity would facilitate rapid f_0 changes. Enhanced neoglottic closure control might permit more rapid voicing onsets and offsets and a higher average SPL. The availability of a large air reservoir may allow both increased SPLs and/or the production of longer utterances. Finally, ability to modulate transneoglottic airflow via changes in intrathoracic pressure and upper vocal tract impedance might well allow a trade-off between increased SPL and increased utterance length.

The finding that some esophageal speakers are able to control f_0, SPL, and duration in a highly natural but somewhat inconsistent manner has significant clinical implications. In light of the data presented, it may be unjustifiable to dismiss patients when intelligible esophageal utterances are produced with relative fluency. Many laryngectomees may have the capability to go well beyond the point of merely functional esophageal speech. With intensive esophageal therapy emphasis on f_0, SPL, and duration, certain esophageal speakers may approximate suprasegmental normalcy more completely, more rapidly, and more consistently.

SOURCE: McHenry, M., Reich, A., & Minifie, F. (1982). Acoustical characteristics of intended syllabic stress in excellent esophageal speakers. *Journal of Speech and Hearing Research*, 25, 564–573.

Implications for Future Research

As we mentioned earlier, no one research article can answer all of the relevant questions on a given topic. In fact, a particular research article may even raise more questions than it answers. Scientific progress depends, then, on the cumulative efforts of a number of investigators and each of their efforts points toward new avenues of research. The Discussion section usually enumerates some of the questions for future research that occur to the author during the course of the investigation.

Future research may be suggested in a number of different areas, including, but not limited to, improvement of internal validity by refinement of the design and execution of the research, extension of external validity, further clarification of the relationship of results to previous research, additional empirical confirmation of theory, and elaboration of practical applications.

Suggestions for future research are often directed toward improvement of the internal validity of the research by refinement of the methods employed. For instance, the author may discuss limitations imposed on his or her conclusions by aspects of the method of investigation (i.e., threats to internal validity). The author may also incorporate suggestions for future research to overcome these limitations. These suggestions may be in the form of general comments or of specific delineations of procedural steps to be taken in a new study. Indeed, the author may already have such an investigation underway at publication time and readers may anticipate its subsequent publication. The suggestions offered may include replication with larger (possibly randomly selected or assigned) samples, use of more homogeneous or heterogeneous groups of subjects depending on the nature of the study, refinements in design or measurement techniques, or improvements in materials or instrumentation. Of course, if too many such suggestions are made, readers may wonder why the study was ever published in the first place! But a few suggestions for improvement are usually warranted because no study can ever be perfectly designed to avoid all of the possible pitfalls of research.

Suggestions for future research may also be directed toward external validity. The author may be concerned with extending the generalizability of results to other populations, other settings, other measures, or other treatments. Procedures that are successful with adults may not necessarily work with children; replication with children would be needed to verify the generality of the procedure. By the same token, results obtained with one type of communication disorder may not necessarily be obtained with another. Results may be limited to a particular setting and a systematic replication may be needed to extend generalization to another setting. Research suggestions aimed at extending external validity are often coupled with caveats discussed in practical implications and readers may be urged to await further research before attempting to generalize results to other subjects, settings, measures, or treatments.

Future research may also be suggested as a result of comparison of the results of a particular study to those of previous research. If there are disagreements between the results of a study and previous research, more research may be suggested to resolve the differences. The different results may be due to sampling or procedural differences that could be overcome by procedural comparisons, replications with different samples, or by control studies designed to evaluate the reliability and validity of different procedures with different samples. Agreement of previous research with the results of a particular study may also prompt suggestions for future research as such agreement may indicate that researchers have been pursuing a fruitful approach to the study of the particular phenomenon.

Suggested future research may also be related to the theoretical implications of the results. More research may be needed to firm up the empirical grounding of a theory supported by the results of a particular investigation. On the other hand, further research may be needed to account for discrepancies between the results of a study and existing theory. If a new or modified theory is advanced to explain the results, the new theory or modifications may contain predictions of behavior or phenomena that would need to be confirmed empirically by future research. Changes in type of subjects, research materials, instrumentation, or procedures might be necessary to test the predictions of the new theory.

As mentioned previously, the practical implications of a particular research study may not be immediately apparent or feasible and, therefore, further research may be suggested before practical applications can be accomplished. Such suggestions may include standardization of tests on larger samples, gathering of normative data on different populations, development of more efficient or less expensive (i.e., more clinically feasible) methods, or refinements in procedure to improve reliability and validity. Sometimes a procedure may be strongly advocated as useful with a well-defined, closely circumscribed clinical population, but caution is necessary regarding application to other populations until future research confirms the applicability of the measure or technique.

The next five excerpts present examples from Discussion sections that illustrate a variety of thoughtful suggestions for future research. The excerpts concern many of the different kinds of suggestions outlined above. Excerpt 9.21 is from an article on programmed instruction of vowel discrimination with hearing-impaired children. It emphasizes the need for future research before practical applications should be initiated and also suggests further research to aid in the theoretical explanation and understanding of memory processes involved in designing such programs.

EXCERPT 9.21

Before practical programs are initiated, it is necessary to determine the extent to which vowel discriminations acquired by PI actually contribute to speech discrimination and language abilities of the hearing-impaired child. The post-tests did not demonstrate any appreciable improvement in the recognition of the words used in training or of other words containing the same vowels. Similar results were obtained in a previous study (Ling & Doehring, 1969), where the consonant discriminations learned by PI did not transfer to words not used in training. A basic principle of PI states that new material must be introduced in small steps (Holland, 1967). Transfer from the narrow context within which the vowel discriminations were learned to the 13-choice word-recognition task probably was too large a step. Because of the restricted verbal experience of the hearing-impaired child, he is likely to show very little generalization of verbal discriminations learned in a narrow context. Further PI research should be aimed at determining whether the child can be taught to generalize auditory verbal discriminations to the point where there is substantial improvement in his comprehension of running speech. Generalization training should involve not only a gradual broadening of verbal context but also, if possible, a generalization of the instructional task to include written and spoken responses that are immediately reinforced.

In considering the type of generalization training that should be planned, it is of interest to analyze further the possible reasons for the poor performance by many of the children on the pre- and posttests. The memory requirements of this type of test may be too stringent. The child's motivation may have been reduced as a consequence of this and also by lack of knowledge of correctness. Because of his imperfect perception of the word and his restricted verbal experience, the child may have had particular difficulty in rehearsing the word for short-term memory storage while searching for the correct picture among 13 alternatives. Conrad (1970) has recently emphasized the problems experienced by deaf subjects on short-term memory tasks even when stimulus material is presented visually. Further research on auditory verbal memory of hearing-impaired children and on the extent to which this type of memory can be improved by PI would be very helpful in the design of programs for improving language comprehension.

SOURCE: Doehring, D. G., & Ling, D. (1971). Programmed instruction of hearing-impaired children in the auditory discrimination of vowels. *Journal of Speech and Hearing Research, 14,* 746–753.

Excerpt 9.22, taken from an article on imitative modeling with language-disordered children, demonstrates a discussion of the need for further research to examine a previously advanced hypothesis and indicates the need for better understanding of this hypothesis in order to incorporate it into a theoretical model upon which therapy could be based. Future research suggestions are integrated with both theoretical and practical implications of the study. Note also the intent to extend generalization to other treatments by examining the effects of other variables on the modeling process (e.g., reinforcement) and thereby broaden external validity with future research.

EXCERPT 9.22

We believe, nevertheless, that the interference hypothesis deserves rigorous empirical investigation. The need for research into this area becomes even more pressing when one considers that many contemporary methods of speech and language instruction involve some form of overt client verbalization. In fact, several authors have explicitly claimed that the amount of client verbalization is positively related to increases in the learning of language structures (Mowrer, 1970). In contrast to these claims, it is possible that modeling could be proven to be a relatively easy, uncomplicated method of instruction—a method that is significantly more effective than others proposed or used for teaching specific types of grammatical rules or overcoming certain language disorders.

Additional research, we believe, should focus on the effects of other variables on the modeling process. As was indicated earlier, a better understanding of the role of reinforcement is clearly requisite before imitative modeling would be suitable for widespread use as an instructional technique (Kent et al., 1972; Miller & Yoder, 1972). Similarly, questions concerning the type of stimuli which could be most efficaciously employed, for example, pictures, verbal stimuli, and so on (Asher, 1972; Mann & Baer, 1971), and whether they should be administered by the clinician or by a separate model (Leonard, 1975) must be investigated and answered.

In conclusion, this study has supplied initial findings about the potential for imitative modeling as a theoretical base for speech and language instruction. Subsequent studies, then, must attempt to determine the exact nature of this potential and the scope of its usefulness with regard to a wide variety of speech and language deficiencies.

SOURCE: Courtright, J. A., & Courtright, I. C. (1976). Imitative modeling as a theoretical base for instructing language-disordered children. *Journal of Speech and Hearing Research, 19,* 655–663.

Excerpt 9.23, taken from the same study of syllabic stress with esophageal speakers that was used in Excerpt 9.20, illustrates several suggestions for research to extend the external validity of the study. Suggestions are made for studying other measures (e.g., variability within-sentences, perceptual verification of stress magnitude, etc.) and comparing them to the measures reported in this study. Also, this study included only excellent esophageal speakers and the suggestion is made to study the abilities of fair to good speakers also.

EXCERPT 9.23

The present study is limited by a number of factors. Three male and two female esophageal speakers with matched normals comprise a relatively small sample. Furthermore, large-sample perceptual evaluation of stress was not performed. For the purpose of this descriptive study of acoustical characteristics associated with intended syllabic stress, experimenter and trained-phonetician verification was considered adequate. The fact that significant stress main effects and nonsignificant group $\times$ stress interactions were found supports the notion that, for the most part, these esophageal speakers produced intended stress in a manner comparable to their matched normals. This, however, does not address the issue of how frequently or to what degree stress was realized. The necessity of excluding 14% of the esophageal but none of the normal productions implies that even excellent esophageal speakers lack consistent volitional control of the mechanisms underlying stress production. Large-sample perceptual verification of stress magnitude currently is underway in our laboratory. The results of the perceived stress-magnitude study will be correlated with dynamic as well as static acoustical characteristics known to be associated with syllable stress. We anticipated that certain dynamic aspects of prosodic patterning, such as rate of f_0 and SPL change within and between syllables, will correlate more highly with perceived stress magnitude than would the more static features investigated in the present study.

In addition, although the subjects did not seem to produce exaggerated contrasts between stimulus pairs, it is unlikely that the utterances are truly representative of ongoing conversational speech. Most subjects uttered each stimulus sentence as a single phrase. This eliminated the need for rapid air injections and releases that might tax their ability to produce longer, appropriately phrased utterances. Since each stimulus sentence was produced only once, within-sentence, intraspeaker variability data are unavailable. Within-sentence f_0, SPL, and durational variability data would provide information regarding the consistency with which esophageal speakers are able to manipulate these acoustical parameters to signal stress.

The need for further research regarding esophageal prosody is apparent. It will be interesting to investigate the ability of fair to good esophageal speakers to manipulate the acoustical characteristics associated with stress. Trading effects, such as signaling contrasts with durational rather than f_0 or SPL changes, may be evident. Research concerning the linguistic aspects of speech after laryngectomy, including studies of contrastive stress and intonation, would appear to be of great interest. Work addressing these questions currently is underway (Weinberg, Note 1).

SOURCE: McHenry, M., Reich, A., & Minifie, F. (1982). Acoustical characteristics of intended syllabic stress in excellent esophageal speakers. *Journal of Speech and Hearing Research, 25*, 564–573.

Excerpt 9.24, from a study of hearing-impaired speakers' intelligibility, includes two specific suggestions for future research. The first suggestion concerns examination of criterion validity of scaling measures in relation to word-identification tests of intelligibility and acoustical characteristics of speech. The second suggestion concerns extension of the external validity of the results to other populations with impaired intelligibility and to other measures (i.e., dimensions of speech that are scaled).

EXCERPT 9.24

Because the results of this study demonstrate the continuum of our hearing-impaired adults' speech intelligibility to be prothetic, we conclude that direct magnitude estimation has more construct validity than interval scaling for assessing this dimension. Future research should address the criterion validity of direct magnitude estimation by examining its functional relation to word identification tests of speech intelligibility and to acoustical parameters of speech (Monsen, 1978) found to be good predictors of intelligibility.

It is important to test the generalizability of these results to the speech intelligibility of hearing-impaired children, to other populations such as dysarthrics and esophageal speakers with impaired intelligibility, and to other dimensions of speech that are commonly scaled. For example, an interesting parallel is apparent between our results for speech intelligibility and the findings of Berry and Silverman (1972) regarding the inequality of intervals on the *Lewis-Sherman Scale of Stuttering Severity*. They used direct magnitude estimation to judge the widths between adjacent samples of stuttering previously scaled along a 9-point interval scale of stuttering severity and found smaller interval widths at the lower end than at the upper portion of the scale. This finding agrees well with Stevens's (1974) prediction for prothetic continua. Because a number of dimensions like stuttering severity, speech intelligibility, articulatory defectiveness, vocal qualities, etc., are commonly assessed with interval scaling in clinical and research work, it seems imperative that these dimensions be explored to determine whether they constitute metathetic or prothetic continua. A serious reconsideration of the widespread use of interval scaling may be necessary if a number of these continua are found to be prothetic.

As Stevens (1974) has stated:

The human being, despite his great versatility, has a limited capacity to effect linear partitions on prothetic continua. He does quite well, to be sure, if the continuum happens to be metathetic, but, since most scaling

> problems involve *prothetic continua, it seems that category and other forms of partition scaling generally ought to be avoided for the purposes of scaling.* (p. 374)
>
> SOURCE: Schiavetti, N., Metz, D. E., & Sitler, R. W. (1981). Construct validity of direct magnitude estimation and interval scaling of speech intelligibility: Evidence from a study of the hearing impaired. *Journal of Speech and Hearing Research, 24,* 441–445.

Excerpt 9.25 is from a study of progressive hearing loss in children in relation to hearing-aid use and other etiological factors. This is a complicated area of research with many potential independent variables (etiological factors) that can cause deterioration in hearing in addition to the effect of high sound levels of hearing-aid output. The paragraphs excerpted indicate a number of variables that need further research in attempts to delineate the nature of progressive hearing loss in children. The first paragraph, taken from the beginning of the discussion, indicates the importance of following the time course of hearing-aid use and the progression of hearing loss, and the next two paragraphs, taken from the end of the discussion, indicate a number of variables that must be considered in clinical case studies and in future research studies. Excerpt 9.25 indicates the difficulty of generalization in this area without more research on a variety of potential independent variables and their interactions in causing progressive hearing loss in children.

EXCERPT 9.25

The potential of powerful hearing aids causing further hearing loss in hearing-impaired children cannot be discounted. However, an incentive to look beyond the hearing aid is provided by the large number of possible etiological factors associated with progressive hearing loss. Unfortunately, specific etiology in the individual case is often unknown. Scrutiny of factors such as the time relations between hearing aid application and the period of progression, therefore, become extremely significant.

. . . .

If progressive hearing loss is verified and not attributed to hearing aid use, immediate attention should be paid to all other possible factors. Careful questioning of illness, virus, allergy, noise exposure, medication, and family history is in order, and it should be verified that a physician is following the child. The gain and SSPL of auditory trainers, if used in the educational setting, need to be ascertained. In this connection, the Academy of Rehabilitative Audiology recommended to the Food and Drug Administration in 1976 that caution be exercised when SSPLs of over 132 dB are used in auditory trainers; but this level may be too high, according to Rintelman (1975).

Research is needed not only on the effects of gain and SSPL but also on the effects of steady stimulation from inherent noise in the hearing aid. Similarly, research is needed on temporary shifts with hearing aid use and their relation to permanent damage. We also need research on etiological factors in progressive hearing loss; for example, given a known causative agent, what is the rate, extent, and pattern of progression that might be expected once a change in hearing is seen. Finally, much greater emphasis should be placed on obtaining informative case history data. Although reflecting the present state of knowledge with respect to hearing impairment in children, any study such as this one is restricted in its comprehensiveness by the lack of adequate etiological information.

SOURCE: Reilly, K. M., Owens, E., Uken, D., McClatchie, A. C., & Clarke, R. (1981). Progressive hearing loss in children: Hearing aids and other factors. *Journal of Speech and Hearing Disorders, 46,* 328–334.

Summary

This chapter has outlined the structural framework of the culmination of the research article in the Discussion and Conclusions section. The important structural elements of the conclusion of a research article include: relationship of the conclusions to the preceding parts of the article, relationship of results to previous research, theoretical implications of the research, practical implications of the research, and implications for future research. The checklist follows for the evaluation of these elements in the concluding section of a research article.

EVALUATION CHECKLIST

Instructions: The four-category scale at the end of this checklist may be used to rate the *Discussion* section of an article. The *Evaluation Items* help identify those topics that should be considered in arriving at the rating. Comments on these topics, entered as *Evaluation Notes*, should serve as the basis for the overall rating.

Evaluation Items   *Evaluation Notes*

1. Discussion was clearly related to research problem.

2. Limitations of the method were discussed.

3. Conclusions were drawn directly and fairly from results.

4. Reasonable explanations were given for unusual,

atypical, or discrepant results.

5. There was thorough and objective discussion of agreements and disagreements of previous research.

6. The section related results to various theoretical explanations.

7. Implications for clinical practice were stated fairly and objectively.

8. Theoretical or clinical speculations were identified and justified.

9. Suggestions for future research were identified.

10. Miscellaneous.

Overall Rating (Discussion):

| Poor | Fair | Good | Excellent |

Part III
Evaluation of the Complete Research Article: Two Examples

Overview

In the previous part, we presented, of necessity, a rather disjointed view of the evaluation process by using a wide variety of articles from the speech pathology and audiology literature. As a result, the evaluation of the Introduction section was disconnected from the evaluation of the Method section, the evaluation of methods was disconnected from the evaluation of results, and so on. In this part, we have attempted to pull the evaluation process together by analyzing two articles that have been reprinted in their entirety. One will be of more interest to speech pathologists (Chapter 10) and the other to audiologists (Chapter 11). Our commentary is enclosed by open squares.

We chose articles we believed would illustrate many of the points discussed in previous chapters. In general, both articles are examples of good research. Our evaluation notes, however, contain both positive and some negative comments. The reason for an occasional negative comment is simply that no article reporting research is perfect. No single research study can completely handle all threats to internal and external validity, given the practical problems of conducting the research. Nor are there articles that are beyond reproach with respect to the other components of a research report. The studies we have chosen, despite some shortcomings, make important contributions to our knowledge. They are used here to illustrate the process of evaluation, the weighing of positive and negative aspects in order to arrive at a reasonable judgment about the overall adequacy of a research report.

10

Annotated Article: Speech and Language

USE OF PROSODY AND SYNTACTIC MARKERS IN CHILDREN'S COMPREHENSION OF SPOKEN SENTENCES

Reprinted from the *Journal of Speech and Hearing Research*, 17, 656–668, (1974).

MARGARET LAHEY

Margaret Lahey is currently affiliated with Hunter College, City University of New York.

A comparison was made of four- and five-year-old children's comprehension of coordinate, center-embedded relative clause, and right-branching relative clause sentences under four conditions of presentation: (1) prosody (P) and syntactic markers (M) intact; (2) P intact and M eliminated; (3) M intact and P eliminated; and (4) M and P eliminated. The number of semantic-syntactic relationships in a sentence that were correctly acted out were analyzed by age, sentence type, and conditions of presentation. More relationships were acted out appropriately by five year olds. Differences between sentence type were significant with coordinate sentence type the easiest and right-branching sentence type the most difficult. Conditions of presentation did not significantly affect responses, although there was a significant interaction between condition and sentence type. Scores were significantly lower for center-embedded sentences when M was intact and P eliminated. It was concluded that word order was the major linguistic cue used by the children to process these sentences.

☐ *The title is clear and concise and identifies the major variables studied. The abstract briefly summarizes the main points of the method and results of the investigation.* ☐

To understand speech one must segment the sound stream into grammatical units and determine the relationships among these units. The linguistic devices that signal the relationships among grammatical units in sentences include word order, syntactic markers (morphological inflections and function words), and prosody (intonation, stress, and durational aspects). The purpose of this study was to investigate the relative importance of these linguistic devices to the young child who is learning his native language.

☐ *The general problem is clearly identified in the first paragraph and the specific purpose is stated in the last paragraph of the introduction. Details about the specific age groups studied, types of sentences, prosody, and syntactic markers are deferred until the Method section.* ☐

Prosody has been described as the earliest linguistic feature acquired by the child (Lenneberg, 1967) and the first linguistic feature to which the child responds (Lewis, 1951). Werner and Kaplan (1963) reported that relationships among words are expressed by prosody before markers. Kaplan (1970) suggested prosody may aid in the discovery of underlying linguistic constituents. A number of studies have found prosody an important variable in children's imitative responses to sentences (Aurnhammer-Frith, 1969; Menyuk, 1969; Scholes, 1969). Both Scholes and Menyuk reported that the effect of prosody diminished with age while the effect of other linguistic devices increased. However, the importance of prosody in the processing of speech cannot be inferred from imitative responses. Prosody may serve as an aid for echoic memory but not be important in the semantic processing of meaning relationships between constituents.

By age four most children produce complex sentences with syntactic markers (Menyuk, 1969). Four year olds had longer latency times and more incorrect reproductions when imitating sentences with ungrammatical or omitted markers than when imitating grammatically correct sentences in a study reported by Freedle, Keeney, and Smith (1970). This evidence suggests that children of this age are aware of markers, but does not give information about their use of markers to determine relationships.

Children's use of word order before syntactic markers in their early syntactic productions has been reported by many (see Bloom [in press] for a review of these studies). Bever (1970) has suggested that word order is the first and primary strategy used by children in the processing of sentences. Sinclair and Bronckart (1972) reported a developmental change in comprehension strategies based on the relative position of nouns and verbs in three-word utterances without markers. How order might be used in longer utterances, and how it might be influenced by prosody and syntactic markers is not clear.

This study was designed to investigate the relative importance, to the nursery school child, of the linguistic devices of prosody (P), syntactic markers (M), and word order. Their importance was inferred from the number of semantic-syntactic relationships children correctly acted out in response to complex sentences presented with prosody and/or markers eliminated, and with both intact. The order of nouns and verbs was constant for all sentence types and overall conditions.

□ *The middle three paragraphs of the introduction include brief reviews of literature concerned with the influence of prosody, syntactic markers, and word order on sentence comprehension. Each of the three paragraphs ends with a brief comment on gaps in current knowledge and the need to study the relative importance of linguistic devices for signaling grammatical relations in sentences. The rationale is logically developed by citing previous research findings and showing that they do not provide a clear explanation of the influence that prosody, syntactic markers, and word order have on children's comprehension of sentences.*

Although a more intensive discussion of these references might have been helpful to readers unfamiliar with the topic, the journal format has forced the author to be succinct. Nevertheless, Lahey has cited important research the interested reader may consult for more background information. This brief introduction is clearly written and well organized. □

METHOD

Subjects

The subjects in this study included 54 children enrolled in private nursery schools in New York City. All were monolingual English-speaking children with language and speech skills, as judged by their teachers, at a level at least commensurate with their chronological age. School records and teacher reports indicated no marked deviance in mental, emotional, or physical development.

In order to examine the question of age as a variable, the group was divided into two age groups. The four-year-old group included 12 males and 15 females ranging in years and months of age from 3-11, to 4-11, with a median of 4-7. The five-year-old group included 11 males and 16 females ranging in years and months of age from 5-2 to 5-11, with a median of 5-6.

□ *Subjects. A relatively large (N = 54) sample of subjects for a study of language development was selected. No mention is made of random selection. As indicated in Chapters 4 and 7, it is desirable, but rarely practical, to obtain a random sample for strengthening external validity.*

Because this study concerned the behavior of normal children, the selection criteria included teacher judgments of the adequacy of speech and language skills and inspection of school records to rule out mental, emotional, and physical deviations. A more thorough description of the specific nature of teacher judgments or school records would have improved this section and strengthened consumers' confidence in the subject-selection criteria. For example, did the school records contain information regarding any language or intelligence tests or hearing screening? Be-

cause the materials and procedures portions of the Method section are long, the subjects portion may have been reduced to save space.

There were approximately the same number of males and females in each age group, so a sex difference did not threaten the internal validity of the comparison of four- and five-year-olds or limit generalization to one sex only. The extraneous variables of native language, geographical location, and type of school were the same for all subjects, thus precluding these subject-selection variables from threatening the internal validity of the age comparison. Generalization, however, would be limited to four- and five-year-old monolingual children in the urban, private nursery school setting. Note, also, that age groups do not overlap but are mutually exclusive. Subjects were not selected on the basis of extreme scores, so, regression was not a threat to internal validity. No mortality occurred, as data on all 54 subjects are shown in Table 1 of the Results section. □

Stimuli

Sentence types studied were coordinate (CO), center-embedded relative clause (CE), and right-branching relative clause (RB). Each of the sentences had the same order of lexical classes and the same order of grammatical relations as schematized in Figure 1. The location and type of marker varied as did the constituent, which was the subject of the second clause for two of the three sentences.

The prosodic grouping used in the production of the stimuli is marked on Figure 1. While pauses occurred in the same location for each type, the pause

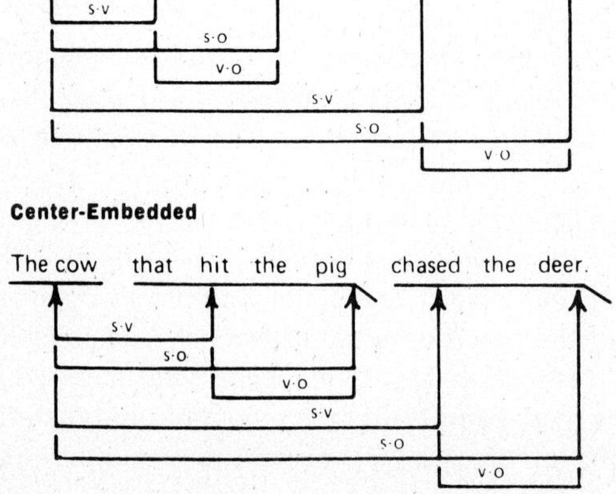

FIGURE 1. Sample of sentence types with grammatical relationships and prosodic groupings marked.

Underlining indicates prosodic groupings. Falling terminal contour is marked with downward slope.

Lines below sentences refer to grammatical relationships between words to which arrows point (s−v= subject-verb. v−o=verb-object. s−o=subject-object.)

Right-Branching

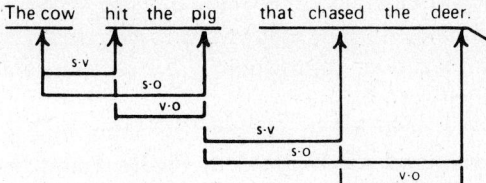

between clauses in RB was shorter than for CE or CO types. The falling terminal contour at the end of the first clause was greatest for CE, less for CO, and not present on RB. The relative clause on CE and RB received less stress than the main clause while both clauses of CO received the same stress.

Each stimulus contained two verbs (hit and chase), and three of a possible five animal names (cow, horse, pig, sheep, and deer). There were 12 different stimuli where the order of the verbs and the selection and order of the animal names varied. The actual stimuli used are listed by condition of presentation in the Appendix.

☐ *The Appendix is reprinted here for convenience.* ☐

APPENDIX

SENTENCE STIMULI

Coordinate

+P+M	The sheep hit the deer and chased the horse.
+P−M	Cow hit horse chase sheep.
−P+M	The horse chased the pig and hit the cow.

Center-Embedded

+P+M	The pig, that chased the cow, hit the sheep.
+P−M	Deer hit horse chase pig.
−P+M	The sheep, that hit the pig, chased the deer.

Right-Branching

+P+M	The horse hit the deer, that chased the cow.
+P−M	Deer chase sheep hit horse.
−P+M	The cow chased the pig, that hit the deer.

Word Order Only

−P−M	Pig chase sheep hit deer.
−P−M	Cow hit deer chase horse.
−P−M	Horse chase cow hit sheep.

Conditions of Presentation

There were four conditions of presentation: (1) normal presentation with sentence prosody and syntactic markers present ($+P+M$), (2) sentence prosody present and syntactic markers eliminated ($+P-M$), (3) syntactic markers present and sentence prosody eliminated ($-P+M$), and (4) sentence prosody and syntactic markers eliminated and only word order retained ($-P-M$). All stimuli were of equal duration, approximately 5.1 seconds, and were recorded in the manner described below.

Condition ($+P+M$). Sentences were recorded in a normal-speaking manner with prosody patterns described above and schematized in Figure 1 and the Appendix.

Condition ($+P-M$). Sentences were spoken without functor words or morphemic endings, but with the same prosody pattern as in condition ($+P+M$). In order to maintain the same total duration of the stimuli the rate was slowed from approximately 1.8 words per second to one word per second.

Condition ($-P+M$). Stimuli were constructed by dubbing words from a master list in the order specified for each sentence type. The master list contained all substantive and functor words recorded with a duration of approximately 300 msec and spoken with similar intonation pattern as in the reading of a list of unrelated words. Normal-speaking effort was used and any marked deviations in loudness among the words were decreased in the dubbing process. After dubbing, a blank piece of tape was spliced between each word to equal a period of 300 msec of silence. The resulting speech pattern of approximately equal duration of speech and silence was quite intelligible and sounded like the reading of a list of words. The resulting prosodic pattern, of word list reading, was unrelated to the grammatical relationships or segments within each sentence.

Condition ($-P-M$). Recording and splicing procedures for this condition were similar to ($-P+M$). However, as noted in ($+P-M$), because of the elimination of markers the rate differed. The duration of both words and silence was increased to approximately 600 msec. The procedure was otherwise similar to ($-P+M$). Increasing the duration of the words did not cause distortion or loss of intelligibility.

☐ *Materials. The materials used in this study are thoroughly described in the sections entitled Stimuli and Conditions of Presentation and also in the Appendix. The Conditions of Presentation section explains how the sentences were tape recorded for the manipulation of prosody and markers and how durational differences between recordings were controlled. The hardware used for recording and timing stimuli is not described in detail, making replication difficult. Any good quality recorder would probably suffice, but a description of timing techniques and hardware would have been helpful. Greater importance may have been given to the description of stimuli than to hardware in order to provide evidence of the content validity of the stimulus items. ☐*

Order of Presentation

The stimuli were arranged in 12 different orders determined by a 12×12 Latin square. Each of these orders formed a list of stimuli which was recorded on a separate tape. The 12 lists were randomly ordered five times to assign presentation order to the subjects.

Manner of Presentation

Each child was seen in a room apart from his classroom. When the experimenter felt certain the child could identify the five toy animals and could demonstrate the actions, the child was told he would hear a lady say some sentences from the tape recorder. His task was to make the animals do what she had said. Four simple sentences with one verb and four stimuli, each containing two simple sentences (for example, "The sheep chased the cow" and "The horse hit the sheep") were used for practice. While the child listened, he had in front of him only the animals that were being named in the stimulus.

Before presenting the experimental stimuli, the child was told that some of the next sentences might sound different or "funny" but that he was still to listen for who hits whom and who chases whom and to demonstrate the actions after the lady finished talking. Again only the animals mentioned in the stimulus were placed in front of him. If the child did not attempt a response, the tape was replayed. As the child acted out the sentences, his responses were hand recorded by the experimenter.

☐ *Procedures. This study may be classified as combined descriptive–experimental research. The author compared the sentence comprehension of four- and five-year-old children. Thus the study had a descriptive (cross-sectional developmental) component. The author also studied the effects of manipulating certain linguistic aspects of the sentence stimuli on children's comprehension. Thus, the study had an experimental component.*

The design of the study is mixed because it incorporates both within-subjects and between-subjects comparisons. The between-subjects aspect of the mixed design is the comparison of the two age groups. The within-subjects aspect of the mixed design is the comparison of the effects of the linguistic variables on sentence comprehension.

Details of the procedures are presented in the sections titled Order of Presentation, Manner of Presentation, and Scoring of Responses. Note the important step that was taken to strengthen internal validity in the within-subjects comparison: presentation order was randomized to minimize sequencing effects and the short-term maturation threat to internal validity. The Manner of Presentation section briefly describes the test environment, instructions to subjects, and the procedure for eliciting responses. Because the task appeared to require a relatively short time to complete, history and maturation would not be serious threats to internal validity, and the absence of pretesting excludes this threat. The separate room and the fact that the experimenter was a stranger to the children probably constituted a reactive arrangement or Hawthorne effect, as is true of most research studies. These were probably reduced somewhat by the researcher's attempts to familiarize the children with the toys and provide them with practice items. ☐

Scoring of Responses

One point was given for each of the six grammatical relationships (schematized in Figure 1) correctly acted out regardless of errors on other relationships or the order in which each clause was demonstrated. When no response was given to a first play of a stimulus sentence, the response to the replay was scored. The no response score of zero was averaged with the replay response and used as a measure of the relationship score for that stimulus item.

Responses to stimuli presented under conditions of ($-P-M$) were handled differently than other responses. Without prosody or markers there was no differentiation with regard to sentence type. In order to compare the use of word order to cue the relationships expressed in each sentence type, the response to each presentation of ($-P-M$) was scored according to the relationships expressed in each sentence type. The three presentations, so scored for each type, were then averaged. The individual's average score for each type was used as an indication of the use of word order to cue relationships expressed in that type. Since in CO and CE types the relationships are expressed by the same constituents, the scores for these conditions were always identical. All scores reported under ($-P-M$) conditions represent an average of each individual's response to the three presentations.

☐ *Particular attention is paid to the description of the method of scoring responses, especially with regard to the complications involved in scoring the "$-P-M$" stimuli. Reference is made to Figure 1 again to illustrate the six grammatical relationships scored in each child's response to each sentence. One shortcoming here is that no mention is made of the examiner's reliability in scoring responses. Presumably, reliability would be high because scoring was a simple notation of what the child did with the toys.*

In summary, the Method section has both merits and demerits, as do all articles. The design appears to be appropriate, the stimuli are described in detail and appear to have content validity, and the procedures have incorporated the important step of randomized presentation. These aspects of the Method section help to reduce threats to the validity of the design. More details on subject selection criteria and hardware would have increased consumers' confidence in the validity of the study. In weighing these positive and negative aspects of the Method section, it appears that the author has succeeded in reducing most of the serious threats to validity in this mixed design. ☐

RESULTS

The mean number of relationships that were acted out correctly with each stimulus are reported in Table 1. To determine the effect of condition of presentation on the comprehension of different sentence types for each age group, a three-way analysis of variance, with repeated measures on two, was computed on the relationship scores.

Five year olds correctly acted out significantly more relationships than did the four year olds (F 11.339, $df = 1,52$; $p < 0.005$). Variations due to sentence type also were significant ($F = 20.90$; $df = 2,104$; $p < 0.001$). A Duncan's Multiple Range Test applied to the ordered pairs of means indicated there

TABLE 1. Mean relationship scores by condition of presentation, sentence type, and age group. Relationship scores listed under "$-P-M$" refer to the average number of times subjects responded to the three presentations of $-P-M$ stimuli with relationships appropriate to each sentence type as cued by order, prosody, and markers. P = prosody and M = markers. Note: maximum possible relationship score = 6.

| | | Condition of Presentation | | | | | | | |
| | Sentence | $+P+M$ | | $+P-M$ | | $-P+M$ | | $-P-M$ | |
Age	Type	Mean	SD	Mean	SD	Mean	SD	Mean	SD
5	Coordinate	4.79	2.1	4.88	1.8	4.79	1.8	4.62	1.7
($N = 27$)	Center-embedded	4.70	1.7	5.11	1.7	3.89	2.5	4.62	1.7
	Right-branching	3.67	1.5	3.87	1.2	3.74	1.2	3.62	0.7
4	Coordinate	3.96	2.1	4.19	1.8	3.46	2.1	3.76	1.7
($N = 27$)	Center-embedded	3.43	3.5	4.19	2.0	2.65	2.0	3.76	1.7
	Right-branching	3.52	1.5	2.65	1.7	3.37	1.5	3.11	0.9

were significant differences between all combinations of sentence types. The mean differences ranged from 1.07 to 3.47 while mean differences of 0.925 and 0.955 were needed to reach significance at the 0.001 level. Thus, the mean score of CO of 17.25 was significantly higher than that of 16.17 on CE and both CO and CE mean scores were significantly higher than the mean score of 13.77 on RB. It was concluded that sentence type was an important factor in the number of relationships acted out correctly with CO the least difficult type and RB the most difficult. There was no overall effect of condition of presentation, indicating condition alone was not an important variable.

☐ *Although the results are somewhat complex, they are generally well organized and thoroughly analyzed. The results are clearly related to the general research problem and the tables and figures help to illustrate the design of the study and the specific subproblems. Tables and figures are well integrated with the presentation of results in the text.*

Appropriate summary statistics are shown in Table 1, which presents the means and standard deviations of the number of grammatical relationships correctly acted out by four- and five-year-olds for each combination of sentence type and condition of presentation. The appropriate mixed design analysis of variance was used: a three-way ANOVA with repeated measures on two factors (i.e., the within-subject comparisons of sentence types and presentation conditions). Significant differences between age groups and sentence types are identified in the text, with size of F, degrees of freedom, and significance levels indicated in parentheses. Duncan's Multiple Range Test was used as the contrast test to examine specific pairs of means as a follow-up to the ANOVA. There is one slight source for confusion in this analysis. The means cited in the text appear to be the means of the three sentence types summed across all four presentation conditions; yet, these combined means are not shown in Table 1. If Table 1 had been enlarged to include all of the combined row and column means, the comparison of sentence types would have been somewhat clearer. ☐

There was a significant interaction between sentence type and condition of presentation (F 3.74; $df = 6,312$; $p < 0.001$). To determine which specific means contributed to the significant interaction, a Duncan's Multiple Range Test was applied to ordered pairs of means for each sentence type under each condition. Mean differences that were significant at the 0.01 level were equal to or greater than 0.856. The means are plotted by type and condition in Figure 2. There was no effect of condition of presentation on relationship scores for CO or RB sentence types. Neither the elimination of prosody nor syntactic markers significantly changed the scores. On sentence type CE significantly lower scores were obtained on ($-P+M$) when compared with ($+P-M$) or ($-P-M$). Thus, it appeared that the elimination of prosody interfered with the determination of relationships only with the CE sentence when markers were present. On all types, scores obtained with order alone ($-P-M$) were not significantly lower than scores with prosody and/or markers present. It was concluded that order was the primary linguistic cue used for the determination of relationships within the sentences.

Comparison of sentence types within condition indicated no significant differences for ($+P+M$) condition. On condition ($-P+M$) scores on CE were significantly lower than on CO, again pointing to the difficulty experienced with CE when prosody was eliminated but markers were present. Within con-

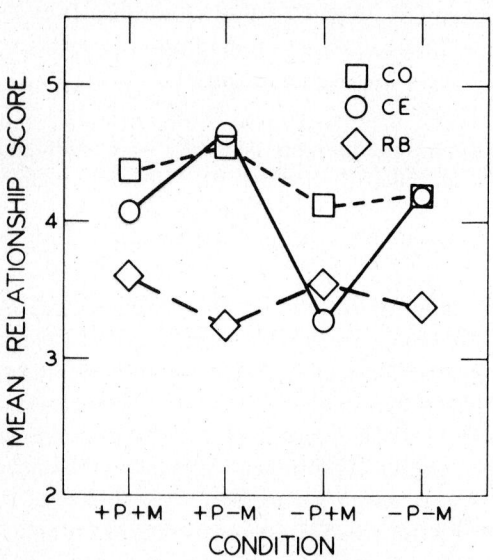

FIGURE 2. Mean relationship score as a function of condition of presentation. The parameter is sentence type (CO represents coordinate; CE, center-embedded; and RB, right-branching). In the condition indicators, the P refers to sentence prosody and the M to syntactic markers. The plus sign ($+$) indicates the presence of markers or prosody, while a minus sign ($-$) indicates their absence.

☐ *The overall effect of condition of presentation was reported as nonsignificant, but there was a significant interaction between sentence type and presentation condi-*

tion. The nature of this interaction was appropriately explored with the Duncan's Multiple Range Test. It is also illustrated in Figure 2, which shows the means for each sentence type and presentation condition (apparently averaged across age groups, because no age-group interaction was reported). The major point of the interaction is that center-embedded sentences are more difficult to comprehend when prosody is absent. Otherwise, removal of prosody and markers had little effect on comprehension of the three types of sentences. This is clearly seen in Figure 2. □

ditions with markers eliminated ($+P-M$ and $-P-M$) scores on RB were significantly lower than scores on CO or CE. Thus, order more effectively cued relationships for CE and CO than for RB.

The number of children obtaining all relationships correct, that is the correct demonstration of a stimulus, is reported in Table 2 by sentence type

TABLE 2. Number of children making correct responses on sentence comprehension task by sentence type, condition of presentation, and age group. Under $-P-M$, responses were judged correct by the average number of times subjects responded to the three presentations of $-P-M$ stimuli with relationships appropriate to each sentence type as cued by order, prosody, and markers. P = prosody and M = markers.

Sentence Type			Condition		Cochran's Q Test
	$+P+M$	$+P-M$	$-P+M$	$-P-M$	
Five-year-old group ($N = 27$)					
Coordinate	19.0	18.0	17.0	16.7	.72
Center-embedded	15.0	20.0	14.0	16.7	3.19
Right-branching	4.0	4.0	4.0	1.3	2.01
Four-year-old group ($N = 27$)					
Coordinate	11.0	11.0	8.0	10.8	1.18
Center-embedded	8.0	13.0	4.0	10.7	8.59°
Right-branching	4.0	2.0	2.0	1.6	1.59

°$p < 0.05$.

and condition. The low number of correct responses for RB sentences regardless of condition again pointed to the difficulty experienced with this sentence type. The effect of conditions of presentation was examined by application of Cochran's Q Test to each sentence type. The only type that was significantly affected by condition of presentation was CE for the four-year-old group. Lower scores were obtained on CE type when markers were present and particularly when markers were present but prosody eliminated. Although not significant, the same pattern was found in the five-year-old group. In general, as many children responded correctly with order alone as a cue as with prosody or markers also present. This appeared to support the conclusion that order was the primary linguistic cue used in the processing of relationships. It also appeared that the presence of markers interfered with the use of order for processing relationships on CE sentences.

Inspection of the pattern of responses indicated that most children took the first noun in the sentence as the agent of both actions and the noun following the verb as the subject of that action. No other predominate pattern was found.

☐ *As a further exploration of the data, the author examined the number of children who correctly acted out all grammatical relationships in each sentence type for each presentation condition. Each child was, therefore, categorized as "all correct" or "not all correct" in his or her responses, and these categories were treated as nominal data. Table 2 shows the number of children in each age group categorized as "all correct" for each sentence type and presentation condition. The Cochran's Q Test, mentioned in Chapter 5 as a nonparametric alternative to ANOVA for use with nominal data, was used in this supplementary analysis. Apparently, the author believed than an analysis of the number of children correctly acting out all grammatical relationships was an important addition to the analysis of the mean number of correct responses and, therefore, appended this supplemental analysis.*

In general, the data of this study are rather complex, particularly because of the nature of the interaction effects. The author has presented a thorough and clear organization and analysis of these complex data. The data presentation might have been improved by (1) the addition of the combined means in Table 1 and (2) the addition of an analysis of variance summary table to display all of the main and interaction effects together. ☐

DISCUSSION

Prosody

The finding that the elimination of prosody did not detrimentally influence the acting out of relationships suggested that the children did not use prosody for sentence processing. This finding supports the view of speech processing as an active search for structure but does not support the contention that children are more "tuned in" to the prosodic patterns of speech than other grammatical aspects, nor the hypothesis that children learn other aspects of grammar through the use of prosody.

One explanation for the difference in the use of prosody between this study and that reported in studies of imitation may relate to the nature of the two response modes. It is not clear that imitation demands an interpretation of semantic relationships as is necessary for the manipulation of objects. In addition, there is a time differential between the stimulus and response for each of the two tasks. Manipulation of objects tends to take longer than imitation and this longer interval between stimulus and response may mean that different memory processes are tapped. Lahey (in preparation) found that young children did not use prosody to recall order information on a task involving the manipulation of objects although Ryan (1969) reported rhythm aided adults' imitation of order information. It has been suggested that short-term memory may be dependent on the physical, or acoustic attributes of the signal while later stages of memory are coded in terms of meaning (Kumar, 1971; Aaronson, 1967). Elicited imitation may be more susceptible to such acoustic variations, as prosodic patterns, than is the ability to demonstrate the meaning of a sentence.

On CE sentence type there was an interaction between the elimination of prosody and the presence of markers. Two questions might be asked: (1) why was the center-embedded sentence type the only type where the presence of markers without prosody appeared to interfere with the order strategy, and (2) why did the presence of markers not interfere with the order strategy when prosody was present on the same sentence type? While the marker was placed after the first noun-verb-noun sequence in both CO and RB sentences, the marker was placed within this sequence in CE. Watt (1970) has suggested that sentence complexity is determined by the number of constituents it takes to assign a deep structure. He attributes this to the amount of unprocessed sentences the listener will have to hold in memory. It is possible that the presence of the marker in the first noun-verb-noun sequence interfered with processing by increasing both the length of time the child must hold the first noun in memory and the number of constituents the child must hold in memory before completing the subject-verb-object relationship. The position of markers after the first s-v-o in CO and RB sentences and the fact that markers did not interfere with processing suggested that the completed s-v-o may be held as a unit thus relieving the memory system for another search for s-v-o.

The presence of prosody on CE in condition (+P+M) appeared to reduce the interference of the markers. In sentence prosody, substantive words are stressed more than function words thereby decreasing the duration of function words relative to substantive words. This is in contrast to (−P) conditions where the duration of all words was equal. Thus, in (−P+M) condition the amount of time needed to hold the first noun before completing s-v-o was longer than in (+P+M). It is also possible that the children may have had a search strategy that ignored unstressed elements that had no referent and held only stressed words in memory—when there was such a stress differential. If so, prosody may play a role in language learning by pointing out the major lexical items upon which to apply an order strategy, and not as a device signaling relationships.

There are other possible linguistic functions of prosody that have not been discussed and were not studied here. Maratsos (1973) reported that 78% of five year olds correctly changed the grammatical role of personal pronouns when they were presented with emphatic stress. It is also possible that distorted prosody would affect processing of relationships. What is reported here is that word order was the primary cue, and normal sentential prosody was not used for the processing of relationships within these complex sentences.

□ *The discussion is divided into four sections: prosody, syntactic markers, word order, and implications. In the section on prosody, the author briefly summarized her results and discussed their relation to previous findings. She attempted to explain discrepancies between her results and those of imitation studies by comparing the tasks of imitation and manipulation of objects and by considering their relation to memory and acoustical attributes of speech. Some interesting questions are raised about her findings regarding the interaction of sentence type and presentation conditions. Some possible explanations and directions for future research are suggested.* □

Syntactic Markers

Since the elimination of syntactic markers did not interfere with the children's determination of relationships on any of the sentences, it was concluded that the children did not use markers to determine relationships among words within these sentences. Children used order as a primary strategy even in the age range during which they produced many markers in their spontaneous speech. During the present experiment it was observed that some children spontaneously imitated sentences reproducing, or adding to a ($-M$) stimulus, a relative pronoun that marked a relationship they subsequently did not demonstrate while acting out the same sentence. Sheldon (1973) reported similar instances. According to Vygotsky (1962) children use subordinate conjunctions long before they grasp the relationships expressed by them. Bloom (1970) reported that one of the children she studied appeared to learn the syntactic function of temporal adverbs before their semantic function. Further support for differences between comprehension and production was found in the comparison of the relative difficulty children in this study had with RB and CE sentences. Menyuk (1969) reported that more nursery school children produced RB type sentences than CE. The production of some aspects of language then may precede comprehension—indicating an attention to surface features incorporated into speech without awareness of the relationships expressed by them.

☐ *In the section on syntactic markers, another brief summary of results is included and some anecdotal remarks are made about some children's behavior during the experiment. Reference is made to previous literature on comprehension and production of syntactic markers that is consistent with her results, and a brief speculation on comprehension and production of markers ends this section.* ☐

Order

It is interesting to speculate as to why an order strategy was used that handled discontinuity between the subject and predicate rather than one that handled contiguous relationships—as for RB sentences where the noun before each verb was the subject of that verb and the noun after each verb was the object of that verb. In such a demonstration, one referent must serve in two different semantic-syntactic functions—both as agent of an action and as object of an action. Bever (1970) has suggested that psychological complexity is added when one word has two different functions. The results of this study suggest that double function of a referent is more difficult for children to handle than discontinuity between subject and predicate. Some support for this would appear to be evident in Sheldon's report (1973) that nursery-school-aged children comprehended relative clause sentences best when the relative pronoun had the same grammatical function as its antecedent. When a relative pronoun has a different grammatical function from its antecedent, the referent must serve in two semantic-syntactic roles. For children then, the order strategy (noun-verb-noun is taken as agent-action-object) suggested by Bever (1970) may be influenced in its elaboration for complex sentences by the number of roles a referent may have.

When do children change order strategies through the use of such other linguistic information as formal syntactic markers? Pilot data indicated that children eight to 12 years of age and adults used the same order strategy as the four- and five-year old children in this study, but changed this strategy for RB sentences under conditions of (+M). This would suggest that some time between six and eight years of age children do incorporate formal markers into their processing strategies. This estimate coincides with reported data on passive construction comprehension—again a situation where an order strategy must be changed on the basis of formal markers (Turner and Rommetveit, 1967). It is also the age range when Karpova (1955) found improvement in children's ability to identify individual words within a sentence. All of these tasks demand attention to linguistic features that have no distinct semantic reference to reality. Maratsos' (1973) finding that five year olds used emphatic stress to change the grammatical role of pronouns may indicate that emphatic prosody can be used to change an order strategy before markers. Further research is needed to answer this question.

☐ *The section on word order begins with a clearly labelled attempt at speculation on why word order appeared to be a major cue in sentence comprehension. The results of previous research are also employed for support in this theoretical discussion. The section ends with the suggestion that future research is needed to clarify the role of word order.* ☐

Implications

In the foregoing discussion a number of points have been made: (1) prosody was not used as a linguistic device to signal relationships, suggesting that such a function for prosody may be acquired after order is established as such a device; (2) the elimination of prosody interfered with processing when a marker was located within the first s-v-o, suggesting differential stress may aid processing by reducing the time or space in storage for elements not considered essential in the search for s-v-o; (3) children did not use syntactic markers to determine relationships among words within these sentences though children in this age range reportedly do produce similar markers in their speech, suggesting the possibility of differing strategies operating for comprehension and production; and, (4) the order of words emerged as the primary linguistic cue used for the determination of relationships among the words—a strategy was used that handled discontinuity between subject and predicate and maintained each referent in one semantic-syntactic function. Since only three sentence types were used and each had the same order of lexical classes, the generalization of the finding of word order as the major linguistic cue to processing other complex sentences is limited. Similar study needs to be carried out with different sentence types and different orders of lexical classes. What the study does suggest is that information about the strategies children employ in the processing of sentences is needed and cannot be inferred from production data, imitation data, or comprehension data presented only in terms of the number of correct responses to sentence stimuli.

Information is also needed on how processing strategies may differ with children who evidence a language disorder. Do children with a language disorder use order as a strategy for processing stimuli—if so, is it the same strategy as is used by the child developing language normally and does prosody influence their use of order? Difficulty with sequential ordering of stimuli has been reported as a problem with populations labeled as aphasic (Efron, 1963; Lowe and Campbell, 1965; Stark, 1967). It has also been reported that differential stress improved the sequencing responses of a group of aphasic children, but not of a control group of normal children (Stark, Poppen and May, 1967). Such reports are, however, based on sequencing of unrelated items. It is an easy, but not necessarily legitimate, jump to assume that if sequencing is a problem with unrelated items the use of order as a liguistic cue may likewise be a problem and that remediation lies in the improvement of sequencing and memory for ordered items. There is an important difference, however, in that the use of order to signal relationships within sentence stimuli involves semantic motivation. Word order in sentences cues semantic relationships and is not just a sequence of words. Certainly if normal performance in language learning is relevant to teaching the child with a language disorder, one point is clear— meaningful stimuli should be used and the use of order as a cue to semantic relationships must be learned. The extent to which prosody may aid in such learning is yet to be determined.

☐ *The last section, titled Implications, begins with a summary of four major points that had been considered previously. The limitations of external validity of the research are clearly identified and further research is suggested to extend generalization to other sentence types and lexical classes. Some interesting questions about sentence comprehension of language-disordered children are posed and some limitations of previous research with language-disordered children are identified. Finally, the author ends with some suggestions for future research with language-disordered children.*

The discussion includes most of the major points covered in Chapter 9. Preceding parts of the article are discussed (mainly results, but also some points on limitations in method). The relationship of results to previous research and theory are discussed, with an objective attempt to consider both agreements and disagreements. Speculations are clearly labelled, and several avenues for future research are suggested. ☐

ACKNOWLEDGMENT

This report is based on part of a doctoral dissertation completed by the author at Teachers College, Columbia University, 1972. Abundant helpful assistance and support was given throughout the study by Lois Bloom, who served as sponsor. A paper based on this study was presented at the Annual Convention of the American Speech and Hearing Association, San Francisco, 1972. Requests for reprints should be addressed to Margaret Lahey, Department of Communication Sciences and Disorders, Montclair State College, Upper Montclair, New Jersey, 07043.

REFERENCES

AARONSON, D., Temporal factors in perception and short memory. *Psychol. Bull.*, **67**, 130-144 (1967).

AURNHAMMER-FRITH, U., Emphasis and meaning in recall in normal and autistic children. *Lang. Speech*, **1**, 29-39 (1969).

BEVER, T. G., The cognitive basis for linguistic structures. In J. R. Hayes (Ed.), *Cognition and the Development of Language*. New York: Wiley (1970).

BLOOM, L., *Language development: Form and function of emerging grammars*. Cambridge: MIT Press (1970).

BLOOM, L., Language development. In F. Horowitz et al. (Eds.), *Review of Child Development Research*. Chicago: Univ. of Chicago Press (in press).

EFRON, R., Temporal perception and deja vu. *Brain*, **86**, 403-424 (1963).

FREEDLE, R. O., KEENEY, T. J., and SMITH, N. D., Effects of mean depth and grammaticability on children's imitations of sentences. *J. verb. Learn verb. Behav.*, **9**, 149-154 (1970).

KAPLAN, E. L., Intonation and language acquisition. *Papers and Reports on Child Language Development*. Stanford, Calif.: Committee on Linguistics, Stanford Univ. **1**, 1-21 (1970).

KARPOVA, S. N., Osonznanie slovesnogo sostava rechi rebenkom doshkol' nogo vozrasta. *Voprosy Psikhol*, **4**, 43-55 (1955). Abstracted by D. I. Slobin, *Abstracts of Soviet studies of child language*. In F. Smith and G. Miller (Eds.), *The Genesis of Language*, Cambridge: MIT Press, 370-371 (1966).

KUMAR, V. K., The structure of human memory and some educational implications. *Rev. educ. Res.*, **41**, 379-418 (1971).

LENNEBERG, E. H., *Biological Foundations of Language*. New York: Wiley (1967).

LEWIS, M. M., *Infant speech, a study of the beginnings of language*. New York: Humanities (1951).

LOWE, A., and CAMPBELL, R., Temporal discrimination in aphasoid and normal children. *J. Speech Hearing Res.*, **8**, 313-314 (1965).

MARATSOS, M., The effects of stress on the understanding of pronominal co-reference in children. *J. psycholing. Res.*, **2**, 1-9 (1973).

MENYUK, P., *Sentences Children Use*. Cambridge: MIT Press (1969).

RYAN, J., Temporal grouping, rehearsal and short-term memory. *Quart. J. exp. Psychol.*, **21**, 148-155 (1969).

SCHOLES, R. J., The role of grammaticality in the imitation of word strings by children and adults. *J. verb. Learn. verb. Behav.*, **8**, 225-278 (1969).

SHELDON, A., The role of parallel function in the acquisition of relative clauses in English. *Univ. of Minnesota Working Papers in Linguistics and Philosophy*. **1**, (1973).

SINCLAIR, H., BRONCKART, J. P., and BRONCKART, V. O., A linguistic universal? A study in developmental psycholinguistics. *J. exp. Child Psychol.*, **14**, 329-348 (1972).

STARK, J., A comparison of the performance of aphasic children on three sequencing tests. *J. commun. Dis.*, **1**, 31-34 (1967).

STARK, J., POPPEN, R., and MAY, M., Effects of alteration of prosodic features on the sequencing performance of children. *J. Speech Hearing Res.*, **10**, 849-855 (1967).

TURNER, E. A., and ROMMETVEIT, R., The acquisition of sentence voice and reversibility. *Child Develpm.*, **38**, 649-660 (1967).

VYGOTSKY, L. S., *Thought and Language*. Cambridge: MIT Press (1962).

WATT, W., On two hypotheses concerning psycholinguistics. In J. R. Hayes (Ed.), *Cognition and the Development of Language*. New York: J. Wiley 137-220 (1970).

WERNER, H., and KAPLAN, B., *Symbol formation*. New York: J. Wiley (1963).

Received Nov. 26, 1973.
Accepted Feb. 7, 1974.

11

Annotated Article: Audiology

CHILDREN'S PERCEPTION OF SPEECH IN REVERBERATION

Reprinted from the *Journal of the Acoustical Society of America, 73,* 2145–2149, (1983).

ARLEEN C. NEUMAN AND IRVING HOCHBERG

Doctoral Program in Speech and Hearing Sciences, Graduate School, City University of New York, New York, New York 10036(Received 8 November 1982; accepted for publication 28 · February 1983)

Recordings of nonsense syllables (VCV construction) were presented to groups of children aged 5, 7, 9, 11, and 13 years and young adults under monaural (reverberation time = 0.6 s) and binaural (reverberation times = 0, 0.4, and 0.6 s) conditions of reverberation. Phoneme identification performance was affected by age, reverberation, and mode of presentation (monaural versus binaural). The major findings were (1) phoneme identification scores in reverberant conditions improved with increasing age and decreased with increased reverberation time; (2) children's performance in reverberant conditions did not reach asymptote until age 13; (3) binaural performance was consistently better than monaural performance for all age groups, with 5-year-olds showing the largest binaural advantage.

PACS numbers: 43.70. Dn, 43.55.Br, 43.50.Qp

☐ *The succinct title clearly identifies the major variables studied. The abstract clearly summarizes the independent variables and their effects on the dependent variable by describing briefly the method and results.* ☐

410

INTRODUCTION

Assumptions are often made about the perceptual abilities of children based on the findings of studies performed on adults, despite documented evidence that developmental changes in auditory performance often occur as a function of age. Studies of children's perception of speech in noise (e.g., Elliott *et al.,* 1979), of dichotic syllables (e.g., Mirabile *et al.,* 1978), and of time-compressed speech (e.g., Beasley *et al.,*1976) all demonstrate an increase in children's ability to perceive degraded speech as a function of age. While some of these experimental forms of degradation bear little relationship to everyday listening conditions, children do listen to a naturally occurring form of degraded speech daily—reverberant speech.

The traditional parameter which has been studied in evaluating the effect of room acoustics on speech perception is reverberation time, which is defined as the time necessary for a steady-state signal to decay by 60 dB once the sound is terminated. The effect of reverberation is to sustain the intensity of the speech signal, as well as prolong it. Short reverberation times may actually be beneficial to the listener if the speech signal is of insufficient intensity. In general, however, reverberation degrades speech identification since the reflected energy overlaps with the direct signal thus introducing a temporal form of masking (Knudsen and Harris, 1950).

One purpose of the present study was to examine whether or not developmental changes in performance occur for reverberant speech materials as they do for other forms of degraded speech. If children are affected more by reverberation than adults, then the acoustic characteristics of classrooms and other learning environments need to be based on data for children and not adults, as is currently the case. For example, Knudsen and Harris' (1950) recommendation of a 0.75-s reverberation time as optimal for normal-hearing listeners in a typical classroom is based on the performance of adults on speech intelligibility tests. If, as Ross (1978) suggests, the criterion of optimal reverberation time be based on maximum speech discrimination ability, then the recommended reverberation time for classrooms may be excessive for children.[1]

☐ *The first two paragraphs of the introduction set the stage for reporting the details of the experiment by presenting a rationale for studying the effects of reverberation on children's speech perception. The main purpose of the study is stated in the third paragraph along with comments on the potential implications of the research as an indication of the importance of studying this particular problem.* ☐

---

[1]An alternate criterion to consider is listener preference. Berkley (1980) points out that listeners may prefer different reverberant conditions, even within a range where speech intelligibility is not degraded. The issue of listener preference was not addressed in this study.

In any event, surveys of reverberation time in schools reveal that many classrooms for normal-hearing children have reverberation times far in excess of those recommended by Knudsen and Harris. Thomas and John (1957), for example, reported measured reverberation times of 1.3 to 3.4 s in classrooms, Tolk (1961) reported average reverberation times of 1.2 s, while Kodaras (1960) reported a range of 0.4 to 1.1 s. In their survey of schools built between 1890 and 1960, McCroskey and Devens (1975) found that classrooms in the more recently constructed schools had shorter reverberation times than those in older buildings. It was not uncommon to find reverberation times in excess of 1.0 s in the older buildings, while the average reverberation time in the new buildings was 0.6 s.

It is likely that normal-hearing young adults would experience some difficulty listening to speech in classrooms with reverberation time in excess of 1.0 s, but would have little difficulty in classrooms where reverberation is less than 1.0 s. But what of children? Finitzo-Hieber and Tillman (1978) examined the effect of reverberation and noise on monosyllabic word intelligibility for normal-hearing and hearing-impaired children, aged 8 to 13. Three reverberation times (0, 0.4, and 1.2 s) and four listening conditions (quiet; + 12, + 6, and 0 dB signal-to-noise ratios) were evaluated. The results of their study follow the same trends observed in studies on adults. That is, increasing reverberation time caused a decrease in word discrimination for both normal-hearing and hearing-impaired children, and the combination of reverberation and noise had a greater effect on hearing-impaired than on normal-hearing children. Discrimination of speech by the normal-hearing children did not decrease significantly in the 0.4-s reverberation condition (quiet), although significant decreases did occur in the 1.2-s reverberation condition. The combined effect of reverberation and noise did, however, affect the normal-hearing children even at the rather short 0.4-s reverberation time.

An interesting observation noted by Finitzo-Hieber and Tillman was that the normal-hearing children in their study seemed to be affected more by reverberation than were a group of normal-hearing adults tested under similar experimental conditions by Crum (1974). While Crum found little decrease in speech discrimination by adults in a 1.2-s reverberation condition (quiet), Finitzo-Hieber and Tillman found significant decreases in discrimination by children. A major difference between the two studies is the fact that Crum's subjects were tested binaurally, whereas the children in the Finitzo-Hieber and Tillman study were tested monaurally. Since binaural hearing can increase speech discrimination under reverberant conditions (e.g., Moncur and Dirks, 1967; Nabelek and Pickett, 1974 a, b), a study designed to directly compare performance by children and adults is necessary to substantiate whether or not age differences affect performance.

Such a comparison was made by Nabelek and Robinson (1982) who included a group of 10-year-old children in their study of reverberation and age. Word-identification scores were obtained on the Modified Rhyme Test in the nonreverberant condition and under three reverberant conditions (0.4, 0.8, and 1.2 s) in quiet. Children's scores were poorer than those of young adults (mean age of 27) in the reverberant conditions, but not in the nonreverberant condition. Furthermore, increasing the reverberation from 0.4 to 0.8 s caused a greater decrease in discrimination for the children than for the young adults. Thus it would seem that children are more affected by reverberation than adults. However, because only one group of children was tested, it remains unclear whether or not the performance of these 10-year-olds is typical of all young children. The age at which children's performance approximates that of adults also remains undetermined.

The purpose of the present study was to determine whether or not children's perception of speech under reverberant conditions typical of modern classrooms would change as a function of age. The nature of the binaural advantage in children under reverberant conditions was also investigated.

☐ *Paragraphs four through seven of the introduction review literature on reverberation time in school rooms, effects of reverberation on speech intelligibility, and monaural vs. binaural hearing in reverberation in order to build a case for why the study of the specific variables that the authors have chosen is necessary. The last paragraph of the introduction states the specific purposes of the study by identifying the independent and dependent variables to be examined.*

As with the Lahey article reviewed in Chapter 10, the discussion of the references is not as extensive as would be found in a literature review article because the journal format forces authors of research articles to be succinct. Nevertheless, the introductory review covers the salient features of the important literature needed to introduce the problem and provides a convincing rationale for undertaking the study. Overall, the introduction is concise, clearly organized, and well written.

The reader should immediately grasp the fact that this study is combined experimental-descriptive research. The experimental part examines the effects of the manipulable independent variables (reverberation time and binaural vs. monaural listening) on the dependent variable (phoneme identification). The descriptive aspect of the research is the developmental study of the effects of independent variables on the dependent variable over the age span of 5 to 13 years. ☐

I. METHOD

A. Experimental Materials

Nonsense syllables were chosen as the experimental stimuli because these materials would be less affected by age factors than meaningful materials.[2]

[2]Lexical knowledge and familiarity with test vocabulary are both factors which can influence speech identification scores (e.g., Broadbent, 1967; Hirsh *et al.,* 1952; Epstein *et al.,* 1968). Special test materials have been designed with items believed to be appropriate to the vocabu-

The stimuli consisted of symmetric VCV (vowel-consonant-vowel) disyllables in which each of three vowels /i/, /a/, and /u/ was combined with each of 19 consonants (all consonants of English with the exception of the semi-vowels /w/, /r/, /l/, and /j/). Since each of the stimuli appeared twice in the experimental material, this resulted in one list of 114 nonsense disyllables (e.g., /ipi/, /apa/, and /upu/) which would be used for each of the experimental conditions. The order of syllables in this list was randomly assigned.

The single list of disyllables was recorded by a male talker with extensive experience in making recordings to be used in studies of speech identification. The recording was made in a sound-treated room. Each disyllable was preceded by the carrier phrase, "say the word," with each syllable of the stimulus receiving equal stress (e.g., /ípí/). The peak level of the key word "word" in each carrier phrase of this master recording was measured using a Brüel and Kjær graphic level recorder with the averaging time set at approximately 25 ms and the pen writing rate at 100 mm/s. Peak levels were found to be constant within ± 2 dB across all utterances. A 1000-Hz calibration tone and a speech-spectrum noise calibration signal were recorded at the beginning of the master recording. The level of each of the calibration signals would produce a deflection on a graphic level recording equal to the measured average peak level of the key word in the carrier phrase. The 1000-Hz tone was used to set the tape recorder level for playback, while the speech-spectrum noise was utilized to set the signal level during the making of the room recordings.

The master recording of the nonsense syllables was played into an empty room (volume 156.5 m³)[3] in which reverberation time was varied by adding or removing acoustically absorbent materials. The master recording was introduced into the reverberation room through a loudspeaker and recordings were made through a KEMAR manikin. Before making the reverberant recordings, reverberation time measurements were obtained by introducing gated white noise bursts (2.5-s duration, 10-ms rise/decay time) into the room and measuring the decay after offset in 1/3-octave bands. The noise signal was introduced into the room through a loudspeaker centrally located at a distance 1.8 m from the front of the room and at an elevation 0.79 m

---

laries of young children (e.g., Haskins, 1949; Ross and Lerman, 1970; Elliott and Katz, 1980). While these materials are more likely to be suitable for children than materials designed for adults, children within particular age ranges will not necessarily be familiar with all the vocabulary items. Lexical items which are unknown to a child are treated as if they are nonsense words. Furthermore, those words known to all of the children will have been used more frequently by the older children and thus be more familiar to them. Meaningful materials could thus be more difficult for younger than older children. If differences in speech identification scores are found between younger and older children on such materials, these differences may reflect cognitive rather than perceptual differences between subjects of different ages. The use of nonsense syllables would minimize the influence of possible cognitive effects.

[3]The room is wedge shaped (the ceiling is slanted). Its dimensions are length 9.3 m, width 5 m, and height 3 m and 3.7 m.

from the floor. The sound level meter/filter set was placed on a tripod at a distance 4.5 m from the speaker at 0° azimuth. Reverberation times were calculated from graphic level recordings with a Brüel and Kjær reverberation time protractor (Broch and Jensen, 1966).

Reverberant recordings were made of the nonsense stimulus materials at two reverberation times, 0.4 and 0.6 s (average of measured reverberation at 500, 1000, and 2000 Hz). Reverberation times varied by less than 0.15 s between 125 and 8000 Hz. The reverberation times chosen for the recordings are shorter than those found in most classrooms (McCroskey and Devens, 1975) and might be considered to represent acceptable, or even desirable classroom acoustics.

The signal source and the microphones used to make the recordings in the reverberation room were arranged to simulate a classroom situation. The loudspeaker (AR12C) was placed in a center position 1.8 m from the front of the room and at an elevation 0.79 m from the floor, a position typical of a teacher standing in the front of the classroom. The KEMAR was placed to approximate the position of a student seated in the back of a classroom, at 0° azimuth and 4.6 m from the loudspeaker. This distance was calculated to be in excess of the critical distance for the room (volume 156.5 m³), loudspeaker (Q= 1.15), and reverberation times (0.4 and 0.6 s) used for the study (Klein, 1971). Since the critical distance is that point in a room where direct and reflected energy are equal (Peutz, 1971), placement of the KEMAR at a distance in excess of the critical distance would assure that the microphones used for recording were located in the reverberant field. The level of the speech signal was set so that the speech-spectrum noise calibration signal was 60 dBA at the center of the manikin's head. The output from each of KEMAR's microphones was amplified, passed through an equalization filter (Killion, 1979), and recorded on a two-track tape recorder set at a speed of $7\frac{1}{2}$ ips. Recording was done at −10 VU.

An additional recording was made through the KEMAR in an anechoic chamber in order to obtain a nonreverberant test tape made in a manner similar to the reverberant tapes.

☐ Materials: *The materials and equipment used in the study are thoroughly described in the section entitled Experimental materials. The test environments, instrumentation, calibration procedures, and speech materials used are all adequately described and descriptions are accompanied by a rationale where necessary. Note particularly the discussion in the next to the last paragraph of the attempt to simulate the classroom situation: this is an excellent example of an attempt to balance the need for rigorous experimental control with the need to generalize results to a more typical setting. Also, note that there is a different emphasis here than in the Lahey article reviewed in Chapter 10. Whereas the Lahey article paid more attention to the description of stimulus material than to hardware, this article does the reverse. The reason should be fairly obvious: the critical point in the language article is the content validity of the stimulus material, whereas instrumental control of stimulus parameters is more important for the audiology article. The reader should also have noticed Footnote 2 in the first paragraph which addresses the issue of the content validity of the speech materials used with this particular age range of subjects.* □

B. Subjects

Twenty-five children ages 5, 7, 9, 11, and 13 (five children per group, mean ages: 5.5, 7.5, 9.5, 11.6, 13.4 years) were the subjects in this experiment. All children had normal hearing for pure tones (*re:* ANSI 1969), speech discrimination scores better than 90% on the CID W-22 lists, normal intelligence (as determined by age-appropriate school placement), and normal articulation skills (as determined on the Goldman-Fristoe Test of Articulation). A group of five normal-hearing young adults (aged 20 to 29, mean: 24 years) was also included in order to obtain asymptotic measures on the experimental stimuli.

□ Subjects: *A reasonably large number of subjects (N = 25) was employed for an experimental study, but the number of subjects in each age group is somewhat small for a cross-sectional developmental study. The small number is a practical compromise because the test environment and equipment required for the research necessitated the expensive and time-consuming process of transporting individual children from their schools to the laboratory. Had the experimenters been able to bring their equipment and test environment to the subjects, they would have been able to test a larger sample. By opting to concentrate their efforts on control of experimental variables rather than on obtaining a larger sample, the experimenters have followed Campbell and Stanley's admonition that strengthening of internal validity has a higher priority than extending external validity. In addition, an interesting practical trade-off in external validity can be seen in comparing the Lahey and Neuman and Hochberg articles. Lahey used a larger number of subjects per age group than Neuman and Hochberg, but she used a smaller number of age groups and a more restricted age range. Because Neuman and Hochberg wished to sample a larger number of ages within a wider range, they reduced their practical ability to test a larger sample in each group. Thus, readers may feel more comfortable about generalization from the Lahey article because of the larger sample, but they would also feel more comfortable about the view of the developmental process in the Neuman and Hochberg article because of the wider age span. Such practical complications are a major constraint in the design of any research.*

The relevant characteristics of the subjects are succinctly, yet thoroughly, described: ages, hearing levels, intelligence, articulation skills. One possibly important subject characteristic not described is the sex distribution within each age group as was specified in the Lahey study. The balancing of the sexes, however, would be more important in the Lahey study because sex differences would be more likely to influence only the younger children and would have more effect on complex language tasks than on a simpler phoneme identification task. □

C. Experimental Procedures

All testing was done in a double-walled IAC sound-treated room. The speech recordings were played on a two-channel tape recorder and presented to the subject via Sennheiser HD 414X headphones.

Testing was done in one or two sessions, depending on the age and attention span of the subject. Binaural testing of the nonreverberant, 0.4- and 0.6-s reverberation conditions was done at 60 dB SPL. The 0.6-s condition was also presented in the monaural mode. Monaural testing was done at 63 dB SPL so that differences in intensity would not account for any monaural/binaural differences. The order of presentation of conditions was randomized. The test ear in the monaural mode was also alternated, so that right and left ears were tested equally.

Subjects were instructed to repeat the stimulus word and the examiner transcribed responses on an answer sheet. Repetition was chosen as the method of response because it would be a simple task for young children and because it would place little load on memory, therefore minimizing cognitive demands. It also allowed ongoing assessment of the subject's attentiveness.

During the experimental session(s), each subject was given a rest period after each experimental list. In order to sustain subject attention and motivation, children were given tangible reinforcement after each 15 test items and were given a "prize" for participation at the end of the test session.

□ Procedures: *This study may be classified as combined descriptive-experimental research. The experimental component is the examination of the effects of reverberation time and mode (monaural vs. binaural) on phoneme identification. Thus, reverberation time and mode are manipulable independent variables and phoneme identification is the dependent variable. The descriptive component is the cross-sectional developmental study of these effects over the age range of 5 years to young adulthood. The design is mixed; the experimental independent variables are manipulated within-subjects, whereas the age comparison is made between-subjects. The reverberation time is a multivalent independent variable, mode is a bivalent independent variable (monaural vs. binaural is a true dichotomy), and the nonmanipulable age variable is examined as a multivalent independent variable.*

An interesting limitation can be seen in the structure of the experimental independent variables: they do not represent a complete parametric experiment. The monaural mode only includes one level of the reverberation time variable: 0.6 second; whereas the binaural mode includes all three levels of the reverberation time variable: 0, 0.4, and 0.6 seconds. Therefore, the complete interaction of reverberation time and mode cannot be examined. This limitation is the result of another practical compromise. Running the complete parametric experiment might be impractical by requiring too much time and attention from the children, thus introducing a short-term maturation threat to internal validity. Thus, the authors have sacrificed the ability to generalize to other treatments (i.e., the interaction of reverberation time and mode) in order to strengthen internal validity, thus following Campbell and Stanley's advice that internal validity is the sine qua non of research. However, because the longer reverberation time is more likely to show the most reduction in phoneme identification and thereby maximize discrimination between binaural and monaural performance, the authors' compromise is the best possible choice for looking at the main effects of these variables and their interactions with age. Also, as mentioned by the authors in the Materials section, the longer reverberation times are more characteristic of actual classrooms and, therefore, are of more immediate interest.

Note the important step that was taken to strengthen internal validity in the within-subjects manipulation of the independent variables: presentation order of the listening conditions was randomized to minimize any possible sequencing effects and short-term maturation problems. The rest periods and the monitoring of subjects' attention and motivation would also help to reduce short-term maturation effects.

The use of a sound treated room and special instrumentation served to standardize the presentation of stimuli to subjects in order to reduce or eliminate instrumental threats to internal validity. As with all experiments, this introduces a certain artificiality relative to the usual classroom listening situation of the children, thereby creating a possible reactive arrangement or Hawthorne effect, which may somewhat limit generalization to other settings. However, this is necessary to ensure proper experimental control of stimuli and environment and is again consistent with Campbell and Stanley's admonition concerning the primacy of internal over external validity.

In summary, the Method section has merits and demerits, as do all articles; but, in weighing these, it appears that the authors have succeeded in reducing most of the major threats to internal validity and have made the appropriate practical compromises where necessary. Possible suggestions to be incorporated in any replications might include: investigation of sex differences at each age level, use of larger samples, and a parametric investigation of reverberation time and mode of listening. □

II. RESULTS

The mean phoneme identification scores (in percentages) are plotted for each of the reverberation conditions as a function of age in Figure 1. It is evident that increasing reverberation caused a decrease in phoneme identification in each age group. This finding has been well documented on adults in the past. The figure also illustrates a tendency for performance to improve as a function of age. In the 0.6-s condition, binaural scores are superior to monaural for all age groups.

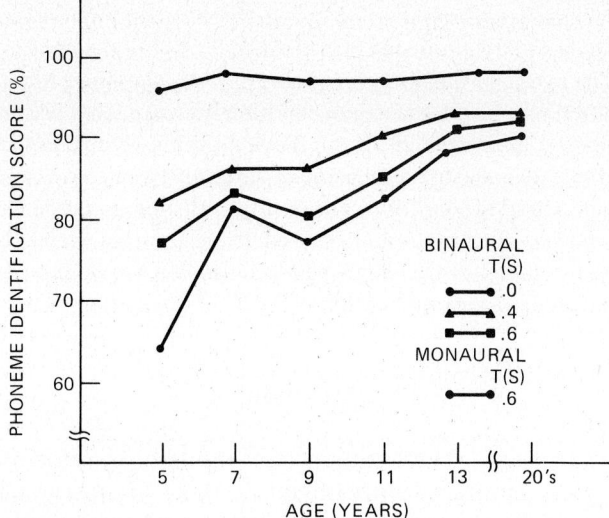

Figure 1.   Mean monaural and binaural phoneme identification scores as a function of age and reverberation time *T*(S).

These phoneme-identification scores were converted to arcsine units in order to stabilize the error variance (Brownlee, 1965). Two analyses of variance were performed. The first to determine the effect of reverberation, age, and their interactions on phoneme identification scores and the second to determine the effect of mode of presentation, age, and their interactions on phoneme identification scores. In both cases, a two factor analysis of variance with repeated measures on one factor was used (Winer, 1971).

The results of the first analysis revealed that the factors of age [F (5,24) = 6.52, $p < 0.001$] and reverberation [F (2,48) = 155.66, $p < 0.001$] were both highly significant. The interaction was only marginally significant [F (10,48) = 2.19, $p < 0.05$].

Mode of presentation (binaural versus monaural) was an additional experimental factor in the 0.6-s reverberation condition. The analysis revealed that the factors of age [F (5,24) = 7.52, $p < 0.001$] and mode of presentation [F (1,24) = 15.75, $p < 0.001$] were both highly significant. The interaction failed to reach significance.

☐ *The results are analyzed in a clear and concise fashion. The figure clearly shows the mean results for monaural and binaural listening at the different reverberation times for each age group and allows immediate comparison of all conditions at each age level. The text clearly describes these results with careful references to the figure. The appropriate analyses of variance are described clearly to show the main effects of the experimental variables and of the age variable. Note the arcsine transformation of the phoneme identification scores that was made; this is necessary whenever an analysis of variance is performed on scores that are percentages or proportions. All F-values, degrees of freedom, and significance levels are reported in the text in a clear fashion. The two separate analyses of variance are necessary because the mode and reverberation time variables were not completely crossed in a parametric experiment. One suggested improvement of the results section would be the addition of standard deviations (or some other measure of variability such as range) for each age group under each listening condition. Variability statistics would have provided an index of the homogeneity of performance of each age group in each listening condition. These statistics may have been omitted because they would crowd the figure or take up too much room in a separate table.* □

III. DISCUSSION

The data show that age, reverberation, and mode of presentation all affect performance on a phoneme identification task. Phoneme identification scores increase with increasing age and decrease with increases in reverberation time, and binaural identification scores are consistently higher than monaural scores for all age groups, with 5-year-olds showing the largest binaural advantage.

Recently, Nabelek *et al.* (1982) reported significant differences between the performance of 10-year-old children and adults under reverberant conditions. Findings of the present study reveal a developmental change in the ability of children to identify speech materials which have been recorded under two conditions of reverberation (0.4 and 0.6 s). The ability to identify speech in reverberant environments improves with increasing age and reaches asymptote at age 13 when performance approximates that of young adults.

A comparison of the data on the 11-year-old subjects in the present study to those for the 10-year-old subjects in the Nabelek and Robinson study reveals essential agreement in the magnitude of the reverberation effect, despite the differences in test materials. The decrement in binaural phoneme identification scores found in the youngest groups (5-, 7-, and 9-year-old children) is larger than that of Nabelek and Robinson's 10-year-olds, but is similar in magnitude to those reported by Nabelek and Robinson for their oldest groups (ages 64 and 72).

□ *The first three paragraphs of the Discussion section briefly summarize the results of the experiment and compare them to previous findings with different age groups and other stimulus materials, noting consistent similarities between the authors' results and those of other investigators.* □

Because nonsense syllables were used as the stimuli in the present study, it is difficult to predict subjects' ability to identify running speech under similar amounts of reverberation. The contribution of contextual cues to speech discrimination is well known (e.g., Miller *et al.,* 1951). Studies of recognition of mispronunciations in running speech, shadowing of speech, and phoneme monitoring tasks reveal that semantic knowledge and contextual cues prevent the listener from identifying errors which have been purposefully introduced by the experimenter, and that the person listening to running speech does not attend to all of the acoustic information in the speech wave (e.g., Cole and Jakimik, 1978). In other words, a certain amount of "noise" does not interfere with the perception of a speech signal, if semantic knowledge and knowledge of context can be used.

In the present study, phoneme identification by adults was still excellent for the 0.6-s reverberation condition, despite the fact that the effect of reverberation was statistically significant. When one considers that nonsense syllables were employed in the study and that in the "real world" semantic and syntactic knowledge would be available to the adult to clarify possible phoneme confusions, it is doubtful that these adults would experience difficulty listening to speech in a room with a 0.6-s reverberation time in quiet. However, it has been demonstrated that younger children are less able to utilize semantic and contextual cues in difficult listening situations than are older children and adults. Elliott (1979) found an age-related change in performance by children aged 9 to 17 on the high-predictability sentences of the SPIN test at the 0 dB signal-to-noise ratio, but not on the sentences in quiet or on the low-predictability sentences in noise. Adultlike performance was not attained until age 15. Marshall *et al.* (1979) also reported that discrimination scores of children ages 5 to 11 were poorer than scores of adults on sentence materials which had been distorted by switching between ears, by interruption, or by low-pass filtering, despite the fact that vocabulary was appropriate for the youngest children included in the study. Thus the children's phoneme identification scores are more likely to predict the effect of reverberation on running speech than are those of adults.

☐ *The next two paragraphs discuss some limitations of the study regarding the stimulus material that was used and consider some external validity problems concerning generalization to other stimuli in other listening situations. References to previous research are made and consideration is given to both theoretical and practical implications of the experimental and developmental aspects of the research.* ☐

The developmental effect found in the present study is in agreement with other findings in auditory development and with the statement by Fior (1972) that adultlike performance on many auditory tasks is achieved by age 13. As has been demonstrated by Fior and by others (e.g., Siegenthaler, 1969; Maxon and Hochberg, 1982), the more complex the task (discrimination versus identification), or the more difficult the task (low redundancy versus high redundancy), the more likely that the child will be older before adultlike performance is demonstrated.

The performance of children cannot be described in incremental stages as a function of age. Performance changes gradually and at different rates for different children. While younger children are more affected by reverberation than older children, there is an overlap in performance between age groups. In fact, the performance of the 7-year-olds in this study was slightly better on the average than that of the 9-year-olds. Chronological age is only one factor in the maturation process. However, the trend of improvement in performance reaching asymptote at age 13 is clear. It is difficult to determine the factors which underlie the differences in performance between the younger and older subjects in the present study. Although minimal demands were placed on memory, other cognitive differences might have contributed to the superior performance of older subjects.

Binaural scores tended to be superior to monaural in each age group. The binaural advantage (difference between binaural and monaural scores) was probably larger in the youngest group than in any other group due to the low mean monaural score for that group. The monaural scores for subjects 7 years and older were all better than 75% and could thus be expected to lie above the linear portion of the speech identification function. The average binaural advantage obtained for subjects age 7 and older is small, but suggests the inferiority of the monaural condition. In this experiment, reverberation times were short and testing was done only in quiet. With longer reverberation times and/or the addition of noise, a larger binaural advantage could be expected.

That children's performance was poorer than adults, despite the fact that the reverberation times employed were relatively short and in quiet, has important implications for the acoustical design of classrooms for normal-hearing children. Children need shorter reverberation times than do adults in order to achieve maximum speech identification, but the specification for design of classrooms has been based on adult performance (Knudsen and Harris, 1950). In order for children to obtain maximum identification of a speech signal, close to anechoic conditions are required. The present study revealed significant decreases in phoneme identification in quiet for children for a reverberation condition of 0.4-s. Even shorter reverberation times would be necessary for maximum identification in noise, since the combined effect of noise and reverberation is more than additive (Finitzo-Heiber and Tillman, 1978). It would seem that the recommendation by Finitzo-Hieber and Tillman that reverberation times in classrooms designed for hearing-impaired children should not exceed 0.4 s should also be applied to classrooms for normal-hearing children, ages 5 to 11.

☐ *The last four paragraphs of the Discussion section consider theoretical implications of the results regarding the developmental effects observed, implications of the* results regarding the differences between binaural and monaural modes, and a number of suggestions for further research that may answer some of the questions raised by the results. Finally, practical implications regarding recommended reverberation times in classrooms are discussed in light of the developmental trends seen in this and other studies.

The discussion covers most of the major points outlined in Chapter 9, including discussion of results in relation to previous research, theoretical implications, limitations of the study, practical implications, and suggestions for future research. □

ACKNOWLEDGMENTS

Reverberant recordings were made at The Auditory Department, United States Naval Submarine Medical Research Laboratory, Groton, CT. The authors express their appreciation to Harry Levitt and Michael Studdert-Kennedy for their assistance throughout this study.

American National Standard Specifications for Audiometers (1969). ANSI 53.6.

Beasley, D. S., Maki, J., and Orchik, D. (1976). "Children's perception of time compressed speech on two measures of speech discrimination," J. Speech Hear. Disord. 41, 216–225.

Berkley, D. A. (1980). "Normal listeners in typical rooms. Reverberation perception, simulation, and reduction," in *Acoustical Factors Affecting Hearing Aid Performance*, edited by G. A. Studebaker and I. Hochberg (University Park, Baltimore, MD), pp. 3–24.

Broadbent, D. E. (1967). "Word frequency effect and response bias," Psychol. Rev. 74, 1–15.

Broch, J. T., and Jensen, V. N. (1966). "On the measurement of reverberation," Brüel and Kjær Tech. Rev. No. 4.

Brownlee, K. A. (1965). *Statistical Theory and Methodology in Science and Engineering* (Wiley, New York), 2nd ed.

Cole, R. A., and Jakimik, J. (1978). "Understanding Speech: How words are heard," in *Strategies of Information Processing*, edited by G. Underwood (Academic, New York), pp. 67–116.

Crum, M. A. (1974). "Effects of speaker to listener distance upon speech intelligibility in reverberation and noise," unpublished Doctoral dissertation, Northwestern University, Evanston, IL.

Elliott, L. L. (1979). "Performance of children aged 9 to 17 on a test of speech intelligibility in noise using sentence material with controlled word predictability," J. Acoust. Soc. Am. 66, 651–653.

Elliott, L. L., Connors, S., Kille, E., Levin, S., Ball, K., and Katz, D. (1979). "Children's understanding of monosyllabic nouns in quiet and in noise," J. Acoust. Soc. Am. 66, 12–21.

Elliott, L. L., and Katz, D. R. (1980). *Development of a New Children's Test of Speech Discrimination* (Auditec of Saint Louis, Missouri).

Epstein, A., Giolas, T., and Owens, E. (1968). "Familiarity and intelligibility of monosyllabic word lists," J. Speech Hear. Res. 11, 435–438.

Finitzo-Hieber, T., and Tillman, T. W. (1978). "Room acoustics effects on monosyllabic word discrimination ability for normal and hearing impaired children," J. Speech Hear. Res. 21, 440–458.

Fior, R. (1972). "Physiological maturation of auditory function between 3 and 13 years of age," Audiology 11, 317–321.

Haskins, H. (1949). "A phonetically balanced test of speech discrimination for children," unpublished Master's thesis. Northwestern University, Evanston, IL.

Hirsh, I. J., Davis, H., Silverman, S. R., Reynolds, E. E., Eldert, E., and Benson, R. W. (1952). "Development of materials for speech audiometry," J. Speech Hear. Disord. 17, 321–337.

Killion, M. C. (1979). "Equalization Filter for eardrum-pressure recording using a KEMAR manikin," J. Audio Eng. Soc. 27, 13–16.

Klein, W. (1971). "Articulation loss of consonants as a basis for the design and judgment of sound reinforcement systems," J. Audio Eng. Soc. 19, 920–922.

Knudsen, V. O., and Harris, C. M. (1950). *Acoustical Designing in Architecture* (Wiley, New York).

Kodaras, M. J. (1960). "Reverberation times of typical elementary school classrooms," Noise-Control 6, 17–19.

McCroskey, R. L., and Devens, J. S. (1975). "Acoustic characteristics of public school classrooms constructed between 1890 and 1960," NOISEXPO Proc., 101–103.

Maxon, A. B., and Hochberg, I. (1982). "Development of psychoacoustic behavior: Sensitivity and discrimination," Ear Hear. 3, 301–308.

Marshall, L., Brandt, J. F., Marston, L. E., and Ruder, K. (1979). "Changes in number and type of errors on repetition of acoustically distorted sentences as a function of age in normal children," J. Am. Audiol. Soc. 4, 218–225.

Miller, G. A., Heise, G. A., and Lichten, W. (1951). "The intelligibility of speech as a function of the test materials," J. Exp. Psychol. 41, 329–335.

Mirabile, P. J., Porter, R. J., Hughes, L. F., and Berlin, C. I. (1978). "Dichotic lag effect in children 7 to 15," Dev. Psychol. 14, 277–285.

Moncur, J. P., and Dirks, D. (1967). "Binaural and monaural speech intelligibility in reverberation," J. Speech Hear. Res. 10, 186–195.

Nabelek, A. K., and Pickett, J. M. (1974a). "Monaural and binaural speech perception through hearing aids under noise and reverberation with normal and hearing-impaired listeners," J. Speech Hear. Res. 17, 724–739.

Nabelek, A. K., and Pickett, J. M. (1974b). "Reception of consonants in a classroom as affected by monaural and binaural listening, noise, reverberation, and hearing aids," J. Acoust. Soc. Am. 56, 628–639.

Nabelek, A. K., and Robinson, P. K. (1982). "Monaural and binaural speech perception in reverberation for listeners of various ages," J. Acoust. Soc. Am. 71, 1242–1248.

Peutz, U. M. A. (1971). "Articulation loss of consonants as a criterion for speech transmission in a room," J. Audio Eng. Soc. 19, 915–919.

Ross, M. (1978). "Classroom acoustics and speech intelligibility," in *Handbook of Clinical Audiology,* edited by J. Katz (Williams and Wilkins, Maryland), 2nd ed.

Ross, M., and Lerman, J. (1970). "A picture identification test for hearing impaired children," J. Speech Hear. Res. 13, 44–53.

Siegenthaler, B. (1969). "Maturation of auditory abilities in children," Int. Audiol. 8, 59–71.

Thomas, H., and John, J. (1957). "Design and construction of schools for the deaf," in *Educational Guidance and the Deaf Child,* edited by A. W. G. Ewing (Manchester U.P., London).

Tolk, J. (1961). "Acoustics, intelligibility of speech and electroacoustic systems in classrooms," in *Proceedings of the 2nd International Course in Paedo-Audiology* (Groningen Univ., Netherlands).

Winer, B. J. (1971). *Statistical Principles in Experimental Design* (McGraw-Hill, New York).

Appendix A

PROTECTION OF HUMAN SUBJECTS IN SPEECH AND HEARING RESEARCH

Reprinted from *Asha*, 27 (3), 25–29, (1985).

DALE EVAN METZ AND JOHN W. FOLKINS

In the view of authors Dale Evan Metz and John W. Folkins, federal regulations regarding human research subjects protect not only the subjects but also investigators and institutions. Issues of concern to speech, language, and hearing researchers are (1) the development, role, and applicability of federal regulations, (2) the structure of Institutional Review Boards (IRBs), (3) the actions of IRBs, (4) risk-benefit determination, (5) subject contact, information to subjects, and informed consent, (6) research and the speech and hearing clinic, and (7) students and research. Metz is associate professor of speech science at the National Technical Institute for the Deaf at Rochester Institute of Technology in Rochester, New York. Folkins is associate professor in the Department of Speech Pathology and Audiology at the University of Iowa in Iowa City. Both have served on Institutional Review Boards, which review research involving human subjects.

Issues relating to the protection of human subjects in experimentation have a history that is linked to the development and growth of medical, behavioral, and social sciences. In the past two decades, ethical, legal, and scientific concerns have resulted in federal regulations designed to safeguard the rights and welfare of human subjects. In accord with a resolution passed by the National Advisory Health Council, in February 1966, the Surgeon General issued a policy statement that required all clinical research funded by the Public Health Service to be independently reviewed by the grantee institution. This review was designed to assure independent determination:

(1) of the rights and welfare of research subjects, (2) of the appropriateness of methods used to obtain informed consent, and (3) of the risks and potential benefits of the research.

In July 1966, this policy was extended from clinical research to all research involving human subjects funded by Public Health Service grants with the additional requirement that grantee institutions ". . . submit with the application, or as soon after submission of the application as possible, a certification that this review and approval has taken place." This policy was further extended in December 1971 to include, not just the Public Health Service, but all research involving human subjects funded by any agency of the Department of Health, Education, and Welfare (currently the Department of Health and Human Services, HHS).

A central event shaping the development of the federal regulations was the enactment of the National Research Act of 1974 (Public Law 93–348), which created the National Commission for the Protection of Human Subjects in Biomedical and Behavioral Research. This commission was to identify basic principles that should underlie biomedical and behavioral research with human subjects. The commission was also charged with the responsibility to develop guidelines to assure compliance with those principles. Basic regulations regarding the protection of human subjects, published in the Federal Register (1974), explicitly defined the responsibilities of the Institutional Review Board (IRB) and detailed the nature of informed consent. Extended provisions regarding IRB review criteria, which provided specific protections for pregnant women, fetuses, and prisoners, were added to the basic regulations in 1975 and 1978. The final code of federal regulations was published in 1981 (Federal Register, 1981). In March 1983, Subpart D was added extending IRB review criteria for research involving children. The current regulations are available from the Office for Protection From Research Risks, National Institutes of Health, 9000 Rockville Pike, Building 31, Room 4B09, Bethesda, Maryland 20205.

THE ROLE OF THE REGULATIONS

It is sometimes asserted that our system for protection of human subjects has been developed in response to abuses of human subjects in research. Certainly, there have been some deplorable abuses and unjust treatments of human subjects in the name of science. Examples of human subject abuse include the involuntary experimentation by the Nazis in World War II, the denial of antibiotics to 300 rural black persons in the Tuskegee syphilis study, and the sterilization of 200 mentally disabled young women with the experimental drug Depo-Provera in Arlington, Tennessee. Such treatment of human beings in some research situations led to the creation, in 1974, of the National Commission for the Protection of Human Subjects in Biomedical and Behavioral Research. However, after four years of investigation, debate, and the publication of nine reports, the commission found a system which could be improved, but not one which was plagued with abuses (Brady & Jonsen, 1982). The fact that widespread abuse of human subjects had not occurred prior to the development of federal regulations is not surprising. Our scientific system has a history of respect for human rights and welfare and our health delivery systems have a history of ethical principles for patient care. Prior to the development of federal regulations, discussion of ethical issues often occurred in scientific meetings. For example, Travis presented a study in 1925 in which the speech of stutterers was studied in a condition of "emotional upheaval" produced by taking them into a darkened room and unexpectedly firing a pistol near them. As might be expected, the discussion following the presentation did not deal with the topic of the presentation. It was a tirade on the inappropriateness of the procedures (Moeller, 1976).

A number of scientists were strongly opposed to the regulations governing human subjects research when they were first proposed. They argued that the scientific system already included safeguards and that specific regulations could stifle academic freedom and undermine the trust between patient (subject) and health-care provider (investigator). It was also felt that development of regulations was a *de facto* admission of widespread abuse. Despite the early objections, the system of federal regulations appears to have gained general acceptance—even for much nonfederally funded research which is not subject to current federal regulations. This is true in spite of the large expense involved in maintaining Institutional Review Boards and the delays and time burdens placed on investigators by the system.

Although the primary purpose of the federal regulations is to protect human research subjects, we believe that there are other purposes which may be important and which help to explain the success and acceptance of the system. These purposes involve the public-science interface, investigator direction, and institutional awareness.

Public-Science Interface

Triumphs of science influence our lives daily. However, along with the power of science, the public is often reminded of the potential to abuse such power. In conjunction with legitimate indictments of human subject abuse such as those cited above, the potential for abuse has been developed in fictional writings. Recent successes with organ transplants seem to bring us closer to Shelley's *Frankenstein,* written in 1818. Recent successes with test-tube fertilization and recombinant DNA seem to bring us closer to Huxley's *Brave New World,* written in 1932. Such concerns are not limited to medical research. Skinner's *Walden Two,* written in 1948, illustrates the power of behavioral conditioning. These fictional examples may overstate the situation, but it is reasonable to assume that the public's perception of what typically happens to subjects in the research process may be inaccurate. Given this climate, it is not surprising that many lay persons may be apprehensive when asked to participate as a research subject.

An important mechanism for alleviating a potential subject's concerns about participation in a research study is adequate communication. However, some investigators may not realize the need for communication with subjects. Institutional Review Boards insure that the investigator (1) properly solicits subject participation, (2) provides sufficient information to the subject so that the subject can give "informed consent," and (3) provides an open channel of communication with the subject throughout the experiment.

In this regard, members of an IRB, by virtue of their familiarity with and sensitivity to the issues, can be an important interface between the subject and investigator. For example, by assisting the investigator with the development of informed consent documents the IRB performs a service that may be difficult to duplicate outside of the regulatory system. Indeed, just the existence of an IRB may help to remove the perception that research is not open to public scrutiny.

Investigator Direction

As mentioned above, some investigators have considered the human subjects regulatory process as an affront to their integrity and judgment. Nonetheless, an investigator's judgment of subject risk relative to the potential benefits of the research may be influenced (often unintentionally) by a variety of conditions. Even the most conscientious investigator might overlook research conditions that could violate the rights and welfare of human subjects. In this regard the IRB provides a service to the investigator. During the IRB's review process, unbiased scrutiny can lead to significant modifications in the experimental procedures.

There are a number of areas (for example, the use of X rays to study normal speech production) in which many scientists hold strong opinions based on a combination of objective evidence, emotion, and research bias. When questions regarding the appropriateness of an experimental procedure are raised during an IRB review, the IRB can question the investigator and also solicit the opinions of experts in the area. Advice and counsel of this nature may be difficult to duplicate outside of the regulatory structure. Thus, the IRB regulatory system is not necessarily a bureaucratic obstacle for the investigator, but rather a resource to allow an unbiased review of proposed experimental procedures.

IRBs also may be in a position to stand behind an investigator who has complied with the regulations. Prior to the development of the regulatory system, it was possible for an overzealous individual to delay or prevent an area of research with an unsubstantiated allegation of subject abuse. With the present system, if a project is approved by an IRB, and then challenged for some reason, an investigator can claim that an IRB has agreed with his/her determination that the procedures are appropriate. This may save the investigator the time and effort involved in defending him/herself. It also minimizes the possibility that a scientist with a competing theory could circumvent scientific discussion by raising an unfounded claim of subject abuse. However, this discussion should be qualified by the fact that investigators and IRBs should always be open to new information concerning the protection of subjects. There may be instances in which new information makes it appropriate to amend or discontinue research activities, even if they have been approved previously.

Institutional Awareness

In some cases, administrators may be in a position to stop research that has been approved by an IRB. This would depend on the type and structure of the institution as well as the reasons for stopping the research. In general, however, administrators may not override an IRB's disapproval of a project. Although IRBs function with autonomy in this respect, they also perform a service for administrators. When a research project is challenged, it may be easier for an administrator to stand behind an investigator if the procedures have been reviewed and approved by an IRB. The minutes of IRB meetings may be a valuable resource when documenting the review procedures followed. The minutes also allow administrators to be more aware of the research conducted in the name of an institution.

THE APPLICABILITY OF FEDERAL REGULATIONS

The federal regulations for the protection of human subjects specifically apply only to research conducted or funded by HHS. At present HHS only "strongly recommends" similar protection mechanisms for other research. As such, one might consider these regulations to be the norm for any human subjects experimentation. The President's Commission for the Study of Ethical Problems in Medicine and Biomedical and Behavioral Research, however, recently recommended that all federal agencies adopt the HHS regulations (45 CFR Part 46, *Federal Register,* March 8, 1983) and that the Secretary of HHS establish an office to coordinate and monitor government-wide implementation of the regulations. Decisions on these matters should be forthcoming soon.

What Is Research?

It is important, yet sometimes difficult, to decide which activities are research and which activities do not qualify as research. The federal regulations define research as "a systematic investigation designed to develop or contribute to *generalizable knowledge*" (our italics). This means the pur-

pose of an activity is what makes it subject to review as research, not the characteristics of the specific procedures. Activities that are research may also have administrative, client care, or educational purposes. It is the presence of any purpose to contribute to generalizable knowledge that determines whether the activities are research; the presence of other purposes does not influence this determination. For example, a reporter might ask questions of a writer about language structures for a newspaper article. This would not be research as the purpose would be to inform the public about a specific writer's style (i.e., it would not add to generalizable knowledge). However, the same questions could be used for a purpose of exploring generalities about effective language structures. In this case the purpose would be to contribute to generalizable knowledge about language structures and the activity would qualify for review as research. This system seems awkward in that, if the purpose of the regulations is to protect human subjects, then the breadth of the regulations should be defined relative to what needs protecting, not relative to an investigator's intentions. However, in practice it would be extremely difficult, if not impossible, to define research on a procedure-by-procedure basis. The purpose definition is more workable.

Even with the above definitions it is often not easy to determine the "boundary" between research and clinical practice. This issue was dealt with by the National Commission for the Protection of Human Subjects in Biomedical and Behavioral Research in the Belmont Report (1979). The boundary problem is especially acute in the areas of innovative therapy or nonvalidated practice. The fact that a new procedure is untested does not place it in the category of research. However, if the therapy works well, the clinician may wish to try it with other clients and to make generalizations as to its effectiveness. At some point in this process a research purpose emerges. This point is not always clear. When in doubt, it is safest for an investigator to consider an activity to be research.

What Is a Human Subject?

The federal regulations are explicit and detailed in the definition of what is "human." While this is not a problem for most research in speech and hearing, it is sometimes difficult to decide who is a subject and who is an investigator. Pilot studies, for example, are research. When an investigator tries something on him herself or colleagues, they are subjects.

In a hearing experiment one usually thinks of the listeners as subjects. One would not consider an investigator who produced a speech sample to be presented to listeners as a subject. However, in a speech experiment the investigators who listen to and judge the speech are not usually thought of as subjects, yet the individuals who produced the speech samples are. Sometimes it is safest if both speakers and listeners are considered as subjects. For example, in a recent experiment (Jones, 1983) six cleft-palate speakers were used as subjects. Their speech was rated for nasality by a pool of listeners who were also considered to be subjects. However, the IRB did not consider the investigator who gave articulation tests to the cleft-palate children as a subject even though he listened to their speech and made judgments. The IRB also did not consider the investigator who made acoustic measurements of the speech to be a subject, even though he made visual judgments when he adjusted a cursor on the screen of a computer terminal.

THE STRUCTURE OF INSTITUTIONAL REVIEW BOARDS

The IRB is a major component of the regulations for protection of human subjects. Each institution applying for HHS funding must provide written assurance that it will comply with the code of regulations. The assurance must specify the IRB members and IRB rules to be followed in the review of research. The requirements for the assurance document are provided in section 46.103 of the code of federal regulations, 45 CFR Part 46. Additionally, the Office for Protection from Research Risks has published a sample assurance document which is available upon request.

Members of an IRB are appointed by a top institutional official. Each IRB must have a minimum of five members, but the number is usually higher. It is required that at least one person have a nonscientific background (e.g., lawyers or members of the clergy). Each IRB also must include at least one member who is not affiliated with the institution. Often the nonscientific member is also the noninstitutional member. The members should reflect a wide variety of backgrounds and interests. For example, in a university IRB membership should include faculty and staff from diverse departments. A student may be included on the IRB. In a hospital, the IRB might be predominately a mix of physicians with different specialties, but it also might include speech-language pathologists, audiologists, nurses, patient representatives, and administrators. A school district might include teachers from various disciplines, administrators, and other professionals such as speech-language pathologists and audiologists.

In most cases each institution has one IRB. However, more than one IRB may be necessary in institutions that have a large volume of research. Also in some universities, it may be desirable to have different IRBs for the teaching hospital and the rest of the university. Some multicampus universities have an IRB for each campus and a supraIRB to set policy and review appeals from the campus based IRBs (Ryan, 1982).

In some cases research may be conducted in clinics, laboratories, or schools that are not a part of a larger institutional (or school) system. These small programs may not have the resources or personnel to set up an IRB. They also may not have the volume of research to warrant an IRB. In these situations it is common for the program to solicit the help of an IRB from a neighboring (or somehow affiliated) institution (Ryan, 1982). For example, an audiologist conducting research in private practice may formally delegate reviews to the IRB of a local hospital. Of course, an institution may also choose to ignore the IRB procedures if federal funding is not used to support the research.

THE ACTIONS OF INSTITUTIONAL REVIEW BOARDS

Prior to contacting potential subjects, investigators must prepare a proposal describing their research procedures (including subject contact, subject information, and consent forms) and submit the proposal to an IRB. IRBs have the authority to approve, require modifications, or disapprove research proposals. Disapprovals are uncommon. When potential risks are identified it is usually possible to modify the proposal to avoid or minimize the risks. Modifications in research procedures are required often when the IRB determines that it is possible to minimize subject discomfort, misunderstanding, coercion, etc. Such minor modifications occur most often in procedures for subject identification and contact, information to subjects, and informed consent procedures.

In general, IRBs review proposed research at convened meetings. When research activities involve no more than a minimal emotional or physical risk to the subjects, an expedited review procedure conducted by the IRB chair alone or by one of the committee members designated by the chair may be used. Projects can only be approved or modified via expedited review: expedited review cannot be used to disapprove a project. The key to expedited review is the determination of minimal risk. Procedures involve more than minimal risk if subjects experience pain, physical danger, emotional arousal, psychological stress, long-term behavior change, embarrassment, deception, or social disadvantage beyond that ordinarily encountered in daily life (*Federal Register,* 46.102g, 1981). Most procedures in speech-language pathology and audiology qualify as less than minimal risk and are eligible for expedited review. Full committee review is required for procedures involving highly personal or sensitive information, X-ray procedures, subcutaneous electrodes, high-level sound exposure, vocal abuse, most types of deception, and so on. Procedures that substitute an experimental therapeutic procedure for a traditional one may present a risk and therefore require full committee review.

An IRB also may determine that a proposed project falls into one of five areas of "exempted" research, for which investigators are not required to submit a written proposal for IRB review. Within a number of restrictions, research involving (1) common educational techniques, (2) educational tests, (3) some survey or interview procedures, (4) observation of public behavior, and (5) the use of existing data may qualify as exempt from review. The categories of research qualifying as exempt from review are described more completely in the *Federal Register,* 46.110 (1981).

When HHS funds are involved in research, the IRB has 60 days after the investigator submits a grant proposal to notify the funding agency that the proposal has been approved. The study sections of peer scientists convened by the funding agency to review the scientific merit of the proposed research also must approve of the procedures for use of human subjects or the grant or contract cannot be funded.

IRBs are additionally obligated to conduct continuing review of HHS funded research at regular intervals. The intervals are to be appropriate to the degree of risk, but not longer than one year. However, as Wollman and Ryan (1982) point out, it is important that the IRB not be thrust into the role of a police force. Although an IRB may be required to keep abreast with changes in, or problems arising from, a research protocol, it must trust the investigator. Allegations of dishonesty should be handled by the institutional administration, not the IRB.

RISK-BENEFIT DETERMINATION

Although other factors may be involved, IRB approval of a project always involves consideration of the benefit of the study in relation to the potential risks to subjects. The potential risks to subjects are many and varied. They might include physical risks from exposure to noise, exposure to radiation, electrical shock, vocal abuse, and so on. A risk from experimental therapy must be a less than optimal clinical result. There are also emotional risks, such as a potential for embarrassment, invasion of privacy, or undue stress. There may be a risk of adverse financial effects on subjects. There is a risk of misleading subjects (and their families) about their health or abilities. Also, risks which are acceptable with some populations may not be allowed with other groups, such as children.

Benefit usually refers to scientific benefit and not benefit to the subject as an individual. However, benefits foreseen for the subject may be a factor in some cases and failure to receive a personal benefit from an alternative procedure may be a risk. The estimation of scientific benefit is often problematic. The benefit of a study will depend on the soundness of the theoretical issues and the experimental design. IRBs are not generally qualified to judge this and therefore must rely on the opinions of the investigators. Certainly many scientifically marginal projects are approved. When substantial risks are foreseen an IRB may take special precautions to insure that the benefits of the study are also substantial. This may include soliciting documentation of the soundness of the research from qualified scientists who are not involved in the research project under review.

It should be emphasized that IRBs do not stop research simply because it is risky. There is always a determination of the risk relative to benefits. It is recognized that research is desirable, and that it inevitably involves some risk. IRBs often explore possible ways to reduce risk and maintain benefits.

SUBJECT CONTACT, INFORMATION TO SUBJECTS,
AND INFORMED CONSENT

Much of the risk of many research projects deals not with the clinical or laboratory procedures, but in the way the investigators communicate (or fail to communicate) with the subjects. IRBs routinely deal with this communication process and modify subject contact, information to subjects, and informed consent to improve the subject's understanding of what will be done and what his/her rights are.

Subject contact has many sources: clinician referral, teacher referral, hospital records, advertisements. IRB approval must be obtained before an investigator approaches potential subjects. In this way IRBs can screen contact procedures for (unintentional) coercion or a misrepresentation of procedures or subject benefits. Subjects should know where an investigator obtained their name. As mentioned above, research may invoke many misconceptions in the eyes of the public which often can be avoided by a few words of explanation.

Subject contact is tied in with information to subjects in that subjects must be given sufficient information to decide whether or not to participate. Sometimes information is provided orally. In many cases it is combined with a formal statement of informed consent.

The informed consent document must be written in language understandable to the subject and cannot contain exculpatory statements which waive the legal rights of the subjects or release the investigator or institution from liability or negligence. Its basic elements include: (1) statements that indicate the study involves research, the purpose of the research, procedures used, and the duration of the subject's involvement; (2) a description of any foreseeable benefits, risks or discomfort to the subject; (3) a disclosure of any alternative procedure or treatments, if any, that might be advantageous to the subject; (4) a statement describing the extent to which confidentiality of records identifying the subject will be maintained; (5) for research involving more than minimal risk, an explanation of whether any compensation or medical treatment is available (for additional information see *Compensating for Research Injuries,* U.S. Government Printing Office, Washington, DC); (6) an explanation of who to contact for pertinent questions about the research, and (7) a statement that indicates participation is voluntary and that the subject is free to discontinue participation at any time without loss of benefits to which the subject is otherwise entitled. The general requirements for informed consent are described in the final regulations (Federal Register, 46.116, 1981).

Research classified as exempt from review does not require a subject consent form. However, even in these cases it is often desirable to provide information to subjects and obtain a written consent form. There are also instances when an IRB may approve research which does not involve informed consent. This might occur if, for some reason, the research project would be compromised if the consent form were not waived.

When subjects are under the age of legal consent (18 years in most states), parents or guardians sign the consent form. When subjects are between 7 years and 18 years, both the child and parent guardian usually sign the form. Technically, the adults provide legal "consent" and children "assent." Care must be taken that information is presented to both children and parents at levels appropriate to their understanding. Parents, guardians, or caretakers may also be involved in the consent process for subjects over 18 years when necessary due to mental or emotional disability.

Special care must be taken with many communication disordered subjects to insure that they understand what they are told and that they freely assent or give consent. Information might be signed to deaf subjects as well as written in a form appropriate to their reading and language abilities. Mentally disabled, language disordered, and emotionally disturbed subjects can present a dilemma; the communication problem that the investigator would like to study may preclude the transfer of information allowing the investigator to study the subject. It is not the intent of the federal regulations that subjects who are difficult to inform should not be studied. Instead, it should be recognized that special risks (which are uniquely determined by the subject population and environment) may be involved with those who are difficult (or impossible) to inform. These risks should be considered in the determination of the risk-benefit relationship. IRBs may help to insure that extraordinary measures are taken to communicate with those who are difficult to inform about what to expect in an experimental procedure and the voluntary aspect of their participation.

RESEARCH IN THE SPEECH AND HEARING CLINIC

As mentioned above, it is sometimes difficult to determine when, in a clinical program, a research purpose emerges in addition to the purpose of serving the particular client under study. Often there is a situation in which an investigator would like to go back over clinic records (either his/her own or those of other clinicians) with a research purpose which was not present when the records were produced. This may require the consent of the clients whose files are to be used. One way to avoid recontacting clients (who may not have been seen for years) is to routinely have new clients sign a release form to allow clinic records to be used in future research.

Even if clients sign a release of clinic records, this does not constitute permission to use experimental procedures with them. Whenever new procedures are tried with a subject, or traditional procedures are withheld with a research purpose in mind, the process is subject to human subjects regulations. However, there is often a fine line determining what is an experimental procedure which may be generalizable, and what is an unusual clinical procedure required by the specific needs of the client. Along these lines it should be pointed out that withholding a common clinical procedure from a subject is not necessarily unethical. This is parallel to using a unique clinical procedure.One must assess the potential risks to the subject in regard to the potential benefits.

When speech, language, or hearing clients are involved in research, subjects should be explicitly told of not just the risks but any therapeutic benefits they might expect. Investigators must be careful when sharing experimental test results with subjects. Tests that are designed for experimental purposes may lead to misunderstanding if they are interpreted diagnostically. Experimental screening procedures are especially vulnerable to misunderstanding. For example, if hearing screening is included in an experimental protocol, it is important that the investigators work out in detail what to tell the potential subjects who fail the screening test. One would not want them to leave with the impression that they have been diagnosed to have a hearing loss. Some screening procedures might warrant referral of subjects who fail for a diagnostic procedure, others might not.

STUDENTS AND RESEARCH

Teaching students about research procedures is not research. There may be many activities performed as class projects or as laboratory demonstrations that are not covered by the regulations on human subjects because the purposes are entirely didactic. Teaching activities may even involve invasive procedures or contact with the public or patient populations. The propriety of these activities is left to the academic judgment of the professor and the college administrative system. In some cases activities have a predominately educational purpose, but there may also be a research purpose which would make these activities subject to IRB review. For example, the students in a class could conduct a survey which would be both a learning experience and a contribution to generalizable knowledge. Theses and dissertations have both an educational and a research purpose and are subject to review.

There is a potential problem with thesis projects involving diagnostic or therapeutic procedures if students have not yet completed clinical training. Even if a student's major purpose is related to research, *in our opinion,* his/her clinical activities should be supervised if clients are receiving clinical services. In some cases this may make research on clinical procedures by students awkward or even impractical.

University faculty involved in research also should be careful when using students as research subjects. The teacher-student relationship may put undue pressure on some students to participate. Teachers must be careful when soliciting subjects in the classroom. Students should not have class grades influenced by research participation. Even though an announcement may be made to this effect and an explanation included in the statement of informed consent, it is difficult to insure that students do not feel they are somehow earning extra credit. In some cases a professor may feel that participation in an experiment is a valuable educational experience. When this is the case, students should be given a number of options as to the kind of research participation they are required to undertake.

SUMMARY

We have reviewed the development of the regulations presently guiding biomedical, behavioral, and social research with human subjects. We have mentioned the specifics of many of the regulations and where to find more information about them. We have explained the operation of the review system and made value judgments as to where and how it should be effective. We have tried to provide some specific examples and applications of the system to issues in speech, language, and hearing. Perhaps most importantly, we have tried to explain the purposes of the system. The purpose of the regulations is not just to protect subjects from physical and mental harm, but also to protect subjects from misunderstanding, and to protect investigators and institutions. In this regard, we see the system of regulations for human subjects review not as a bureaucratic hurdle but as a resource to be used by all individuals involved in speech, language, and hearing research.

Acknowledgement

This paper was prepared under the auspices of the Committee on Scientific Affairs of the American Speech-Language-Hearing Association. We would like to thank the other members of the Committee on Scientific Affairs for advocating the writing of this paper and commenting on the manuscript. The Committee members are Robert C. Bilger, Lawrence L. Feth (Chair), Sharon L. James, Jerry L. Punch, J. Buckminster Ranney, Tens K. Schery, Arnold M. Small, Jr. and Diane J. Van Tasell. The authors thank David Doyle of the Office for Protection from Research Risks, Bethesda, Maryland, for his assistance in the preparation of this manuscript. We also thank William H. Trease of the Office of the Vice President for Educational Development and Research, University of Iowa; Dean E. Williams, University of Iowa; John F. Brandt, University of Kansas; Susan Fischer and Ross Stuckless, National Technical Institute for the Deaf at Rochester Institute of Technology for commenting on the manuscript. This review represents the perspectives of the authors. Many of our opinions were developed during service on IRBs. Dale Metz is a member of the IRB at the National Technical Institute for the Deaf at Rochester Institute of Technology. John Folkins is chair of one of the four University of Iowa IRBs. This review should not be interpreted as a philosophical or policy statement of the American Speech-Language-Hearing Association.

References

Annas, G. J., Glantz, L. H. & Katz, B. F. (1977). *Informed consent to human experimentation: The subject's dilemma.* Cambridge, MA: Ballinger Publishing Company.

The Belmont Report: Ethical principles and guidelines for protection of human subjects of research. (1979). *Office for Protection from Research Risks Reports,* Bethesda, MD.

Brady, J. V. & Jonsen, A. R. (1982). The evaluation of regulatory influences on research with human subjects. In R. A. Greenwald, M. K. Ryan, & J. E. Mulvihill (Eds.), *Human subject's research: A handbook for institutional review boards,* New York: Plenum Press.

Final regulations amending basic HHS policy for the protection of human subjects. (1981). *Federal Register, 46,* 16, pp. 8366–8392.

Huxley, A. (1965). *Brave new world.* New York: Harper and Row.

Implementing human research regulations. Second biennial report on the adequacy and uniformity of federal rules and policies, and their implementation, for the protection of human subjects. (1983). Washington, DC. U.S. Government Printing Office.

Jones, D. L. (1983). *The effect of utterance rate on speech production in cleft palate speakers.* Unpublished Master's thesis. University of Iowa.

Moeller, D. (1976). *Speech pathology and audiology: Iowa origins of a discipline.* Iowa City: The University of Iowa Press.

Protection of Human Subjects. Code of federal regulations 45 CFR 46. *O.P.R.R. Reports.* (1983). Washington, D.C. U.S. Government Printing Office.

Ryan, M. K., General organization of the IRB. (1982). In R. A. Greenwald, M. K. Ryan, & J. E. Mulvihill (Eds.), *Human subjects research: A handbook for institutional review boards.* New York: Plenum Press.

Shelley, M. W. (1961). *Frankenstein or the Modern Prometheus.* New York, MacMillan.

Skinner, B. F. (1948). *Walden two.* New York: MacMillan.

Wollman, S. & Ryan, M. K. (1982). Continuing review of research In: R. A. Greenwald, M. K. Ryan, & J. E. Mulvihill (Eds.), *Human subjects research: A handbook for institutional review boards.* New York: Plenum Press.

Author Index

Abbs, J. H., 67, 221, 222, 236, 304
Adams, M. R., 7, 22, 37, 38, 40, 41, 48, 53, 68, 135, 139, 141, 186, 264, 322, 342, 343, 354, 361
Allen, D. V., 67
American Psychological Association (APA), 13, 16, 100, 102, 189, 194, 195, 216
American Speech-Language-Hearing Association (ASHA), 4, 8, 12, 14, 15
Andrews, G., 102, 136, 137, 141, 229, 230, 260, 261
Arndt, W. B., 101, 252, 304
Auer, J. J., 6, 7, 22
Ayukawa, H., 50, 68

Babbie, E. R., 295, 296, 304
Bacon, H. M., 31, 69
Badia, P., 144, 188
Baken, R. J., 28, 57, 68, 69, 287, 289, 290, 314
Baltaxe, C. A. M., 284
Bankson, N. W., 258, 259
Bar, A., 338
Barber, T. X., 253, 304
Barefoot, S. M., 203, 208
Barlow, D. H., 14, 23, 133, 135, 138, 142, 300, 304

Barlow, S. M., 236, 304
Barrett, L. S., 96, 102
Barzun, J., 28, 68
Beasley, D. S., 44, 45, 68, 140
Bendel, R. B., 96, 102
Benson, R. W., 69
Bergman, M., 55, 68
Bess, F. H., 140
Binder, A., 19, 22
Blanton, R. L., 339
Bless, D., 236, 304
Blom, E. L., 67
Bloom, L. M., 5, 22, 55, 56, 63, 68
Bolders, J. G., 357
Boothroyd, A., 362
Borden, G., 358
Boring, E. G., 28, 68
Bosler, S., 120, 141
Bounds, W. G., 80, 103, 104, 142
Boyle, W. F., 64
Bracht, G. H., 90, 102
Brandes, P., 50, 69
Brannon, J. B., 52, 53, 69
Brennan, D. G., 221
Brewer, D. W., 332, 335
Brinton, B., 96, 103
Brooks, A. R., 342
Brookshire, R. H., 65, 69, 91, 101, 102, 131, 141

Brutten, G., 63, 69
Buros, O. K., 100, 102, 241, 242, 304

Campbell, D. T., 2, 72, 74, 75, 80, 81, 83, 84, 87, 89, 90, 93, 101, 102, 103, 104, 109, 121, 122, 125, 127, 130, 131, 132, 134, 135, 138, 141, 300
Campbell, T. F., 247, 249
Capella, J. N., 60, 69
Carhart, R., 59, 63, 69, 294, 295, 334, 336
Carpenter, R. L., 289
Carver, R. P., 161, 188
Casby, M. W., 247
Castle, W. E., 18, 22
Chaiklin, J. B., 64, 69, 96, 102, 254
Chapey, R., 243, 370
Chaplin, J. P., 10, 22
Chermak, G. D., 96, 102
Chomsky, N., 9, 22
Christensen, J. M., 319
Christensen, L. B., 106, 107, 109, 114, 134, 135, 141, 218, 253, 304
Clarke, R., 389
Cohen, J., 162, 188
Cohen, R. L., 66, 69, 318
Colburn, N., 63, 69, 199, 208

Cole, K. J., 236, 304
Coleman, R. O., 334
Conrad, R., 187
Conture, E. G., 196, 257, 265, 266, 271, 332, 335
Cook, T. D., 135, 138, 141
Cormier, W. H., 80, 103, 104, 142
Cosker, L., 18, 23
Costello, D. G., 14, 22
Costello, J., 120, 141
Costello, J. M., 277, 281
Cottrell, I. A. W., 120, 141
Courtright, I. C., 120, 141, 194, 246, 385
Courtright, J. A., 120, 141, 194, 246, 385
Crawford, S., 321
Cronbach, L., 100, 102
Cullinan, W. L., 221
Curlee, R. F., 61, 69

Danhauer, J. L., 321
Daniloff, R. G., 46, 51, 69
Darley, F. L., 241, 304
Davey, B., 140
Davidson, P. O., 14, 22
Davis, H., 69
Davis, J. A., 295, 304
Davis, J. M., 241, 243, 299
Dever, R. B., 98, 102, 377, 378
Dodds, E., 62, 69
Doehring, D. G., 385
Doherty, J. E., 67, 139
Dorman, M. F., 348, 349
Downs, D. W., 213
Drew, C. J., 19, 22, 72, 87, 88, 102
Duffy, J. R., 7, 23, 222, 225, 263, 329
Duffy, R. J., 7, 23, 222, 225, 262, 263
Dunn, J., 360

Edgerton, B. J., 321
Eilers, R. E., 220, 221
Eldert, E., 69
Elliott, L. L., 91, 103
Elzey, F. F., 25, 69, 72, 103
Emerick, L. L., 13, 23
Engebretson, A. M., 205, 209
Erber, N. P., 43, 44, 69, 369, 371, 376, 377
Erickson, R. L., 308

Farb, J., 120, 141
Fein, D. J., 61, 69, 140
Ferguson, G. A., 106, 112, 141

Fisher, H. B., 67
Folkins, J. W., 67, 139, 221, 222, 355, 425
Fowler, C. G., 194
Fox, C. M., 311
Fox, D. J., 12, 23
Fristoe, M., 339, 340
Fucci, D., 272
Fujiki, M., 96, 103

Giles, H., 7, 23
Giles, J. A., 7, 23
Giolas, T. G., 329
Girardeau, F. L., 131, 141
Gladstein, K. L., 67
Glass, G. V., 90, 102
Goldman, M. D., 234, 235
Goldman, R., 68, 339, 340
Goldsmith, H., 102
Goldstein, D. P., 21, 312
Goodwin, P. E., 21
Gorga, M. P., 299
Graff, H. F., 28, 68
Guilford, J. P., 150, 154, 167, 188
Guillemin, B. J., 236, 304
Guitar, B., 68, 98, 103, 120, 136, 141, 142, 251
Gutkin, B., 196

Haber, A., 144, 188
Hagen, E., 94, 95, 97, 100, 103
Hamre, C. E., 345
Hanley, J. N., 374
Hansen, W. R., 141
Harford, E., 62, 69
Haroldson, S. K., 135, 141, 142
Harris, J. D., 12, 15
Harvey, R., 102, 229, 230
Hatten, J. T., 13, 23
Hawkins, D. B., 301
Hawley, J. L., 236, 304
Hayden, P., 186
Hayes, C. S., 21
Healey, E. C., 196, 354, 361
Hersen, M., 14, 23, 133, 135, 138, 142, 300, 304
Hill, W., 262, 305
Hipskind, N. M., 253, 304
Hirsh, I. J., 42, 69
Hixon, T. J., 3, 23, 234, 235, 236, 304, 305
Hochberg, I., 65, 69, 410
Hoemann, H. W., 327
Hollien, H., 57, 58, 69
Holloway, M. S., 51, 69
Hoock, W. C., 100, 103
Hoops, H. R., 293

Horii, Y., 214, 358
Horner, J., 301
Howie, P. M., 136, 141, 256
Hubbard, D. J., 187
Huck, S. W., 80, 103, 104, 142
Humes, L. E., 200, 201, 208
Hunter, J. E., 120, 121, 135, 136, 137, 142
Huntington, D. A., 187
Hurst, M. R., 277, 281
Hutchinson, J., 41, 53, 68, 139

Ingham, R. J., 131, 142, 260, 261
Isaac, S., 25, 69, 72, 80, 103

Jackson, G. B., 120, 142
Jaeger, C. G., 31, 69
Jerger, J., 6, 14, 15, 21, 23, 63, 69
Jerger, S., 63, 69
Johnson, K. O., 18, 22
Johnson, W., 62, 69
Jordan, E., 60, 69, 98, 103

Kahn, J. V., 256
Kaplan, A., 25, 69
Karsh, D. E., 50, 69
Kazdin, A. E., 134, 142
Kearns, K. P., 131, 142
Keith, R. W., 66, 69, 318
Kelly, J. F., 140
Kennard, K. L., 186
Kent, R. D., 195, 211, 251, 252
Kerlinger, F., 10, 23, 25, 29, 30, 31, 32, 33, 60, 69, 73, 94, 97, 99, 103, 104, 142
Kidd, K. K., 67
Kirk, S. A., 101
Kirk, W. D., 101
Kling, J. W., 36, 69
Koenigsnecht, R. A., 137, 142
Koh, S. D., 344
Konkle, D. F., 140
Krawiec, T. S., 10, 22
Kushner, D., 187
Kushnirecky, W., 137, 142

Lahey, M., 65, 69, 393
Lane, H., 28, 69
Lapointe, L. L., 251, 252, 301
Lasasso, C., 140
Leach, E. A., 55, 56, 69
Lee, B. S., 140
Lee, L. L., 137, 142, 252, 305

Leonard, L. B., 357
Lerman, J., 354
Levine, S., 25, 69, 72, 103
Levitt, H., 235, 236, 305
Lilly, D. J., 233, 367
Ling, D., 385
Lloyd, L. L., 67, 131, 139, 316
Lodge, D. N., 55, 56, 69
Lombardi, L., 186
Lubinski, R., 209
Ludlow, C. L., 313

Macauley, B. D., 131, 142
Macready, G., 140
Mahshie, J. J., 196, 257
Mallard, A. R., 354, 361
Manning, W. H., 364, 365
Margolis, R. H., 311
Martin, D. E., 293
Martin, F. N., 61, 69
Martin, R. R., 135, 141, 142, 275, 277
Marx, M., 10, 23
McCall, G. N., 332, 335
McCauley, R., 100, 101, 103, 244, 246, 305
McClatchie, A. C., 389
McClean, M., 326
McClellan, M. E., 37, 38, 39, 69
McGlone, R. E., 21, 240, 241
McGough, W. E., 140
McHenry, M., 382, 387
McMahan, D. A., 369, 371, 376, 377
McReynolds, L. V., 131, 142
Mead, J., 234, 235
Metter, E. J., 141
Metz, D. E., 100, 103, 139, 207, 240, 388, 425
Michael, W. B., 25, 69, 72, 80, 103
Miller, J. A., 357
Miller, J. F., 273, 275, 346, 348
Minifie, F. D., 3, 23, 220, 221, 382, 387
Moll, K., 91, 103
Monge, P. R., 60, 69
Monsen, R. B., 120, 142, 198, 205, 209
Montague, J., 120, 141
Montanelli, D. S., 68
Moore, W. H., 37, 38, 40, 41, 48, 68, 322, 342, 343
Morris, H., 91, 103
Morrison, E. B., 209, 243, 370
Mulhern, S. T., 137, 142

Muma, J., 100, 103
Mysak, E. D., 63, 69, 199, 208

Netsell, R., 236, 304, 305
Neuman, A. C., 410
Newman, P. W., 18, 22
Nguyen, D. T., 236, 304
Noffsinger, D., 194
Nunnally, J. C., 339

Ochs, M. G., 200, 201, 208
Odom, P. B., 339
Olswang, L. B., 289
Owens, E., 225, 227, 228, 229, 389

Panagos, J. M., 47, 69
Parasnis, I., 53, 54, 69, 320
Parsons, H. M., 88, 103
Pashek, G. V., 65, 69
Pearson, K. L., 222, 225, 263
Pederson, C. M., 96, 102
Pedhazur, E. J., 60, 69
Peins, M., 140
Pennington, C. D., 61, 69
Perkins, W., 13, 23
Petrosino, L., 272
Plutchik, R., 19, 23, 36, 37, 40, 43, 48, 62, 67, 69, 72, 103, 232, 305
Porter, L. S., 59, 63, 69, 294, 295, 334, 336
Prelock, P. A., 47, 69
Price, J. G., 316
Prosek, R. A., 213
Punch, J., 4, 23

Quigley, S. P., 68, 219, 220

Raffin, M. J. M., 233
Ramig, P., 264
Reed, C. R., 140
Reich, A., 140, 382, 387
Reilly, K. M., 389
Rettaliata, P., 64, 69
Reynolds, E. G., 69
Richards, A. M., 360
Riensche, L., 364, 365
Riggs, L. A., 36, 69
Rigrodsky, S., 187, 209, 243, 370
Ringel, R., 14, 15, 21, 23
Rintelmann, W. F., 44, 45, 68, 253, 304
Robbins, J., 67
Robinson, D. O., 67
Rosenbeck, J. C., 195, 211
Rosenthal, R., 82, 103, 230, 252, 305

Rosnow, R. L., 230, 252, 305
Ross, M., 354
Roth, F. P., 102
Rubin, M., 262, 305
Ruder, K. F., 247
Rudmin, F., 50, 68
Rummel, R. J., 10, 23
Runyan, C. M., 213
Runyon, R. P., 144, 188

Sacco, P. R., 207
Samar, V. J., 186, 207, 260, 359, 365
Sanders, J. W., 236, 238
Sands, E., 267, 269, 270
Santo Pietro, M. J., 187
Sarno, M. T., 267, 269, 270
Saxman, J. H., 273, 275, 346, 348
Schiavetti, N., 100, 103, 388
Schiff, N. B., 212
Schiff-Myers, N., 63, 69
Schmidt, F. L., 120, 142
Schwartz, A. H., 68
Schwartz, D. M., 236, 237
Schwartz, M. F., 22
Schwartz, R. D., 80, 103
Schwimmer, S., 44, 45, 68
Seaton, W. H., 18, 23
Sechrest, L., 80, 103
Seider, R. A., 67
Shanks, J. C., 293
Shanks, J. E., 367
Sharbrough, F. W., 63, 69
Shaughnessy, J. J., 35, 69, 115, 142
Shearer, W. M., 7, 23
Shelton, R. L., 342
Shepard, N. T., 299
Sherman, D., 16, 23, 38, 69
Shipp, T., 21, 57, 58, 69, 240, 241
Shriberg, L. D., 247, 249
Shriner, T. H., 46, 51, 52, 69
Sidman, M., 10, 23, 119, 142
Siegel, G. M., 22, 186, 275, 277
Siegel, S., 150, 171, 175, 184, 186, 188
Silver, M. J., 253, 304
Silverman, E. M., 7, 23, 120, 142
Silverman, F. H., 7, 23
Silverman, M., 267, 269, 270
Silverman, S. R., 69
Simpson, M. E., 238
Sims, D. G., 186, 260, 359, 365
Singer, M. I., 67
Sitler, R. W., 100, 103, 388

Sivarajan, M., 67
Skinner, B. F., 9, 10, 23, 24, 27, 28, 69
Sloane, H. N., 131, 142
Slonim, M. J., 295, 305
Small, L. H., 272
Smith, N. C., 119, 142
Smith, N. L., 219, 220
Smitheran, J. R., 236, 305
Sokol, S., 186
Speaks, C., 21
Spekman, N. J., 102
Spradlin, J. E., 131, 141
Spriestersbach, D. C., 14, 91, 103
Stanley, J. C., 2, 72, 74, 75, 80, 81, 83, 84, 87, 89, 90, 93, 101, 102, 104, 109, 121, 122, 125, 127, 130, 131, 132, 134, 141, 300
Starkweather, C. W., 131, 135, 142
Starr, C. D., 135, 141, 142
Stassen, R. A., 64, 69
Stelmachowicz, P. G., 299
Stevens, S. S., 9, 10, 22, 24, 100, 103, 121, 142, 144, 188
Stitt, C. L., 187
Sweeting, P. M., 287, 314

Swisher, L. P., 100, 101, 103, 244, 246, 305, 313

Thorndike, R. L., 94, 95, 97, 100, 103
Thornton, A. R., 233
Throne, J. M., 120, 141
Till, J., 140
Toler, S. A., 258, 259
Trammel, J. L., 21
Tranel, B., 28, 69
Tweney, R. D., 327

Uken, D., 389
Underwood, B. J., 35, 69, 115, 142

Van Dalen, D. B., 109, 142
Ventry, I. M., 50, 64, 69, 96, 102, 254, 262, 305
Vernon, M., 344

Waltzman, S., 65, 69
Watt, J., 7, 23
Webb, E. J., 80, 103
Weber, J. L., 137, 142
Webster, L. M., 63, 69
Webster, R. L., 348, 349
Weikers, N. J., 63, 69
Weinberg, B., 319

Weiner, P., 100, 103, 328, 330, 331
Weinrod, H., 18, 23
Whitehead, B. H., 240
Whitehead, R. L., 140, 203, 208, 240
Wilbur, R. B., 68, 219, 220
Wilder, C. N., 57, 69, 289, 290
Williams, F., 3, 23
Wilson, F. B., 269, 270, 271
Wilson, K. J., 236, 304
Wilson, R. H., 198, 208
Wingate, M. E., 310, 345
Wingfield, A., 186
Witter, H. L., 312
Wood, G., 20, 24, 218, 305
Wood, K. S., 14, 15
Woodford, C. M., 381
Woods, C. L., 243, 244
Woods, R. W., 262, 305

Young, M. A., 7, 24, 54, 60, 62, 69, 203, 204, 208
Youngstrom, K. A., 342

Zimmer, C. H., 7, 23
Zimmermann, G. N., 64, 69, 102, 374

Subject Index

A - B design. *See* Time-series designs
A - B - A design. *See* Time-series designs
Abstract of the article, 193, 195–197, 393, 410
Active variable, 32–33
Alpha. *See* Significance level
American Speech-Language-Hearing Association (ASHA), 4, 11, 16, 18, 61, 189
Analysis of covariance, 185
Analysis of variance, 175–185, 345–350
  analysis of covariance, 185
  conceptual framework of, 175–177, 345–346
  contrast tests for, 183–184, 349–350
  examples of, 345–350, 400–403
  F-ratio in, 175–179, 346–349
  interaction effects in, 179–183, 346–349
  main effects in, 175–182, 345–350
  nonparametric alternatives to, 184–185
  significance levels in, 177–182, 346–350
  summary table format for, 175–176, 179, 181, 346–348
  See also Excerpts 8.27, 8.28
ANOVA. *See* Analysis of variance
Applied research, 8
Applied scientist, 13–15
Attribute variable, 32–33, 291

Baseline. *See* Time-series designs
Basic research, 8
Behavioral instruments, 241–249
  appropriateness of, 249–252
  instructions as, 261–264
  nonstandardized instruments, 245–249
  standardized instruments, 241–244
  validity and reliability of, 94–100
  See also Instrumentation threat; Excerpts 7.15, 7.16, 7.17, 7.18, 7.19, 7.21, 7.23, 7.24, 7.25, 7.30, 7.31

Behavioral science, 8
Between-subjects designs, 105–113, 266–273, 281–284
  combined matching and randomization in, 109–110
  control of threats to internal validity in, 106–110, 266–273, 281–284
  in descriptive research, 111–113, 281–284
  in experimenal research, 105–111, 266–273
  matching of subjects in, 106, 107–110, 112–113, 269–270
  random assignment of subjects in, 106–107, 266–273
  See also Excerpts 7.5, 7.6, 7.7, 7.33, 7.34, 7.39
Bimodal distribution, 153
Bivalent experiments, 37–40, 48
  analogy with comparative research, 51–52, 111
  between-subjects designs for, 106–110
  compared to multivalent experiments, 40–43
  defined, 37
  examples of, 37–40
Bonferroni t-test, 350

Carry-over effect, 114–115, 265
Case study research, 62–64, 300–301
Categorical variable, 33–34, 53
Cause-and-effect relations, 30, 35
  cautions in descriptive research, 49–51, 54, 60, 169
  in experimental research, 35–36
Central tendency, 149–155, 315–322
  See also Excerpts 8.7, 8.8, 8.9, 8.10, 8.11, 8.12

Chi square, 170–172, 184–185, 332, 335, 344–345
  in analysis of differences, 172, 184–185, 344–345
  in analysis of relationships, 170–172, 332, 335
  See also Excerpts 8.18, 8.25, 8.26
Classification variable, 50, 51–55, 62, 111, 273
Clinical enterprise in speech pathology and audiology, 4–7
Clinician as applied scientist, 13–15
Clinician-researcher dichotomy, 13–15
Cochran Q test, 184–185, 403–404
Combined experimental-descriptive research, 64–66, 117, 273–275, 399, 417
Comparative research, 51–55, 281–284
Concurrent validity, 98. See also Validity of tests and measurements
Construct validity, 99–100. See also Validity of tests and measurements
Content validity, 97–98. See also Validity of tests and measurements
Contingency coefficient, 170–172
Contingency table, 170–172
Continuous variable, 33–34, 53
Contrast tests for analysis of variance, 183–184, 346–347, 349–350
Control groups, 105–111, 266–271
  ethics of using, 137–138
  in therapy research, 121–138, 266–271
Correlational analysis, 162–172, 325–337
  Chi square used in, 170–172, 332, 335
  contingency coefficient, 170–172
  contingency table, 170–172
  index of determination, 167–169
  intercorrelation matrix, 166–167, 328–331
  Pearson product-moment correlation coefficient, 164–167, 184, 325–331
  regression analysis, 169–170, 184, 334–337
  scattergrams, 57–58, 164–166, 325–327, 332–334
  significance levels in, 167, 328–332
  Spearman Rank-order Correlation Coefficient, 164, 166, 167, 184, 332–334
  See also Excerpts 8.13, 8.14, 8.15, 8.16, 8.17, 8.18, 8.19
Correlation Coefficients. See Correlational analysis; Correlational research
Correlational research, 51, 57–60, 290–293
  correlation coefficients in, 57–58
  graphic displays in, 57–58
  predicted variable in, 50–51, 58–60, 169
  predictor variable in, 50–51, 58–60, 169
  regression analysis in, 58–60
  threats to validity of, 291
  See also Excerpt 7.43
Counterbalancing, 79, 114–115
  control of short-term maturation, 79
  in within-subjects designs, 114–115
Criterion validity, 98–99. See also Validity of tests and measurements
Criterion variable, 50, 52, 62
Cross-sectional research. See Developmental research
Cumulative frequency distribution, 146–149, 307–309

Data analysis procedures, 155–185, 324–352
  characteristics of, 350–351
  summary table of, 184
Data organization procedures, 146–155, 306–324
  characteristics of, 323–324
Deductive reasoning, 9
Degrees of freedom, 162
Dependent variable, 29–32, 48, 73–75, 78
  defined, 30
  in descriptive research, 30, 50–51, 59, 73–75
  in experimental research, 30, 37–48, 73–75
Descriptive research, 9, 49–64, 73–75
  between-subjects designs for, 111–113, 281–287
  compared with experimental research, 49–51
  defined, 49
  design objectives in, 73–75
  internal and external validity of, 74–75
  mixed designs for, 117, 289–290
  within-subjects designs for, 113, 116, 287–289
  See also Comparative research; Correlational research; Developmental research; Survey research
Developmental research, 51, 55–57, 284–290
  between- and within-subjects designs for, 55, 111, 116, 284–290
  cross-sectional research, 55–56, 111, 285–287
  longitudinal research, 56, 116, 287–289
  semilongitudinal research, 56–57, 289–290
  threats to validity of, 116
  See also Excerpts 7.40, 7.41, 7.42
Differential selection of subjects threat, 84–86, 222–230
  control of, 85, 106–110
  defined, 84
  descriptive research and, 85–86
  examples of, 85–86, 222–230
  experimental research and, 84–85
  See also Threats to internal validity
Direct replication, 119, 120
Discussion and conclusions, 353–390, 404–408, 420–423
  relation to method of investigation, 355–359
  relation to research problem, 354–355
  relation to results, 359–362
  See also Future research implications; Practical research implications; Previous research, relation of results to; Theories; Excerpts 9.1, 9.2, 9.3, 9.4, 9.5, 9.7, 9.8, 9.9, 9.10
Distribution of data, 146–155
Duncan multiple range test, 183, 402

Editorial process, 15–18
Empiricism, 9
  common steps in empirical research, 25–29
Error of misplaced precision, 122
Ethics of using control groups, 137–138
Evaluation checklist, 190
  for discussion section, 389–390
  for introduction section, 216

for method section, 302–304
for results section, 352
Experimental group, 105–111
Experimental research, 9, 35–48, 73–75
  bivalent experiments, 37–40
  cause-and-effect relations in, 35–36
  compared with descriptive research, 49–51
  control and manipulation of variables in, 36
  defined, 35–36
  dependent variables in, 35–48
  design objectives in, 73–75, 105–111, 113–116
  independent variables in, 35–48
  internal and external validity of, 74–75
  multivalent experiments, 40–43
  parametric experiments, 43–48
  See also Excerpts 7.32, 7.33, 7.34, 7.35, 7.36, 7.37, 7.38
Experimenter bias. See Instrumentation threat
External validity, 74–75, 89–94, 117–121, 356, 358–359, 383, 387–388
  definition of, 74, 89
  and random sampling, 118
  and replication, 118–121
  See also Threats to external validity
Extraneous variables, 73–75

Frequency distribution, 146–149, 307–315
  See also Excerpts 8.1, 8.2, 8.3, 8.4, 8.5, 8.6
Frequency histogram, 146–149, 309–314
  See also Excerpts 8.2, 8.4, 8.6
Frequency polygon, 146–149, 311–313
  See also Excerpt 8.5
Frequency table, 146–149, 307–309, 311–313
  See also Excerpts 8.1, 8.3
F-ratio. See Analysis of variance
Friedman two-way ANOVA 184–185
F-test. See Analysis of variance
Functional relationship, 31–32, 40–43, 45–48, 55, 57
Future research implications, 382–389
  See also Excerpts 9.21, 9.22, 9.23, 9.24, 9.25

Generalizability. See External validity
Graphic display of results, 31–32, 34, 57–58, 146–155, 307–324, 402–403, 418–420
  abscissa, 31
  functional relation, 31–32, 40–43, 45–48, 55, 57
  ordinate, 31
  scattergram, 57–58, 162–166, 325–327, 332–334
  summary statistics, 149–155, 317–322
  See also Excerpts 8.2, 8.4, 8.5, 8.6, 8.8, 8.9, 8.11, 8.13, 8.14, 8.17, 8.27

Hardware instrumentation, 81, 110, 231–241, 413–416
  appropriateness of, 249–252
  calibration of, 81, 238–241
  evaluation of, 231–238
  purposes of, 231–232
  reasons for using, 232
  See also Instrumentation threat; Excerpts 7.9, 7.10, 7.11, 7.12, 7.13, 7.14

Hawthorne effect, 87–89, 92–93, 129
  defined, 87–88
  and external validity, 92–93, 129
  and internal validity, 87–89
  as a reactive arrangement, 92–93, 129
  See also Threats to external validity; Threats to internal validity
Histogram. See Frequency histogram
History threat, 75–77
  defined, 75
  examples of, 76
  See also Threats to internal validity
Hypothesis, 10, 158–162, 210–214. See also Null hypothesis

Independent variable, 29–32, 73–75
  in combined experimental-descriptive research, 64–66
  defined, 30
  in descriptive research, 30, 50–51, 55, 59, 73–75
  in experimental research, 30, 37–48, 73–75
Index of determination, 167–169
Inductive reasoning, 9
Instructions to subjects, 261–264
  See also Excerpts 7.30, 7.31
Instrumentation threat, 81–83, 110–111, 123, 231–264
  calibration, 81, 238–241
  defined, 81
  examples of, 81–83
  experimenter bias, 82–83, 252–259
  human instrumentation, 82–83, 252–259
  Rosenthal effect, 82–83, 111, 123, 252–259
  test environment, 83, 259–261
  See also Threats to internal validity; Excerpts 7.23, 7.24, 7.25, 7.26, 7.27, 7.28, 7.29
Interaction effect, 43–48. See also Analysis of variance
Interaction of internal validity threats, 89
  defined, 89
  examples of, 89
  See also Threats to internal validity
Intercorrelation matrix, 166–167
Interjudge reliability, 239–240, 246–249, 257–259
  See also Excerpts 7.13, 7.19, 7.20, 7.26, 7.27
Internal validity, 74–89, 356–359, 382–383, 399, 417–418
  defined, 74, 75
  See also Threats to internal validity
Interval level of measurement, 144–146
Interviews. See Survey research
Intrajudge reliability, 239–240, 246–249, 257–259
  See also Excerpts 7.13, 7.19, 7.20, 7.26, 7.27
Introduction section, 193–216
  components of, 193–194
  definition of terms in, 214–215
  evaluation checklist for, 216
  limitations of the study, 215
  See also Rationale for the study; Review of literature; Statement of problem; Statement of purpose, research questions, and hypothesis

Kruskal-Wallis one-way ANOVA, 184–185
Kurtosis, 151–155

Leptokurtic distribution, 151–155
Letters to the editor, 7, 17
Levels of measurement, 144–146
Longitudinal research. See Developmental research

Main effect, 43–48. See also Analysis of variance
Mann-Whitney U test, 173–175, 178, 184, 340–342. See also Excerpt 8.23
Matching of subjects, 107–110, 269–270
  advantages and disadvantages, 109–110
  combined with randomization, 109–110
  overall matching, 108, 269–270
  pair matching, 108–109
Materials, 231–264. See also Behavioral instruments; Hardware instrumentation; Instrumentation threat
Maturation threat, 77–79
  control of, 77–79
  defined, 77
  examples of, 77–79
  long-term, 77
  short-term, 77
  See also Threats to internal validity
Mean, 149–155, 173, 316–322. See also Summary statistics
Measurement, 144–146, 231–264
  appropriateness of, 249–252
  defined, 144
  levels of, 144–146
  See also Excerpts 7.21, 7.22
Median, 149–150, 152–153, 155. See also Summary statistics
Mesokurtic distribution, 151–155
Meta-analysis, 135–137
Missing data, 315
Mixed designs, 117, 273–275, 399, 417
  between-subjects component, 117, 273
  within-subjects component, 117, 273
  See also Excerpt 7.36
Mode, 149–150, 152–153
  See also Summary statistics
Mortality threat, 86–87
  defined, 86
  example of, 86–87
  experimental research and, 86–87
  follow-up studies and, 87
  See also Threats to internal validity,
Multiple regression, 169–170, 334–337
  See also Correlational analysis; Excerpt 8.19
Multiple-treatment interference threat, 93–94
  See also Threats to external validity
Multivalent experiments, 40–43, 48
  analogy with comparative research, 52–53, 111
  compared with bivalent experiment, 40–43
  defined, 40
  example of, 40–43

Newman-Keuls test, 183, 350
Nominal level of measurement, 144–146

Nonequivalent control group design, 124–125
Nonparametric statistics, 157–158, 164, 170–172, 173–175, 184–185, 331–335, 340–345
Nonreactive measures, 80
Nonstandardized tests. See Behavioral instruments
Normal distribution, 151–155, 156–157
Nuisance variables, 73–75
Null hypothesis, 158–162, 172–185

One-group pretest-posttest design, 76, 78, 122–123
"One-shot" case study, 121–122
One-tailed tests, 161–162
Order effect, 114, 399, 417–418. See also Within-subjects designs
Ordinal level of measurement, 144–146

Parameter, 43–48, 144
  defined, 43
  experimental meaning of, 43–48
  statistical meaning of, 43, 144
  See also Statistic
Parametric experiment, 43–48
  analogy with comparative research, 53–54, 111
  defined, 43
  examples of, 43–48
  interaction effects in, 43–48
  main effects in, 43–48
Parametric statistics, 157–158, 162–170, 172–185
Pearson product-moment correlation coefficient, 162–170, 184, 325–331. See also Correlational analysis
Placebo, 88, 129
Platykurtic distribution, 151–155
Polygon. See Frequency polygon
Population, 144
Practical implications of research, 374–382
  See also Excerpts 9.17, 9.18, 9.19, 9.20
Predictive validity, 98–99. See also Validity of tests and measurements
Previous research, relationship of results to, 362–368
  See also Excerpts 9.11, 9.12, 9.13
Protection of human subjects, 138–139. See also Appendix A

Questionnaire. See Survey research

Random assignment of subjects, 78, 85, 106–110, 266–273
  advantages and disadvantages of, 109–110
  in between-subjects designs, 106–107
  combined with matching, 109–110
  control of threats to internal validity by, 78, 85, 106–107
  and sample size, 109
  See also Excerpts 7.2, 7.3, 7.34
Random selection of subjects, 118, 217–222
  See also External validity; Excerpt 7.1
Randomized pretest-posttest control group design, 125–130
Randomizing conditions, 79, 114–115, 399, 417–418. See also Within-subjects designs

Range, 150–155. *See also* Summary statistics
Rationale for the study, 193, 200–207
  defined, 200
  evaluation of, 200–207
  examples of, 200–207
  importance of, 200, 207
  See also Excerpts 6.9, 6.10, 6.11, 6.12, 6.13
Ratio level of measurément, 144–146
Rationalism, 9
Reactive arrangements threat, 92–93, 259–261
  test environment as, 259–261
  See also Threats to external validity
Reactive or interactive pretesting threat, 92. *See also* Threats to external validity
Reactive measures, 80
Regression analysis, 57–60, 169–170, 334–337. *See also* Correlational analysis; Correlational research; Excerpts 8.14, 8.19
Reliability of tests and measurements, 94–97
  defined, 94
  and nonstandardized tests, 96–97
  odd-even, 95
  parallel or equivalent forms, 95
  reliability coefficients, 96
  split-half, 95
  standard error of measurement, 95–96
  test-retest, 95
  See also Excerpts 7.15, 7.16, 7.17, 7.19, 7.20, 7.26, 7.27
Replication, 118–121
Research design, meaning of, 73–75
Research enterprise in speech pathology and audiology, 8–13
Retrospective research, 62–64, 294–295. *See also* Excerpts 7.44, 7.45
Reversal design. *See* Time-series designs
Review of literature, 193, 207–210, 394–395, 412–413
  evaluation of, 209–210, 395, 413
  examples of, 208–209, 394–395, 412–413
  purpose of, 207–208
Rosenthal effect, 82, 111, 123, 252–259. *See also* Instrumentation threat

Sample, 144
Sample size, 218–222
  adequacy of, 218–219
  in between-subjects designs, 218, 266–273
  criteria for, 218
  examples of, 219–222, 395–396, 416–417
  and random assignment, 220–221
  and random selection, 219–220
  in within-subjects designs, 218, 265–266
  See also Excerpts 7.1, 7.2, 7.3, 7.4
Scattergram. *See* Correlational analysis; Graphic display of results
Schemapiric, 9, 10
Science, 8
Scientific method, 8
Semi-interquartile range, 150–155, 322. *See also* Summary statistics
Semilongitudinal research. *See* Developmental research
Sequencing effect, 114–115, 399, 417–418. *See also* Within-subjects designs

Sheffé contrasts, 183
Significance level, 159–162
Single-subject experiments, 14. *See also* Time-series designs
Skewness, 151–155
Solomon randomized four-group design, 130–131
Spearman Rank-order Correlation Coefficient, 164, 166–167, 331–334. *See also* Correlational analysis
Standard deviation, 150–155, 315–322. *See also* Summary statistics
Standard error of measurement, 95–96. *See also* Reliability of tests and measurements
Standardized tests. *See* Behavioral instruments
Statement of problem, 193, 197–199, 394, 411, 413
  evaluation of, 197–199, 394–395, 411
  examples of, 197–199, 394–395, 411
  restatement in discussion section, 354
  See also Excerpts 6.6, 6.7, 6.8, 9.1, 9.2
Statement of purpose, research questions, and hypothesis, 193, 210–214, 394, 411, 413
  as culmination of rationale, 210
  evaluation of, 210–214, 413
  example of, 210–214, 413
  and null hypothesis, 212
  See also Excerpts 6.15, 6.16, 6.17, 6.18, 6.19
Static group comparison, 123–124
Statistic, 144. *See also* Parameter
Statistical analysis procedures, 155–185
  summary table of, 184
Statistical regression threat, 83–84
  control of, 84
  defined, 83
  examples of, 83–84
  See also Threats to internal validity; Excerpt 7.8
Subject selection criteria, 222–230, 395–396, 416–417
  exclusion criteria, 222, 228
  and statistical regression threat, 229–230
  See also Excerpts 7.5, 7.6, 7.7, 7.8
Subject selection threat, 90–91, 222–230
  defined, 90
  in descriptive research, 90–91
  examples of, 91, 222–230
  in experimental research, 90–91
  See also Threats to internal validity
Summary statistics, 149–155, 315–322
  described, 149–155
  examples of, 315–322
  use of, 151–155
  See also Excerpts 8.7, 8.8, 8.9, 8.10, 8.11, 8.12
Survey research, 61–62, 295–299
  appropriateness of, 295–296
  example of, 297–299
  interviews in, 61, 62, 296–297
  questionnaires in, 61–62, 296–297
  sampling in, 61, 296
  threats to internal validity of, 295–297
  See also Excerpt 7.45
Systematic replication, 119, 120

Test practice threat, 79–81. *See also* Threats
    to internal validity
Theories, 10
    theoretical implications of research,
      368–374
    See also Excerpts 9.14, 9.15, 9.16
Therapy research designs, 121–138,
    266–271, 275–281
    equivalent control groups, 125–131,
      266–271
    ethical considerations in, 137–138
    meta-analysis of, 135–137
    nonequivalent control groups, 124–125,
      266–271
    one-group pretest-posttest, 122–123
    "one-shot" case study, 121–122
    randomized pretest-posttest control group,
      125–130, 266–271
    Solomon randomized four-group, 130–131
    static group comparison, 123–124
    time-series, 131–135, 275–281
Threats to external validity, 89–94
    Hawthorne effect, 92–93
    multiple-treatment interference, 93–94
    reactive arrangements, 92–93
    reactive or interactive threat of pretesting,
      92–93
    subject selection, 90–91
Threats to internal validity, 75–89
    differential selection of subjects, 84–86
    Hawthorne effect, 87–89
    history, 75–77
    instrumentation, 81–83
    interaction of factors, 89
    maturation, 77–79
    mortality, 86–87
    statistical regression, 83–84
    test practice, 79–81
Time-series designs, 131–135, 275–281
    See also Excerpts 7.37, 7.38
Title of the article, 193, 194–195, 393, 410
    See also Excerpts 6.1, 6.2, 6.3
t-test, 173–176, 184, 338–340
    See also Excerpts 8.20, 8.21, 8.22

Tukey test, 183
Two-tailed tests, 161–162
Type I and Type II errors, 159

Unobtrusive measures, 80

Validity of tests and measurements, 97–100
    concurrent, 98
    construct, 99–100
    content, 97–98
    criterion, 98–99
    defined, 97
    predictive, 98–99
    See also Excerpts 7.15, 7.16, 7.17, 7.18,
      7.20
Variability measures, 150–155
    See also Excerpts 8.7, 8.8, 8.9, 8.10, 8.11,
      8.12
Variables, 29
Variance, 73, 150–155
    control of, in research design, 73
    See also Summary statistics
Volunteer subjects, 230

Wilcoxon matched-pairs, signed-ranks test,
    173–175, 177, 341–343
    See also Excerpt 8.24
Within-subjects designs, 113–116, 265–266,
    275–281, 287–289
    carry-over effect, 114–115, 265
    control of threats to internal validity,
      113–116, 265–266
    counterbalancing conditions, 114–115
    in descriptive research, 113, 116, 287–289
    examples of, 265–266, 275–281
    in experimental research, 113–116,
      265–266, 275–281
    order effect, 114
    randomizing conditions, 114–115
    sequencing effect, 114–115
    See also Excerpt 7.32

Zeitgeist, 28–29
z-ratio, 173–175